Functional foods

Related titles from Woodhead's food science, technology and nutrition list:

Benders' dictionary of nutrition and food technology Seventh edition (ISBN: 1 85573 475 3)

David A Bender and Arnold E Bender

The seventh edition provides succinct, authoritative definitions of over 5000 terms in nutrition and food technology (an increase of 25% from the previous edition). In addition there is nutrient composition data for 287 foods.

'This valuable book continues to fulfil the purpose of explaining to specialists in other fields the technical terms in nutrition and food processing.' *Chemistry and Industry.*

Food labelling (ISBN: 1 85573 496 6)

Edited by J Ralph Blanchfield

Food labelling has become a complex and controversial area. This collection draws on the experience of key experts in their field to provide food manufacturers with a framework within which to plan labelling effectively. It covers both the key legislation they need to be aware of, and the issues they need to take account of in successful labelling.

Functional foods (ISBN: 1 56676 487 4)

G Mazza

This text brings together key research on the nature and physiological effects of biologically-active components of major plant foods. It also reviews the major processes for extraction, purification, concentration and formulation of functional products, and the functional characteristics of end products.

Phytochemicals as bioactive agents (ISBN: 1 56676 788 1)

W R Bidlack and M S Meskin

This book focuses on the mechanisms of action of phytochemicals identified as displaying bioactivity in the prevention of cancer, heart disease and other diseases, and the prospects for developing functional foods containing these bioactive compounds.

Details of these books and a complete list of Woodhead's food science, technology and nutrition titles can be obtained by:

* visiting our web site at www.woodhead-publishing.com
* contacting Customer Services (e-mail: sales@woodhead-publishing.com; fax: +44 (0)1223 893694; tel.: +44 (0)1223 891358 ext. 30; address: Woodhead Publishing Ltd, Abington Hall, Abington, Cambridge CB1 6AH, England)

If you would like to receive information on forthcoming titles in this area, please send your address details to: Francis Dodds (address, tel. and fax as above; e-mail: francisd@woodhead-publishing.com). Please confirm which subject areas you are interested in.

Functional foods

Concept to product

Edited by
Glenn R. Gibson and Christine M. Williams

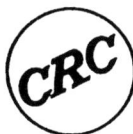

CRC Press
Boca Raton Boston New York Washington, DC

WOODHEAD PUBLISHING LIMITED
Cambridge England

Published by Woodhead Publishing Limited
Abington Hall, Abington
Cambridge CB1 6AH
England
www.woodhead-publishing.com

Published in North and South America by CRC Press LLC
2000 Corporate Blvd, NW
Boca Raton FL 33431
USA

First published 2000, Woodhead Publishing Limited and CRC Press LLC

Reprinted 2001

British Library Cataloguing in Publication Data
A catalogue record for this book is available from the British Library.

Library of Congress Cataloging-in-Publication Data
A catalog record for this book is available from the Library of Congress.

Woodhead Publishing Limited ISBN 1 85573 503 2
CRC Press ISBN 0-8493-0851-8
CRC Press order number: WP0851

Cover design by The ColourStudio
Project managed by Macfarlane Production Services, Markyate, Hertfordshire
Typeset by MHL Typesetting Limited, Coventry, Warwickshire
Printed by TJI Digital, Padstow, Cornwall, England

The Editors and Publisher dedicate this book to
Nicholas Jeremy Jardine
1945–2000

Contents

Contributors

Chapter 1

Professor Marcel Roberfroid
Université Catholique de Louvain
Faculté de Medicine
Dépt des Sciences Pharmaceutiques
Avenue E Mounier 73
UCL/BCTC 7369
B-1200 Bruxelles
Belgium

Fax: 32-2-764-7359
E-mail: roberfroid@pmnt.ucl.ac.be

Chapter 2

Mr Peter Berry Ottaway
Berry Ottaway & Associates
1a Fields Yard
Plough Lane
Hereford HR4 0EL

Tel: +44 (0)1432 270886
Fax: +44 (0)1432 270808
E-mail: berry.ottaway@dial.pipex.com

Chapter 3

Professors Mary K Schmidl and
Theodore P Labuza
Department of Food Science and Nutrition
University of Minnesota
1354 Eckles Avenue
St Paul
MN 55108
USA

Tel: 612 624 9701
Fax: 651 483 3302
E-mail: tplabuza@tc.umn.edu
E-mail: mschmidl@tc.umn.edu

Chapter 4

Professor Glenn R Gibson
The University of Reading
Department of Food Science &
Technology
PO Box 226
Whiteknights
Reading RG6 6AP

Tel: +44 (0)118 931 8700
Fax: +44 (0)118 931 0080
E-mail: g.r.gibson@reading.ac.uk

Chapter 5

Drs Julie Lovegrove and Kim Jackson
Department of Food Science & Technology
University of Reading
PO Box 226
Whiteknights
Reading RG6 6AP

Tel: 0118 931 8700

Fax: 0118 931 0080
E-mail: food@afnovell.reading.ac.uk

Chapter 6

Professor Ian Johnson
Institute of Food Research
Norwich Research Park
Colney
Norwich NR4 7UA

Tel: +44 (0)1603 255000
Fax: +44 (0)1602 507723
E-mail: ian.johnson@bbsrc.ac.uk

Chapter 7

Dr Erika Isolauri and Professor Seppo
Salminen
Department of Pediatrics
University of Turku
Finland

Tel: +358 2 2612433
Fax: +358 2 2611460
E-mail: Erika.isolauri@utu.fi

Chapter 8

Dr David Lindsay
Institute of Food Research
Norwich Research Park
Colney
Norwich NR4 7UA

Tel: +44 (0)1603 255224
Fax: +44 (0)1603 505671
E-mail: david.lindsay@bbsrc.ac.uk

Chapter 9

Professor Ann-Sofie Sandberg
Department of Food Science
Chalmers University of Technology
SE-402 29 Göteborg
Sweden

Tel: +46 (0) 31 3355630
Fax: +46 (0) 31 3355630
E-mail: ann-sofie.sandberg@
fsc.chalmers.se

Chapter 10

Dr Emile de Deckere
Unilever Nutrition Centre
Unilever Research Vlaardingen
Olivier van Noortlaan 120
3133 At Vlaardingen
The Netherlands

Tel: +31 10 4606367
Fax: +31 10 4605993
E-mail: Emile-de.Deckere@unilever.com

Chapter 11

Dr Emma Pickford
Nestlé Product Technology Centre
PO Box 204
Haxby Road
York YO91 1XX

Tel: +44 (0)1904 603194
Fax: +44 (0)1904 604887
E-mail: emma.pickford@rdyo.nestle.com

Chapter 12

Professor Tiina Mattila-Sandholm
VTT Biotechnology
Box 1500
FIN-02044-VTT
Finland

Tel: +358 9 4565200
Fax: + 358 9 455 2028
E-mail: tiina.mattila-sandholm@vtt.fi

Chapter 13

Professor Fabienne Guillon
URPOI-Micro-Macrostructure
INRA Nantes
Rue de la Geraudiere BP 71 627 44 316
Nantes Cedex 03
France

Tel: +33 (0) 2 40 67 50 38
Fax: +33 (0) 2 40 67 50 06
E-mail: guillon@nantes.inra.fr

Abbreviations

AFLP	amplified fragment length polymorphism
ALP	atherogenic lipoprotein phenotype
AOAC	American Organization of Agricultural Chemists
APA	Administrative Procedure Act 1946
BATF	Bureau of Alcohol, Tobacco and Firearms
BMI	body mass index
CARET	carotene and retinol efficacy trial
CCA	Circuit Court of Appeals
CETP	cholesterol ester transfer protein
CFSAN	Center for Food Safety and Applied Nutrition
CFR	Code of Federal Regulations
CHD	coronary heart disease
CM	chylomicron
CPGM	Compliance Policy Guides Manual
CV	conventional
CVD	cardiovascular disease
DHA	docosahexaenoic acid
DRV	daily recommended value
DSHEA	Dietary Supplement Health and Education Act 1994
ELISA	enzyme-linked immunosorbant assay
EPA	eicosapentaenoic acid
ERH	equilibrium relative humidity
FA	fatty acid
FAIR	Food and Agro-Industrial Research
FDA	Food and Drug Administration
FDAMA	Food and Drug Administration Modernization Act 1997

FFDCA	Federal Food, Drug and Cosmetic Act 1938
FISH	fluorescent in situ hybridisation
FOS	fructo-oligosacccharides oligosaccharides
FOSHU	food for specified health use
FR	Federal Register
FSIS	Food Safety and Inspection Service
FTC	Federal Trade Commission
FUFOSE	Functional Food Science in Europe
GALT	gut associated lymphoid tissue
GF	germ-free
GFP	green fluorescent protein
GI	gastrointestinal
GIP	glucose-dependent insulinotropic polypeptide
GLP	glucogon-like peptide
GM	genetically modified
GOS	galacto-oligosaccharide
GRAS	generally recognized as safe
HACCP	hazard analysis and critical control point
HDL	high density lipoprotein
HL	hepatic lipase
HMG-CoA	hydroxy-methyl-glutaryl CoA
HPLC	high performance liquid chromatography
IBD	inflammatory bowel disease
IDL	intermediate density lipoprotein
ILSI	International Life Science Institute
IMO	isomalto-oligosaccharide
LAB	lactic acid bacteria
LCAT	lecithin cholesterol acyltransferase
LDL	low density lipoprotein
LPL	lipoprotein lipase
LPS	lipopolysaccharide
LS	lactosucrose
MAFF	Ministry of Agriculture, Fisheries and Food
MLN	mesenteric lymph nodes
MUFA	monounsaturated fatty acid
NIDDM	non insulin dependent diabetes mellitus
NLEA	Nutrition Labeling and Education Act 1990
NSP	non-starch polysaccharide
ODA	Orphan Drug Act 1988
OFS	oligofructose
PER	protein efficiency ratio
PUFA	polyunsaturated fatty acid
RDA	recommended daily allowance; recommended dietary allowance (US)
RDI	recommended daily intake

RNI	reference nutrition intake
ROS	reactive oxidative species
RS	resistant starch
SC	Supreme Court
SCFA	short chain fatty acid
SDS-PAGE	sodium dodecyl sulfate-polyacrylamid gel electrophoresis
SFA	saturated fatty acid
SOS	soybean oligosaccharide
SPE	sucrose polyester
TAG	triacylglycerol
TCM	traditional Chinese medicine
TDF	total dietary fibre
TH	T helper
USC	United States Code
USDA	United States Department of Agriculture
USP	United States Pharmacopeia
VLDL	very low density lipoprotein
WBC	water binding capacity
XOS	xylo-oligosaccharide

Introduction

Defining functional foods

What are functional foods? The complexities involved in definition are a key theme in Chapter 1 of this book. This suggests the following working definition which seeks to isolate the significance of both 'functional' and 'food' in our understanding of the term:

> A food can be regarded as 'functional' if it is satisfactorily demonstrated to affect beneficially one or more target functions in the body, beyond adequate nutrition, in a way that improves health and well-being or reduces the risk of disease.

This definition suggests that a product must remain a food to be included within the category. On this basis a functional food can be:

- a natural food
- a food to which a positive component has been added, or from which a deleterious component has been removed
- a food where the nature of one or more components has been modified.

The idea of 'functionality' reflects a major shift in attitudes to the relationship between diet and health. Nutritionists have traditionally concentrated on identifying a 'balanced' diet, that is one ensuring adequate intakes of nutrients and avoiding certain dietary imbalances (for example, excessive consumption of fat, cholesterol and salt) which can contribute towards disease. It is important that this lies behind all sound nutritional principles and guidelines. However, the focus is now on achieving 'optimised' nutrition, maximising life expectancy and quality by identifying food ingredients which, when added to a 'balanced' diet, improve the capacity to resist disease and enhance health. Functional foods are one of the outcomes of this.

The functional foods market

Functional foods first emerged in Japan in the early 1980s. Estimates of the value of the functional foods market vary enormously, depending on how the category is defined. Some estimates suggest the world market has grown from US$7–10 billion in 1995 to over US$15 billion in 2000, with annual growth rates averaging 10%. Japan has traditionally accounted for around half of all functional food sales (an estimated US$3–4 billion in 1996), although this proportion is decreasing as the European and US markets expand. The US market was worth about US$8 billion in 1997 with growth at around 5% per annum. Sales of functional foods in Europe in 1997 have been estimated at US$1.7 billion, growing to around US$2 billion by 2000.

There have been a number of important forces driving this growth. These include:

* new research on the links between diet and the prevention of chronic disease
* ageing populations in many developed countries, and an increasing concern about managing the health of this age group who are more prone to disease (and particularly such degenerative disorders as cancer, heart disease, osteoporosis, diabetes and stroke)
* growing pressure on public health spending, leading to a greater emphasis on prevention and more individual responsibility for health care provision
* increased health consciousness among consumers and concern about their dietary intake
* improvements in food science and technology
* changes in the regulatory framework governing this area.

Classifying functional foods

As a result of increasing market growth, there is a huge possible range of functional foods. These include:

* soft drinks such as energy and sports drinks
* cereal and baby foods
* baked goods
* confectionery
* dairy products, especially yoghurts and other fermented dairy products
* spreads
* meat products
* animal feeds.

These functional foods offer varying types of benefit and act in differing ways. One way of categorising their mode of operation is as follows:

- vitamin and mineral fortification
- cholesterol reduction
- dietary fibre
- probiotics, prebiotics and synbiotics
- antioxidants
- phytochemicals
- herbs and botanicals.

Examples of products fortified with vitamins and minerals include calcium-fortified confectionery and fruit drinks, and calcium-enriched milk with folic acid. Folic acid, for example, is documented as a vital nutrient in early pregnancy that guards against spina bifida, while the importance of calcium has been recognised in counteracting osteoporosis. Given the prevalence of osteoporosis among the increasing proportion of elderly people in developed countries, improving calcium intake has been seen as particularly significant in this sector of the functional foods market. Research has concentrated not just on ways of increasing levels of calcium intake but also in improving the efficiency of calcium absorption.

A number of ingredients are associated with inhibiting the absorption of cholesterol which is thought to be a major factor in cardiovascular disease. This category includes omega-3 fatty acids and plant sterols. Examples of products in this area include a margarine containing plant sterol fatty acid esters designed to reduce cholesterol absorption, and omega-3 enriched eggs produced by chickens fed a micoalgal feed ingredient.

Dietary fibre comprises the non-digestible structural carbohydrates of plant cell walls and associated lignan. Consumption of fibre has been linked to a reduced risk of certain types of cancer, for example consumption of wheat bran which has been linked to a reduced risk of colon cancer. High-fibre products include a whole-wheat pasta with three times the fibre of regular pasta.

A probiotic can be defined as a live microbial food supplement which beneficially affects the host by improving its intestinal microbial balance. Probiotics are thought to have a range of potential health benefits, including cholesterol-lowering, cancer chemopreventative and immune-enhancing effects. Probiotics are viewed currently as the world's biggest functional food products. This sector of the functional foods market has been stimulated in recent years by the development of prebiotics, short chain oligosaccharides which enhance the growth of beneficial bacteria already in the gut, and synbiotics which combine pro- and prebiotic characteristics. The field of gut health is now an area of intense research in functional food science.

Cancerous and other mutations can occur as a result of oxidative damage to DNA caused by free radicals generated as a damaging side-effect of aerobic metabolism. Plant and animal cells defend themselves against these effects by deploying so-called antioxidant compounds to trap or quench free radicals and hence arrest their damaging reactions. Antioxidants thus play a role in the body's defence against cardiovascular disease, certain (epithelial) cancers, visual impairments, arthritis and asthma. Antioxidants include vitamin E, carotene, vitamin C and certain phytochemicals. Functional products incorporating antioxidant supplements include sports bars containing vitamins C and E as well as a blend of several carotenoids (alpha- and gamma-carotene and lycopene).

Plant foods are rich in micronutrients, but they also contain an immense variety of biologically active, non-nutritive secondary metabolites providing colour, flavour and natural toxicity to pests and sometimes humans. These 'phytochemicals' have been linked to reducing the risk of chronic diseases such as cancer, osteoporosis and heart disease. They include glucosinolates and phenolic compounds like flavonoids which are very effective antioxidants. Examples of products including phytochemicals are children's confectionery containing concentrates of vegetables such as broccoli, Brussels sprouts, cabbage and carrots.

More recently, herbs and botanicals such as ginkgo, ginseng and guarana have been linked to improved physical and mental performance. These may lead to a new generation of 'performance' functional foods including these and other components such as creatin, caffeine and tryptophane. Products in this area include beverages, chewing gum and sports bars. One product that combines a range of functional claims is a fruit juice designed for the sports market containing carnitine, an amino acid to assist the body in producing energy and in lowering cholesterol, calcium to improve skeletal strength and chromium picolinate to help build lean muscle mass.

Key issues in functional foods: the structure of this book

The functional food industry and interested scientists face a number of key challenges:

- agreeing standards for the validation of claims about the health benefits of functional foods
- ensuring a regulatory framework which balances consumer protection in the way that functional claims are validated and communicated with the freedom for the industry to develop functional products profitably and effectively
- identifying and screening potential functional ingredients for development
- assessing the technological and commercial feasibility of new product ideas
- building in appropriate systems for validating product safety and functional benefits, for example through clinical human trials
- scaling up for commercial production.

This collection of chapters addresses this range of issues. Chapter 1 looks at the key issues of definition and an appropriate methodology for substantiating functional claims. It outlines the idea of identifying 'markers' in demonstrating the impact of a functional ingredient on a target function in the body, and also addresses the problem of how the results of such verification procedures can be communicated effectively to consumers. Chapters 2 and 3 then consider the current regulatory framework in the EU and the US respectively, including current controls on making health claims for functional products.

Part II of this book consists of a series of chapters summarising the current state of research on the links between functional foods and health. An understanding of this is obviously critical to the claims that manufacturers can make about functional products. Chapter 4 looks at colonic functional foods: probiotics, prebiotics and synbiotics. It describes current research on their mode of operation and health benefits. Chapter 5 considers the contribution of functional foods to the prevention of coronary heart disease, identifying the role of dietary factors and considering the impact of antioxidants, probiotics, prebiotics and synbiotics. In Chapter 6, the role of functional foods in preventing cancer is discussed, looking particularly at antioxidants, phytochemicals and dietary fibre. Finally, Chapter 7 looks at the effects of functional foods on acute disorders, assessing the role of probiotics in enhancing the immune system and in prevention and treatment of gastrointestinal disorders.

In Part III the focus shifts to product development issues. Chapter 8 considers the range of plant sources of functional compounds and the impact of processing on these compounds. It also discusses methods of enhancing functional properties such as genetic modification, and includes case studies illustrating improvements to plant macronutrient and micronutrient content. Building on this, Chapter 9 provides a case study of the identification of a functional plant ingredient, preparation and processing issues, applications in food and measurement.

Two chapters assess the issue of selecting a functional ingredient. Chapter 10 considers the research and processing issues involved in identifying a target functional ingredient from the range on offer, concentrating on functional fats and spreads. In Chapter 11, the functional confectionery market is used to analyse the process of product development from market analysis through to formulation, testing and marketing. The final chapters look at processing issues. Chapter 12 discusses probiotic foods and such issues as selecting strains, pilot testing in clinical trials and commercial production. Chapter 13 looks at dietary fibre functional foods, discussing sources, processing and measurement of functional properties.

Part I

General issues

1

Defining functional foods

M.B. Roberfroid, Université Catholique de Louvain, Brussels

1.1 Introduction

To understand functional food it is first necessary to understand how the science of nutrition itself has changed. Nutrition has progressed from the prevention of dietary deficiency and the establishment of nutrition standards, dietary guidelines and food guides, to the promotion of a state of well-being and health and the reduction of the risk of disease.

1.1.1 Nutrition: a science of the twentieth century[1]

Even though 'diet' and 'food' are very old terms, probably as old as human beings, the term 'nutrition' is rather modern, appearing for the first time in the nineteenth century. Nutrition is multidisciplinary as it integrates and applies broad and available knowledge (including basic science) about foods and/or nutrients and their effects on body physiology with the aim of improving the state of well-being and health.

During the twentieth century, essential nutrients have been discovered and nutrient standards, dietary guidelines and food guides established, mainly if not exclusively with the aim of preventing deficiencies and supporting body growth, maintenance and development. More recently, in the last 30 years, recommendations have also been made that we should aim to avoid excessive consumption of some of these nutrients since their potential role in the etiology of miscellaneous (mostly chronic) diseases has been recognised.[2] These advances are reflected in:

- Nutrient standards,[3] the recommended daily allowances (RDAs) or reference nutrition intakes (RNIs) which are the 'average daily amounts of essential

nutrients estimated on the basis of available scientific knowledge to be sufficiently high to meet the physiological needs of nearly all healthy persons'.
- Dietary guidelines,[4] which are 'advice on consumption of foods or food components for which there is a related public health concern', mostly when RDAs or RNIs are not available. These are expressed in relation to total diet, often in qualitative terms (more/less/increased/reduced ...), based on consensus research findings relating diet and health.
- Food guides,[5] which are 'the translation of nutritional standards and dietary guidelines in terms of recommendations on daily food intake'. These form a conceptual framework for selecting the kinds and amounts of foods of various types that, together, provide a nutritionally satisfactory diet. They are based on nutrient standards, composition of foods, food intake patterns and factors influencing food choice.

Through these developments, one of the major contributions of nutritional science in the twentieth century has been the concept of the balanced diet, 'an appropriate mixture of food items that provides, at least, the minimum requirements of nutrients and a few other food components needed to support growth and maintain body weight, to prevent the development of deficiency diseases and to reduce the risk of diseases associated with deleterious excesses'.[6]

1.1.2 Nutrition: a science for the twenty-first century
At the turn of the twenty-first century, the society of abundance, which characterises most of the industrialised world, faces new challenges from an uncontrollable increase in the costs of health care, an increase in life expectancy, improved scientific knowledge and development of new technologies to major changes in lifestyles (Table 1.1). Nutrition has to adapt to these new challenges. As a consequence, nutrition as a science will, in addition to keeping an emphasis on balanced diet, develop the concept of optimum (optimised) nutrition.[7]

Optimum (optimised) nutrition will aim at maximising the physiological functions of each individual, in order to ensure both maximum well-being and health but, at the same time, a minimum risk of disease throughout life. In other words, it will have to aim at maximising a healthy lifespan. At the same time, it will have to match an individual's unique biochemical needs with a tailored selection of nutrient intakes for that individual. Such a selection will be based on

Table 1.1   The challenges for nutrition at the beginning of the twenty-first century

---

- Application of new scientific knowledge in nutrition
- Improved scientific knowledge on diet–disease relationships
- Exponential increase of health-care costs
- Increase in life expectancy
- Consumer awareness of nutrition and health relationships
- Progress in food technology

---

a better understanding of the interactions between genes and nutrition.[8] These interactions include: polymorphism and interindividual variations in response to diet, dietary alteration and modulation of gene expression, and dietary effects on disease risk. These interactions play a role both in the modulation of specific physiological functions and/or pathophysiological processes by given food components, as well as in their metabolism by the body. They control the responsiveness of a particular individual to both the beneficial and deleterious effects of their diet.

Even though a balanced diet remains a key objective to prevent deficiencies and their associated diseases and to reduce the risk of the diseases associated with excess intake of some nutrients, optimum (optimised) nutrition will aim at establishing optimum (optimised) intake of as many food components as possible to support or promote well-being and health, and/or reduce the risk of diseases, mainly for those that are diet-related. At the beginning of the twenty-first century, the major challenge of the science of nutrition is thus to progress from improving life expectancy to improving life quality/wellness.

On the road to optimum (optimised) nutrition, which is an ambitious and long-term objective, functional food is, among others, a new, interesting and stimulating concept inasmuch as it is supported by sound and consensual scientific data generated by the recently developed functional food science aimed at improving dietary guidelines by integrating new knowledge on the interactions between food components and body functions and/or pathological processes.

1.2 Functional foods: defining the concept

Functional food cannot be a single well-defined/well-characterisable entity. Indeed, a wide variety of food products are or will, in the future, be characterised as functional food with a variety of components, some of them classified as nutrients, affecting a variety of body functions relevant to either a state of well-being and health and/or to the reduction in risk of a disease. Thus no simple, universally accepted definition of functional food exists. Especially in Europe, where even the common term 'dietary fibre' has no consensual definition, it would be unrealistic to try to produce such a definition for something as new and diverse as functional food. Functional food has thus to be understood as a concept. Moreover, if it is function driven rather than product driven, the concept is likely to be more universal and not too much influenced by local characteristics or cultural traditions.[9]

1.2.1 Functional food: an international overview

Japan is the birthplace of the term 'functional food'.[10] Moreover, that country has been at the forefront of the development of functional foods since the early 1980s when systematic and large-scale research programmes were launched and funded by the Japanese government on systematic analysis and development of food functions, analysis of physiological regulation of function by food and analysis of functional foods and molecular design. As a result of a long decision-making process to establish a category of foods for potential enhancing benefits as part of a national effort to reduce the escalating cost of health care, the concept of foods for specified health use (FOSHU) was established in 1991. These foods, which are intended to be used to improve people's health and for which specific health effects (claims) are allowed to be displayed, are included as one of the categories of foods described in the Nutrition Improvement Law as foods for special dietary use. According to the Japanese Ministry of Health and Welfare, FOSHU are:

- foods that are expected to have a specific health effect due to relevant constituents, or foods from which allergens have been removed, and
- foods where the effect of such an addition or removal has been scientifically evaluated, and permission has been granted to make claims regarding the specific beneficial effects on health expected from their consumption.

Foods identified as FOSHU are required to provide evidence that the final food product, but not isolated individual component(s), is likely to exert a health or physiological effect when consumed as part of an ordinary diet. Moreover, FOSHU products should be in the form of ordinary foods (i.e. not pills or capsules).

In the meantime, but mainly in the 1990s, a variety of terms, more or less related to the Japanese FOSHU, has appeared worldwide. In addition to functional foods, these include more exotic terms such as 'nutraceuticals', 'designer foods', 'f(ph)armafoods', 'medifoods', 'vitafoods', etc., but also the more traditional 'dietary supplements' and 'fortified foods'. According to Hillian[11] these terms intend to describe 'food substances that provide medical or health benefits including the prevention and treatment of disease'. As discussed in an editorial of the *Lancet*,[12] these are 'foods or food products marketed with the message of a benefit to health' and they 'sit in the murky territory between food and medicine'.[13] For the editors of two other books entitled *Functional Foods*, these terms cover 'foods that can prevent or treat disease'[14] or 'foods or isolated food ingredients that deliver specific nonnutritive physiological benefits that may enhance health'.[15] For these authors, these terms are interchangeable. But it appears that these terms either describe quite different entities that cannot be covered by a single heading or are formulated in such a general and broad sense that they lose specificity and become too vague to be really useful.

- *Nutraceuticals* have been described as 'any substance that is a food or part of a food that provides medical and/or health benefits, including the prevention and treatment of disease'[16] or 'a product produced from foods but sold in powders, pills and other medicinal forms not generally associated with food and demonstrated to have physiological benefits or provide protection against chronic disease'.[17]

- *Vitafoods* are defined by the Ministry of Agriculture, Fisheries and Food (MAFF) as 'foods and drinks to meet the needs of modern health conscious consumers which enhance the bodily or mental quality of life, enhance the capacity to endure or flourish or to recover from strenuous exercise or illness. They may also increase the healthy status of the consumer or act as potential deterrent to health hazard'.[18]
- *Dietary supplements* have, at least in the USA, a more elaborate definition which covers 'a product intended to supplement the diet and that bears or contains one or more of certain specified dietary ingredients (vitamins, minerals, herbs or other botanicals, amino-acids, a dietary supplement) to supplement the diet by increasing total dietary intake, a concentrate, metabolite, constituent, extract or combination. It is a tablet, capsule, powder, softgel, gelcap or liquid droplet or some other form that can be a conventional food but is not represented as a conventional'.[19] However, in France the definition is more restrictive, being 'a product to be ingested to complement the usual diet in order to make good any real or anticipated deficiencies in daily intake'.[20]

Functional food has as many definitions as the number of authors referring to it. These definitions go from simple statements such as:

- foods that may provide health benefits beyond basic nutrition[21]
- foods or food products marketed with the message of the benefit to health[12]
- everyday food transformed into a potential lifesaver by the addition of a magical ingredient[13]

to very elaborate definitions such as:

- food and drink products derived from naturally occurring substances consumed as part of the daily diet and possessing particular physiological benefits when ingested[11]
- food derived from naturally occurring substances that can and should be consumed as part of the daily diet and that serve to regulate or otherwise affect a particular body process when ingested[22]
- food similar in appearance to conventional food, which is consumed as part of a usual diet and has demonstrated physiological benefit and/or reduces the risk of chronic disease beyond basic nutritional functions[17]
- food that encompasses potentially helpful products including any modified food or food ingredient that may provide a health benefit beyond that of the traditional nutrient it contains[23]
- food similar in appearance to conventional food that is intended to be consumed as part of a normal diet, but has been modified to subserve physiological roles beyond the provision of simple nutrient requirements.

Whatever definition is chosen, 'functional food' appears as a quite unique concept that deserves a category of its own, a category different from nutraceutical, f(ph)armafood, medifood, designer food or vitafood, and a category that does not include dietary supplement. It is also a concept that belongs to nutrition and not to pharmacology. Functional foods are and must be foods, not drugs, as they have no therapeutic effects. Moreover their role regarding disease will, in most cases, be in reducing the risk of disease rather than preventing it.

1.2.2 Functional food: a European consensus[9, 24, 25]

The unique features of functional food are:

- being a conventional or everyday food
- to be consumed as part of the normal/usual diet
- composed of naturally occurring (as opposed to synthetic) components perhaps in unnatural concentration or present in foods that would not normally supply them
- having a positive effect on target function(s) beyond nutritive value/basic nutrition
- may enhance well-being and health and/or reduce the risk of disease or provide health benefits so as to improve the quality of life including physical, psychological and behavioural performances
- have authorised and scientifically based claims.

It is in that general context that the European Commission's Concerted Action on Functional Food Science in Europe (FUFOSE), which actively involved a large number of the most prominent European experts in nutrition and related sciences, has been coordinated by the International Life Science Institute – ILSI Europe. It developed in early 1996 to reach a European Consensus on 'Scientific Concepts of Functional Foods' in 1998.[9] To reach that final objective, three major steps were undertaken:

1. Critical assessment of the science base required to provide evidence that specific nutrients and food components positively affect target functions in the body.
2. Examination of the available science from a function-driven perspective rather than a product-driven one.
3. Elaboration of a consensus on targeted modifications of food and food constituents, and options for their applications.[24]

In that context, 'target function' refers to genomic, biochemical, physiological, psychological or behavioural functions that are relevant to the maintenance of a state of well-being and health or to the reduction of the risk of a disease. Modulation of these functions should be quantitatively evaluated by measuring change in serum or other body fluids of the concentration of a metabolite, a specific protein or a hormone, change in the activity of enzymes, change in physiological parameters (e.g. blood pressure, gastrointestinal transit time, etc.), change in physical or intellectual performances, and so on.

The major deliverables of that Concerted Action are three publications:

1. *Functional Food Science in Europe* reviews the published literature to define the state of the art with respect to specific body systems, the methodologies to characterise and quantify specific related functions, the nutritional options modulating these functions, the safety implications related to these nutritional options, the role of food technology in nutritional and safety aspects and the science base required for providing evidence that specific nutrients positively affect function.[24]
2. *Technological Aspects of Functional Food Science* reviews the impact of processing, the importance of the source of materials to prepared food products, processing options to modulate functionality, safety implications of materials and processes, and process monitoring of functions.[25]
3. *Scientific Concepts of Functional Foods in Europe*: a consensus that proposes, for the first time, a consensual framework for the development of functional foods and for the elaboration of a scientific basis for claims.[9]

As already indicated above, because functional food is a concept rather than a well-defined group of food products, that consensus document proposes a working definition:

> A food can be regarded as functional if it is satisfactorily demonstrated to affect beneficially one or more target functions in the body, beyond adequate nutritional effects, in a way that is relevant to either improved stage of health and well-being and/or reduction of risk of disease. A functional food must remain food and it must demonstrate its effects in amounts that can normally be expected to be consumed in the diet: it is not a pill or a capsule, but part of the normal food pattern.[9]

The main aspects of this working definition are:

-   the food nature of functional food that is not a pill, a capsule or any form of dietary supplement
-   the demonstration of the effects to the satisfaction of the scientific community
-   the beneficial effects on body functions, beyond adequate nutritional effects, that are relevant to improved state of health and well-being and/or reduction of risk (not prevention) of disease
-   the consumption as part of a normal food pattern.

The definition encompasses all main features of functional foods identified above; it is aimed at stimulating research and development in the field of nutrition so as to contribute adequately to the scientific knowledge that will be required to define optimum (optimised) nutrition by elaborating new dietary guidelines. However, it should be emphasised that a functional food will not necessarily be functional for all members of the population, and that matching individual biochemical needs with selected food component intakes may become a key task as we progress in our understanding of the interactions between genes and diet.[8] From a practical point of view, a functional food can be:

- a natural food
- a food to which a component has been added
- a food from which a component has been removed
- a food where the nature of one or more components has been modified
- a food in which the bioavailability of one or more components has been modified, or
- any combination of these possibilities.

1.3 Functional food science

Being foods, functional foods need to be safe according to all criteria defined in current food regulations. But in many cases, new concepts and new procedures will need to be developed and validated to assess functional food risks. In Europe, some, but certainly not all, functional foods will be classified as 'novel foods' and consequently will require the decision tree assessment regarding safety that is described in the EU Novel Food Regulation.[26]

However, it must be emphasised that this regulation does not concern the nutritional properties or the physiological effects of these novel foods. It is strictly a safety regulation. The requirement for safety is a prerequisite to any functional food development. Indeed, the risk versus benefit concept, which is familiar to pharmacologists developing new drugs, does not apply to functional foods except perhaps in very specific conditions for disease risk reduction when the scientific evidence is particularly strong. As described in the European consensus document:[9]

> The design and development of functional foods is a key issue, as well as a scientific challenge, which should rely on basic scientific knowledge relevant to target functions and their possible modulation by food components. Functional foods themselves are not universal and a food-based approach would have to be influenced by local considerations. In contrast, a science-based approach to functional food is universal ...
> The function-driven approach has the science base as its foundation – in order to gain a broader understanding of the interactions between diet and health. Emphasis is then put on the importance of the effects of food components on well-identified and well-characterized target functions in the body that are relevant to well-being and health issues, rather than, solely, on reduction of disease risk.

By reference to the new concepts in nutrition outlined above, it is the role of *Functional Food Science* to stimulate research and development of functional foods (see Fig. 1.1).

By reference to basic knowledge in nutrition and related biological sciences, such a development requires the identification and, at least partly, an understanding of the mechanism(s) by which a potential functional food or functional food component can modulate the target function(s) that is/are

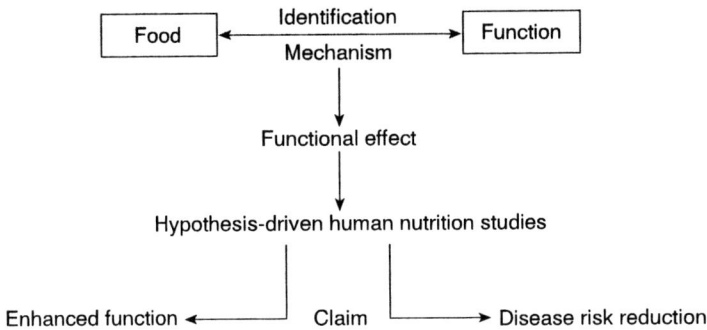

Fig. 1.1   The strategy for functional food development

recognised or proven to be relevant to the state of well-being and health, and/or the reduction of a disease risk. Epidemiological data demonstrating a statistically validated and biologically relevant relationship between the intake of specific food components and a particular health benefit will, if available, be very useful. The conclusion of that first step will be the demonstration of a functional effect that should serve to formulate hypotheses to be tested in a new generation of human nutrition studies aimed to show that relevant (in terms of dose, frequency, duration, etc.) intake of the specified food will be associated with improvements in one or more target functions, either directly or indirectly in terms of a valid marker of an improved state of well-being and health and/or reduced disease risk. If well supported by strong scientific evidence, the conclusion could be a recommendation for improved or new dietary guidelines.

The new-generation human nutrition studies should be hypothesis driven but, in many cases, they will differ quite substantially from what is classically referred to as clinical studies.The main differences are that nutrition studies aim at testing the effect of a food as part of the ordinary diet; they may concern the general population or generally large, at-risk target groups; they are not diagnostic; or symptom based; and they are not planned to evaluate a risk versus benefit approach. Most of these studies will rely on change(s) in validated/ relevant markers to demonstrate a positive modulation of target functions after (long-term) consumption of the potential functional food. A (double) blind type of design based on parallel groups rather than crossing-over will generally be appropriate. Data from these studies should be collected and handled according to good standards for data management, and data analysis should prove statistical as well as biological significance. Finally, the long-term consequences of interaction(s) between functional foods and body function(s) will have to be carefully monitored.

1.3.1 Markers: key to the development of functional foods
The development of functional foods will, in most cases, rely on measurements of 'markers'. These markers need to be identified and validated for their

predictive value of potential benefits to a target function or the risk of a particular disease. Markers of correlated events are 'indicators' whereas markers representing an event directly involved in the process are 'factors'.[9] When related to the risk of disease, indicators and even factors might, in some instances, be equivalent to 'surrogate markers' defined as a biological observation, result or index that predicts the development of chronic disease.[27] The more that is known about the mechanisms leading to health outcomes, the more refined will be the identification of the markers and their appreciation. The markers should be feasible, valid, reproducible, sensitive and specific. They can be biochemical, physiological, behavioural or psychological in nature. However, dynamic responses might be as useful as, or more useful than, static or single point measurements. In many cases, a battery of markers might be needed in order to create a decision tree from multiple tests (see Fig. 1.2).

These markers, most of which still need to be identified and validated, will relate to:

- Exposure to the food component under study by measuring serum, faecal, urine or tissue level of the food component itself or its metabolite(s), or the concentration of an endogenous molecule that is directly influenced by the consumption of the food component.
- Target function(s) or biological response such as change in serum or other body fluids of the concentration of a metabolite, a specific protein, an enzyme, a hormone, etc.

These first two markers are either indicators or factors.

- An appropriate endpoint of an improved state of well-being and health and/or reduction of a disease risk. Such a marker is likely to be a factor rather than an indicator.
- Individual susceptibility or genetic polymorphism controlling the metabolism and/or the effect of the food component under study.[8]

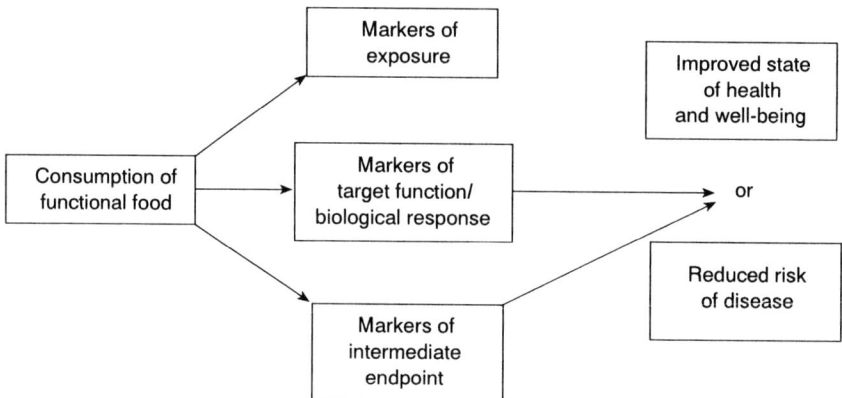

Fig. 1.2   Markers for functional food development

To further develop these markers, a state-of-the-art literature review will be necessary to identify, define and characterise potential markers. Furthermore, the basic scientific knowledge underpinning these markers will be evaluated. The next step will include assessment of their relevance to physiological function, to well-being and health and eventually to disease risk. A validation will then be necessary both for the methodology and biological relevance. Finally, classification as indicator or factor will be made and potential dietary modulations demonstrated. New techniques such as those used by molecular and cellular biologists will be useful in identifying target groups who could benefit from the consumption of specific functional foods.

1.4 Communicating functional claims

1.4.1 A communication challenge
As stated in the European consensus on scientific concepts of functional foods:[9]

> As the relationship between nutrition and health gains public acceptance and as the market for functional foods grows, the question of how to communicate the specific advantages of such foods becomes increasingly important. Communication of health benefits to the public, through intermediaries such as health professionals, educators, the media and the food industry, is an essential element in improving public health and in the development of functional foods. Its importance also lies in avoiding problems associated with consumer confusion about health messages. Of all the different forms of communication, those concerning claims – made either directly as a statement on the label or package of food products, or indirectly through secondary supporting information – remain an area of extensive discussion.

It is also the opinion of C.B. Hudson that 'the links between nutrition science and food product development will flow through to consumers only if the required communication vehicles are put in place'.[28] However, the communication of health benefits and other physiological effects of functional foods remains a major challenge because:

- science should remain the driving force;
- messages – claims – must be based on sound, objective and appropriate evidence; and
- evidence must be consistent, able to meet established scientific standards and plausible.

Moreover, communication in nutrition generally comes from multiple sources that are sometimes contradictory, creating an impression of chaos. And chaotic information often generates ignorance and easily becomes misinformation (see Fig. 1.3).

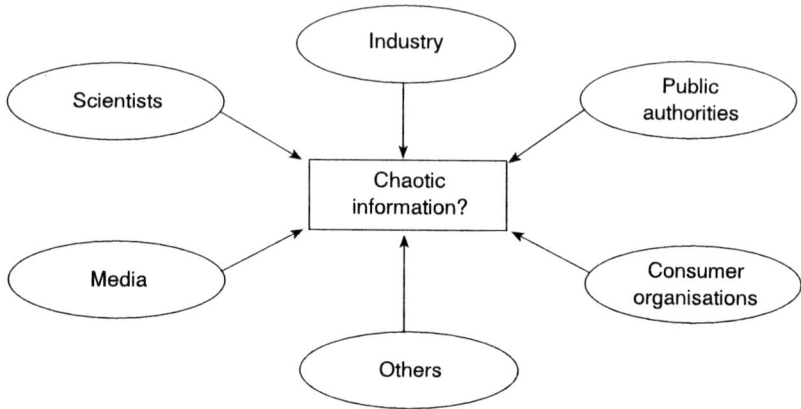

Fig. 1.3   The communication challenge for functional food development

1.4.2 The scientific challenge

Regarding functional foods, claims associated with specific food products are the preferable means of communicating to consumers. In application of the fundamental principle, any claim must be true and not misleading; it must be scientifically valid, unambiguous and clear to the consumer. However, these basic principles should be safeguarded without becoming a disincentive to the production of functional foods or to their acceptance by consumers. Even though a general definition of 'claim' is widely accepted in the field of nutrition as 'any representation, which states, suggests or implies that a food has certain characteristics relating to its origin, nutritional properties ... or any other quality',[29] one of the difficulties in communicating the benefits of functional foods is that distinct types of claims exist, and that in particular the term 'health claims', which is traditionally used to communicate the benefits of foods, is defined differently in different parts of the world.

Seeking clarity, Codex Alimentarius[29] has recently classified and defined four different categories of claims, but excluding the term 'health claim':

1. Relate to dietary guidelines.
2. Relate to nutrient content.
3. Are comparative (reduced, less, more ...).
4. Describe nutrient function (contains ..., that contributes to the development of ...).

These claims refer to known nutrients and their role in growth, development and normal functions as well as to the concept of adequate nutrition. They are based on established, widely accepted knowledge but they do not refer to a particular effect over and above that expected from consuming a balanced diet. These claims are thus not really helpful to communicate the specific benefits of functional foods. Indeed, the claims for functional foods should be based on the scientific classification of markers (indicators and/or factors) for target functions and on the effects on these markers. If such an effect, which goes beyond what could be expected from the established role of diet in growth, development and other normal functions in the body, concerns a target function or a biological activity without direct reference to a particular disease or pathological process, claim will be made for an *enhanced function*. But, if the benefit is clearly a reduction of the risk of a disease or pathological process, claims will be made for *disease risk reduction*. These two types of claims, which are specific for functional foods, are the *type A* and *type B* claims respectively as they are described in the European consensus on scientific concepts of functional foods.[9] The type A claim is similar to the 'structure/function claim', whereas the type B claim can be regarded as equivalent to 'health claim' in the USA respectively. The type B claim also corresponds to 'health claim' in Sweden.[30] In its last proposed draft recommendations for the use of health claims, Codex Alimentarius has included type A and type B claims and defined them as:[31]

• Type A or claims that concern specific beneficial effects of the consumption of foods and their constituents on physiological or psychological functions or biological activities but do not include nutrient function claims. Such claims relate to a positive contribution to health or a condition linked to health, to the improvement of a function or to modifying or preserving health.
• Type B or 'risk of disease reduction claims' that concern the reduction of a disease risk related to the consumption of a food or a food constituent in the context of the daily diet that might help reduce the risk of a specific disease or condition.

One of the major issues still to be resolved, especially with these two types of claims, concerns the biological level at which evidence can be accepted as 'satisfactorily demonstrating' an enhanced function or reduction of disease risk. This evidence should rely on all data available that can be grouped into three categories:

• biological observations,
• epidemiological data, and
• intervention studies, mostly based on markers.

For any given specific food product, supporting evidence for enhanced function or reduction of disease risk might not be available or even not necessary from all three areas.[9] All supporting evidence should, however, be:

• consistent in itself;
• able to meet accepted scientific standards of statistical as well as biological significance, especially dose–effect relationship, if relevant;
• plausible in terms of the relationship between intervention and results, especially in terms of mechanism(s) of action;
• provided by a number of sources (including obligatory human studies) that give consistent findings able to generate scientific consensus.

1.5 Case studies

This section is aimed at illustrating the concepts of functional food by focusing on three major target functions for which relevance to the state of well-being and health as well as the reduction of risk of disease is established or very likely. It summarises the conclusions of expert groups that have recently reviewed the published literature to define the state of the art with respect to these specific body functions; they have identified and reviewed nutritional options modulating these functions and have critically assessed the science base required for providing evidence that specific nutrients positively affect target functions.[9, 24]

1.5.1 Gastrointestinal functions[9, 32]

The gastrointestinal target functions which are associated with a balanced microflora together with an optimal gut associated lymphoid tissue (GALT) are relevant to the state of well-being and health and to the reduction of the risk of diseases. The colonic microflora is a complex ecosystem, the functions of which are a consequence of the combined action of the microbes that, besides interacting with the GALT, contribute to salvage of nutrient energy and produce end-metabolic products like short chain fatty acids (SCFAs) that play a role in cell differentiation, cell proliferation and metabolic regulatory processes. It is generally assumed that the group of potentially health-promoting bacteria includes principally bifidobacteria, and lactobacilli which are and possibly should remain the most important genera in humans. Changes in the composition of the faecal flora, a recognised surrogate marker of the residual colonic microbiota, can be considered as a marker, indicator and factor, of large bowel functions. They might play a role in gastrointestinal infections and diarrhoea, constipation, irritable bowel syndrome, inflammatory bowel diseases and colorectal cancer.

Probiotics (e.g. lactobacilli or bifidobacteria) and prebiotics (like chicory inulin and its hydrolysate oligofructose) are recent concepts in nutrition that have already and will in the future be used to support the development of functional foods targeted towards gut function. Their effects include:

- stimulation of the activity of the GALT (e.g. increased IgA response, production of cytokines);
- reduction in the duration of episodes of rotavirus infection;
- change in the composition of the faecal flora to reach/maintain a composition in which bifidobacteria and/or lactobacilli become predominant in number, a situation that is preferred;
- increase in faecal mass (stool bulking) and stool frequency;
- increase in calcium bioavailability via colonic absorption (e.g. inulin).

1.5.2 Defence against reactive oxidative species[9, 33]

The generation of reactive oxidative species (ROS) is a general feature of any aerobic organism both during development and normal functions or pathological changes. These ROS can damage essential macromolecules like DNA, lipids and proteins by initiating or promoting oxidative processes. Many of these (bio)chemical reactions are thought to be involved in miscellaneous pathological processes such as cataract, some cancers, cardiovascular diseases, rheumatoid arthritis and some neurodegenerative conditions. But it is becoming more and more evident that ROS also play an essential role in regulating gene expression and in participating in cell signalling. Maintaining a balance between production and destruction of ROS is thus a key element in well-being and health and it is likely to play a role in reducing the risk of disease. Examples of target functions for functional food development in relation to the maintenance of such a balance are:

- preservation of the structure and functional activity of DNA that can be evaluated by measuring DNA integrity (COMET assay), damaged DNA bases (e.g. 8 OH desoxyguanine) or specific gene expressions;
- preservation of structural and functional integrity of circulating lipoproteins by measuring either lipid hydroperoxides or their derivatives (e.g. malondialdehyde) or oxidised low-density-lipoproteins in plasma;
- preservation of structural and functional integrity of proteins.

The major functional foods to rebalance oxidative processes are:

- vitamins (especially tocopherols, ascorbic acid and carotenoids);
- polyphenols such as flavonoids.

1.5.3 Psychological and behavioural functions[9, 34]

Some foods or food components provide an important function by changing mood or mental state. They are involved in creating more a sense of 'feeling well' than 'being well'. Target functions for such foods and food components are:

- appetite, satiation and satiety, the most widely used markers of which are either visual analogue scales to evaluate subjectively sensations such as hunger, desire to eat and fullness or quantitative assessment of energy and/or nutrient intake;
- cognitive performance for which several markers are used like reaction to single stimulus test or complex interactive inputs;
- mood and vitality by focusing on behaviours such as sleep and activity, as well as feelings of tension, calmness, drowsiness, alertness assessed either subjectively (e.g. with questionnaires) or objectively (e.g. with electro-physiological measurements);
- stress and distress management based on changes in physiological markers like heart rate, blood pressure, blood catecholamines, blood opioid levels.

The development of functional foods aimed at beneficially affecting behavioural and psychological functions has in the past and will in the future rely on:

- modulation of the intake of macronutrients especially by substitution (e.g. fat substitutes or intense sweeteners);
- use of components like caffeine with the aim of improving cognitive performance;
- use of specific amino acids like tryptophan or tyrosine to reduce sleep latency and promote feelings of drowsiness;
- activation of endogenous opioids (β-endorphins) to reduce pain perception in the general population.

1.6   Food technology and its impact on functional food development[9, 25]

From the point of view of food processing, the development of functional foods will often require an increased level of complexity and monitoring of food processing because the following will have to be considered carefully:

- new raw materials including those produced by biotechnologies;
- emerging thermal and non-thermal technologies;
- new safety issues;
- integration throughout the entire food chain especially to ensure preservation and/or enhancement of functionality.

The main areas for technological challenge that have been identified are as follows:

- The *creation* of new food components in traditional and novel raw materials that add or increase functionality. Examples of such challenges are: genetic modifications, use of under-utilised or unconventional natural sources (e.g. algae, seaweeds), development of bioreactors based on immobilised enzymes or live micro-organisms.
- The *optimisation* of functional components in raw material and in foods to ensure maximal preservation of the component(s), to modify function, to increase their bioavailability. Examples of such challenges are: development of membrane-processing techniques, use of controlled and modified atmospheres, use of high hydrostatic pressure, high-intensity electric field pulse technology or ultrasound treatments.
- The *effective monitoring*, throughout the entire food chain, of the amount and functionality of the component(s) in raw materials and foods. Examples of such challenges are: monitoring of microbial viability and productivity for probiotic functions, development of sensitive markers to record changes in speciation and interactions with food components during processing, especially fermentation.

1.7 Future trends

By reference to the conclusions of the FUFOSE concerted action,[9] future trends are as follows:

- Components in foods have the potential to modulate target functions in the body so as to enhance these functions and/or contribute towards reducing the risk of disease, and functional food science will contribute to human health in the future provided that evidence is supported by sound scientific, mostly human, data.
- Nutritionists and food scientists have the possibility through the development of functional foods to offer beneficial opportunities related to well-being and health and reduction of risk of disease. Such a new approach in nutrition is strongly dependent upon the identification, characterisation, measurement and validation of relevant markers as defined above. The design of such studies still needs to be carefully analysed and specifically developed by reference to, but differently from, classical clinical studies that have been elaborated to help in developing drugs, not food products.
- Major target functions in the body that are or can be modulated by specific food products will have to be identified or characterised. The basic science to understand these functions and how they relate to well-being and health or a particular pathological process needs to be developed so as to give the necessary scientific base to develop new functional food products.
- Progress in food regulation, which is the means to guarantee the validity of the claims as well as the safety of the food, will have to be made.

Optimised nutrition is a major challenge for nutritional science in the twenty-first century. The development of functional foods is part of this challenge but elaboration of claims should remain basically a scientific challenge, and not primarily a marketing one. The proper scientific validation of functional claims is critical to the success of functional foods, both for the benefit of human health and of the food industry.

1.8 References

1 WELSCH, S. 'Nutrient standards, dietary guidelines and food guides'. In *Present Knowledge in Nutrition*, E.E. Ziegler and L.J. Filer eds, Washington DC, ILSI Press, 1996.
2 Food and Nutrition Board *Diet and Health, Implications for Reducing Chronic Diseases*, Washington DC, National Academy Press, 10th edn, 1989.
3 Food and Nutrition Board *Recommended Daily Allowances*, Washington DC, National Academy Press, 10th edn, 1989.
4 US Department of Agriculture/Department of Health and Human Services *Nutrition and Your Health: Dietary Guidelines for Americans*, Home and

Guide Bulletin No. 232, Washington DC, US Government Printing Office, 4th edn, 1990.

5 US Department of Agriculture/Department of Health and Human Services *The Food Guide Pyramid*, Home and Guide Bulletin No. 252, Washington DC, US Government Printing Office, 1992.

6 JAMES, W.P.T. *Healthy Nutrition: Preventing Nutrition-related Diseases in Europe*, WHO, Regional Publications European Series, 1988, **24**, 4–6.

7 MILNER, J. 'Functional foods: the US perspective', 17th Ross Conference on Medical Issues, *Am J Clin Nutr*, 2000, **71**, 1654S–59S.

8 KOK, F.J. 'Functional foods: relevance of genetic susceptibility'. In *Proceedings of Forum on Functional Food*, Council of Europe Publications, Strasbourg, 1999, 217–29.

9 DIPLOCK, A.T., AGGETT, P.J., ASHWELL, M., BORNET, F., FERN, F.B., ROBERFROID, M.B. 'Scientific concepts of functional foods in Europe: consensus document', *Br J Nutr*, 1999, **81** supp. 1 S1–S28.

10 KUBOMARA, K. 'Japan redefines functional foods', *Prepared Foods*, 1998, **167**, 129–32.

11 HILLIAN, M. 'Functional foods: current and future market developments', *Food Technol Internat Europe*, 1995, 25–31.

12 RIEMERSMA, R.A. 'A fat little earner', *Lancet*, 1996, **347**, 775–6.

13 COGHLAN, A. 'A plateful of medicine', *New Scientist*, 1996, **2054**, 12–13.

14 GOLDBERG, I. *Functional Foods, Designer Foods, Pharmafoods, Nutraceuticals*, New York, Chapman & Hall, 1994.

15 MAZZA, G. *Functional foods: Biochemical and Processing Aspects*, Lancaster PA, Technomic, 1998.

16 DEFELICE, S.L. 'The nutraceutical revolution, its impact on food industry research and development', *Trends Food Sci Technol*, 1995, **6**, 59–61.

17 Health Canada. *Policy Options Analysis: Nutraceuticals/Functional Foods*, Health Canada, Health Protection Branch, Therapeutic Products Programme and Food Directorate, Ottawa, 1997.

18 Ministry of Agriculture, Fisheries and Food *Food Advisory Committee Review of Functional Foods and Health Claims*, London, 1996.

19 Federal Register 'Diet Supplement Health Education Act (DSHEA)', *Publ L*, Washington DC, 1994, 103–417.

20 Ministère de la Santé Publique, République Française *Décret Définissant et Réglementat les Compléments Alimentaires*, 14 October 1997, 97–964.

21 IFIC Foundation 'Functional foods: opening the door to better health' *Food Insight*, November/December 1995.

22 SMITH, B.L., MARCOTTE, M., HARMAN, G. *A Comparative Analysis of the Regulatory Framework Affecting Functional Food Development and Commercialization in Canada, Japan, the European Union and the United States of America*, Ottawa, Intersector Alliance Inc., 1996.

23 Food and Nutrition Board, Institute of Medicine, National Academy of Sciences. In *Opportunities in the Nutrition and Food Sciences*, P.R. Thomas and R. Earl eds, Washington DC, National Academy Press, 1994.

24   BELLISLE, F., DIPLOCK, A.T., HORNSTRA, G., KOLETZKO, B., ROBERFROID, M., SALMINEN, S., SARIS, W.H.M. 'Functional food science in Europe', *Br J Nutr*, 1998, **80**, supp. 1 S1–S193.

25   KNORR, D. 'Functional food science in Europe' *Trends in Food Sci Technol*, 1998, **9**, special issue, 295–340.

26   European Commission *Novel Food Directive*, 97/258/CEE.

27   Keystone 'The Keystone national policy dialogue on food nutrition and health: executive summary', *J Nutraceuticals, Functional and Medical Foods*, 1997, **1**, 11–32.

28   HUDSON, C.B. 'The food industry's expectation', In *Health Claims: Substantiation and Research Needs*, ILSI–Australasia, 1994, 9–11.

29   Codex Alimentarius *Codex General Guidelines on Claims*, 1991, CAC/GL 1–1979 Revision 1.

30   Swedish Nutrition Foundation *Health Claims in the Labelling and Marketing of Food Products: The Food Industry's Rules (Self-Regulatory Programme)*, Lund, 1996.

31   Codex Alimentarius. *Proposed Draft Recommendation for the Use of Health Claims*, Geneva, WHO, 1999.

32   SALMINEN, S., BOULEY, C., BOUTRON-RUAULT, M.C., CUMMINGS, J.H., FRANCK, A., GIBSON, G.R., ISOLAURI, E., MOREAU, M.C., ROBERFROID, M., ROWLAND, I. 'Functional food science and gastrointestinal physiology and function', *Br J Nutr*, 1998, **80**, supp. 1 S147–S171.

33   DIPLOCK, A.T., CHARLEUX, J.L., CROZIER-WILLY, G., KOK, F.J., RICE-EVANS, C., ROBERFROID, M., STAHL, W., VINA-ROBES, J. 'Functional food science and defense against reactive oxidative species', *Br J Nutr*, 1998, **80**, supp. 1 S77–S112.

34   BELLISLE, F., BLUNDELL, J.E., DYE, L., FANTINO, M., FERN, E., FLETCHER, R.J., LAMBERT, J., ROBERFROID, M., SPECTOR, S., WESTENHÖFER, J., WESTERTERP-PLANTENGO, M.S. 'Functional food science and behaviour and psychological functions', *Br J Nutr*, 1998, **80**, supp. 1 S173–S193.

2

EU legislation and functional foods
A case study

P. Berry Ottaway, Consultant, Berry Ottaway and Associates Ltd, Hereford

2.1 Introduction

Food law always lags behind innovation and developments, sometimes by more than a decade. This was particularly true in the late 1990s with advances in nutritional science and the general acceptance that some aspects of foods can contribute to health in other ways than by an adequate supply of classical nutrients.

From a relatively slow start, the concept of a functional food has been gaining ground world-wide, and has also been attracting the attention of the major multinational food companies. Within Europe there has been increasing recognition of functional foods by the national authorities, particularly in the area of health claims for foods.

The composition and proposed marketing of many functional foods can introduce a number of anomalies in the application of current EU food legislation and the following is a case study of the proposed introduction of such a product.

2.2 Product description

The product, which was in an advanced stage of development in a country outside the EU, was also being considered for the European market. The concept of the product was a powdered beverage mix which could be made up with milk, water or fruit juices and which provided not only protein, carbohydrate and fat, but also a wide range of micronutrients, added fibre sources and fructo-oligosaccharides. The fructo-oligosaccharides were added for their prebiotic benefits.

The micronutrients included all those listed in the directive on nutrition labelling (90/496/EEC)[1] plus a number of other trace minerals such as selenium, copper and manganese. The antioxidant vitamins C, E and beta-carotene were present at levels of daily intake above the recommended daily allowances (RDAs) used for nutrition labelling purposes in Europe. In addition the formulators of the product wanted to add other carotenoids such as lycopene and lutein as additional *in vivo* antioxidants.

The product was to be available in three flavours with the appropriate colours. The marketing objective in the country of origin was to market the product not only as a nutritious beverage but also to position it for convalescents, athletes and as a meal replacement for weight control purposes.

2.3 Product positioning in the European market

The definition of the product from the marketing point of view was found to be critical. Some of the recommended uses fell into the definition of dietetic as given in the directive on foods for particular nutritional uses (89/398/EEC)[2] known as the PARNUTS directive. There is a specific directive in force, 96/8/EC,[3] which controls both the composition and labelling of foods marketed as meal replacements for use in weight control diets. The composition of such meal replacements must comply with very detailed criteria with respect to the energy, protein, carbohydrate, fat and micronutrient content. The product as developed did not meet all the criteria so the decision had to be made to market it as a convenient healthy beverage applicable to a range of lifestyles.

2.4 Product composition

A detailed investigation had to be carried out on every component, whether ingredient or additive, to ensure compliance with the various European laws.

2.4.1 Protein

The protein contribution was made up of both isolated soya protein and casein (milk protein). The specifications and origins of both had to be checked. To comply with the Council Regulation (EC) No. 1139/98 on the labelling of genetically modified soya or maize,[4] the provenance of the soya had to be traced and certification obtained that it did not contain genetically modified protein or DNA.

There is a European Directive 83/417/EEC laying down the specification and quality criteria for caseinates and the ingredient had to be checked for compliance.[5]

2.4.2 Fat

The fat contribution was supplied from an oil high in polyunsaturated fatty acids plus some lecithin. The specification and typical analyses of the oil were obtained to ensure that permitted maximum levels of erucic acid in the oil were not likely to be exceeded. Erucic acid is a normal constituent of seed oils which has been shown to have detrimental effects on health if consumed in large quantities. There is a limit for erucic acid from oils used in compounded foods where the overall fat content of the food exceeds 5%. The details are given in Directive 76/621/EEC,[6] with the method of analysis in Directive 80/891/EEC.[7]

Directive 76/621/EEC also gives a derogation for member states to apply the provisions of the directive to foods where the total fat content is equal to or less than 5%.

Due to the high polyunsaturated content of the oil it was more susceptible to oxidation (rancidity) than many oils used in such products. The presence of a number of mineral salts in the product also increased the risk of rapid rancidity. Permitted antioxidants for fats and oils are given in the directive on additives other than colours and sweeteners (95/2/EC).[8] As the proposed source of the oil was North America, discussions had to be conducted with the suppliers to ensure that the oil was adequately protected using only the antioxidants and permitted levels given in the directive. As European law in this area differs significantly from that in the USA, this caused considerable problems which were only resolved by changing to a different grade of oil to that originally preferred.

Legal complications were also encountered with the lecithin. In early 1999, when the work was being carried out, Regulation (EC) No. 1139/98 on the labelling of genetically modified (GM) soya and maize was in force but the proposed exclusion list for highly processed soya and maize derivatives had not been adopted. The original source of lecithin proved positive when tested for DNA from GM soya. Alternative supplies were offered from South America but these were found to have differences in their functional characteristics from the original source. The legal requirement to label the lecithin containing the GM DNA was based on its primary function in the product. At that time, the regulation only covered food ingredients from GM soya and maize and specifically excluded additives and flavourings. Lecithins are approved additives and appear in Annex 1 to Directive 95/2/EC as being generally permitted in foodstuffs.

According to the formulator of the product, the lecithin had been included for two reasons: the first was technological, to improve wetting-out characteristics when the powder was mixed into the liquid; and the second was nutritional, to provide a source of phospholipids. This situation, where substances can have dual roles in foods as additives and nutrients, is not uncommon in European food law. The decision was originally made in early 1999 that the primary function of lecithin in the product was as a technological additive and the marketing department had the option not to make the label statement on the GM source. This option was negated in January 2000 when the European Regulation (EC) 50/2000 on the labelling of additives and flavourings from GM sources was adopted.[9] However, while the decision was made to specify the lecithin as an additive, its contribution had to be added to the total fat content given in the nutrition information on the label. Directive 90/496/EEC on nutrition labelling specifically includes phospholipids in the definition of fat.

2.4.3 Carbohydrate

The main carbohydrate component of the product consisted of a mixture of dextrose, fructose and maltodextrin. As these ingredients can be produced from maize, the GM status of each had to be determined. The product was also found to contain relatively small amounts of sorbitol, principally as a component of some compounded ingredients. Under European law the definition of carbohydrates for labelling purposes includes the polyols, of which sorbitol is one, but requires the energy calculation for the contribution from sorbitol to be made with a different factor. Carbohydrates (excluding polyols) must be calculated on the basis of 4kcal/g whereas polyols are at 2.4kcal/g. Also, for the purposes of nutrition labelling, the statement of carbohydrate content had to be subdivided into sugars, polyols and starch. The legal definition of sugars includes all monosaccharides and disaccharides in the foods, but excludes polyols.

2.4.4 Fibre

The added fibre and fructo-oligosaccharides presented a number of legal problems, particularly in the quantification of the fibre content. There is no formal definition of dietary fibre in European food law. When Directive 90/496/EEC was adopted, the definition of fibre was given as follows:

> fibre means the material to be defined in accordance with the procedure laid down in Article 10 (of Directive 90/496/EEC) and measured by the method of analysis to be determined in accordance with that procedure.

This statement resulted from a major disagreement in 1990 among the member states as to what constituted dietary fibre. Almost ten years later this had not been resolved. The debate has revolved around the specific components of non-digestible plant matter that collectively contribute to the dietary fibre content and should be included in the analysis. An early definition of dietary fibre was 'the plant polysaccharides and lignin which are resistant to hydrolysis by the digestive enzymes of man'. There are more recent schools of thought that fibre should be defined more closely as 'non-starch polysaccharides (NSP)'. NSPs are the major fraction of fibre and are chemically identifiable. The British authorities are in favour of the definition being NSP as measured by the Englyst method, while some other member states prefer to use a concept of fibre that includes other substances such as lignin. There are a number of ways of chemically determining the fibre content of foods depending on the definition used and the components included in the definition.

The British authorities have consistently insisted that the quantitative declaration of fibre content given on the label should be based on NSP measured by the Englyst method. Since the adoption of the directive on nutrition labelling in 1990, they have been persistent in trying to persuade the other member states to agree to accept a definition based on NSP. This has not succeeded and in 1996 the British Ministry of Agriculture, Fisheries and Food issued a statement saying that although they still regarded the Englyst method, or one giving the same results, as the official method in UK law, manufacturers could label with fibre content determined by other methods such as the AOAC, provided the method of analysis was declared on the label.[10] However, it was also stated that claims for fibre could only be made on values determined by the Englyst method. This meant that in order to make a claim for a high fibre content for the product in the UK, it had to contain at least 6g per 100g of NSP measured by the Englyst method. If the AOAC method, commonly accepted by other EU countries, had been used, the actual declaration of fibre content on the label would have been much greater, but no claim for it could be made on the pack or in advertising. In 1999 the British government issued proposals for the labelling of fibre to be based on the AOAC method. Unfortunately, as a result of a long consultation period, these proposals had not been introduced into law by the time the product was launched.

A further complexity surrounding the fibre claim was that the product contained significant amounts of inulin and other fructo-oligosaccharides which have been shown to have a beneficial (prebiotic) effect on the gut microflora. The status of these substances in terms of labelling have been the subject of considerable debate in Europe, particularly in the UK. In 1997 the British government Committee on the Medical Aspects of Food Policy (the COMA Committee) was asked to consider the inclusion of inulin and oligofructose in the UK definition of dietary fibre for labelling purposes. In a statement in April 1998 the committee reported that it had agreed to retain the existing definition based on NSPs, but to consider additional categories for declaring resistant starch and non-digestible oligosaccharides on product labels. A year later the committee was asked to reconsider its decision and reported again in April 1999 that, having reviewed submissions in support of the application, the committee was not convinced by the evidence presented and concluded that inulin and oligofructose should not be included in the definition.[11] This decision meant that these substances could not be added to the fibre content for the UK label and had to be declared separately on the statement of nutritional information. These differences in the definition of fibre meant that there would have to be a dichotomy in the marketing strategy between the UK and the rest of Europe.

2.4.5 Micronutrients

The proposed addition of a wide range of micronutrients caused considerable problems. The fortification of foods with vitamins and minerals is one aspect of European food law that is still under discussion and has not yet reached the stage of a draft directive. The complexities of legislating in this area were outlined in a European Commission discussion paper in 1997.[12]

Across Europe there has been no consistent approach to the addition of vitamins and minerals to foods. Some countries, such as the UK and the Netherlands, have relatively liberal policies while others, such as Spain and Ireland, impose very strict controls. Throughout the EU, there are 15 different sets of laws covering the addition of vitamins and minerals to foods and they all differ in detail from each other. Some of these differences are very significant.

Many countries use the RDA as a basis for the legal control of vitamins or minerals. For example, Germany permits vitamins, excluding vitamins A and D, to be added to foods up to 3 × RDA per daily intake of the food. The addition of vitamins A and D to foods is prohibited, with only some specific exceptions. Belgium has complex legislation with vitamins A and D at 1 × RDA, the B vitamins, C and E at 3 × RDA and most others at 2 × RDA, and formal notification is required. Spain and Ireland both impose an upper limit of 1 × RDA on micronutrients in foods. In addition, French law does not permit the addition of micronutrients to foods but permits restoration of vitamins at levels between 80% and 200% and minerals at between 80% and 120% of the natural content of the food before processing, although the addition of micronutrients to foods for particular nutritional uses (PARNUTS products) is allowed in France. Some countries only permit micronutrient addition to foods on the basis of individual product authorisations. A further complication was that some of the countries only allowed the addition to foods of the 12 vitamins and 6 minerals that appear in the Annex to Directive 90/496/EEC. This list does not include the trace elements copper, manganese and selenium which appear in the specific PARNUTS directives and are recognised as being essential in these foods.

These complexities meant that the added micronutrient content of the product either had to be reduced to the lowest common denominator from each country's requirements or a marketing decision had to be made to market the product initially in those countries where the legislation was most compatible with the original product concept. Eventually, the latter option was preferred as the first substantially reduced both the number of micronutrients that could be added to the products and also their level of input.

Once the list of micronutrients had been determined, the chemical forms in which they could be added also had to be checked. This was important as, for the minerals particularly, some of the salts and organic forms of the nutrients are not officially recognised in many countries in Europe. The only guideline that was available was the draft list and opinion of the European Commission's Scientific Committee on Food relating to approved nutrient sources for PARNUTS foods.[13] This draft was published in May 1999, almost exactly ten years after the requirement for such a list was given in Article 4(2) of the PARNUTS Directive 89/398/EEC.

2.4.6 Novel foods and novel ingredients

The original proposal for the product included a number of substances, such as the carotenoids lutein and lycopene, that were to be added for their *in vivo* antioxidant functions. The list of those to be considered consisted of a number of plant extracts including some with high levels of polyphenols.

The first task was to check each proposed substance on the list for acceptability, both in terms of their status with regard to the Council Regulation (EC) No. 258/97 on novel foods and novel ingredients,[14] and to the national situation in the countries of intended sale.

Although the Regulation 258/97 had been in force for over two years at the time the review was carried out, the situation was found to be very confused. The main criterion for classification as a novel food or ingredient is that the substance had not previously been used for human consumption in the European Community *to a significant degree*. Unfortunately, no formal definition of the phrase 'to a significant degree' had been agreed between the European Commission and the 15 member states. Interpretations varied from that which accepted evidence that the substance had been on sale in a food product in one member state before 15 May 1997 (the date that the regulation came into force), to evidence of a large distribution and sales in more than one member state.

The main problem encountered was that although evidence of prior sale in the UK and the Netherlands could be found for some of the substances, enquiries determined that they were not considered acceptable for use in food products in other countries such as Germany and France. The investigations highlighted a major weakness in the system. The intention of Regulation 258/97 is that novel foods and novel ingredients are reviewed and approved by the competent authority in the member state of intended first sale. This is carried out with the knowledge of the other 14 member states who are notified of the application by the European Commission. Once approved, the substance should be accepted throughout the EU. No provision was made in the regulation or in any other European food legislation for mutual recognition of foods and ingredients that have been introduced into one of the national markets a few years before the regulation came into force. This has left a number of ingredients, including some on the proposed list for the product, in a situation where approval for use still has to be obtained on a country-by-country basis.

The lutein and lycopene were an anomaly. Both carotenoids have been approved for use as food colourings in Europe, but with restricted levels of input. They both appear in Annex V of Directive 94/36/EC on colours for use in foodstuffs and their permitted use is restricted to specified categories of food and drink.[15] The category that most closely defined the product was 'non-alcoholic flavoured drinks' and the maximum level given for lutein and lycopene was 100mg/l either individually or in combination. The calculation is based on the pure dye content of the colour. Therefore, if both carotenoids were used in compliance with the directive, the maximum allowable level of each would be 50mg/l of the ready-to-consume drink. There is no official recognition of either lutein or lycopene in any other area of European food law. In terms of the proposed formulation, an acceptable level of both carotenoids could be achieved within the limits given in the directive on colours but it was noted that, in order to comply with the legislation in some countries, these ingredients would have to be listed as colours in the declaration of ingredients on the label.

2.4.7 Colours and flavours

Both food colours and food flavourings are controlled by European directives. The proposed colours and the levels of use had to comply with Directive 94/36/EC. As many of the proposed colours were carried on a base or were in the form of a lake, details of the pure dye content of each had to be obtained to enable the appropriate calculations to be made.

The situation with flavourings was that the flavouring components and source materials used in their production came under the requirements of Directive 88/388/EEC as amended.[16] This directive includes a list of substances that are considered undesirable from the point of view of human health and are therefore restricted.

As most food flavourings are compounded proprietary mixtures, certification had to be obtained from each of the proposed suppliers that their flavouring complied with the requirements of the directive.

2.5 Functional claims

One of the important aspects of the product concept was that both nutrition and health claims could be made for the product. This is a very difficult legal area and the problems have been highlighted by recent developments in the functional food market.

European food legislation in the form of the directive on food labelling 79/112/EEC[17] specifically prohibits the attribution to any foodstuff of the property of preventing, treating or curing a human disease, or any reference to such properties. In this context, human disease has been interpreted as any ailment, injury or adverse condition, whether in body or mind. Under EU Directive 65/65/EEC,[18] the medicines directive, any claim expressed or implied that a product can prevent, treat or cure a disease or condition is regarded as a medicinal claim and the product has to be treated in law as a medicine. Similar legislation applies in most countries of the world.

As there is often a very fine line dividing medical claims and health claims, much rests on the semantics and presentation. A statement that folic acid helps prevent neural tube defects in the foetus would be considered a medical claim if made for a food or food supplement. By saying that folic acid helps with the development of a healthy nervous system in the foetus, the claim becomes a health claim. Both claims are scientifically correct, but the first relates to the prevention of an adverse condition and can only be made for an authorised medicine.

Since 1980 there have been a number of abortive attempts by the European Commission to introduce pan-European legislation on health claims. After a series of fruitless meetings through the early 1990s with no agreement reached by the then smaller number of member states, the European Commission abandoned its plans for a European directive on claims. This meant that the individual national regulations have continued to remain in force, resulting in a diversity of approaches across the EU.

In the absence of pan-European legislation on claims, there has been considerable activity in a number of member states of the EU. For complex legal reasons these developments have been either in the production of Codes of Practice or agreements between the food industry and the national regulatory authorities. Codes of Practice on health claims have been introduced into Sweden,[19] Belgium,[20] the Netherlands[21] and the UK.[22]

In Spain, a voluntary agreement on health claims has been signed between the Spanish food industry and the Ministry of Health.[23] In France, the French Conseil National de l'Alimentation (National Dietary Council) has been considering evidence from consumer groups, scientists and industry and in 1998 drafted an opinion and proposals on claims linking diet and health.[24] While all six countries have taken slightly different approaches to obtain the same objectives, all the codes and agreements agree on the major points.

There is general consensus that some provision should be made to allow health claims for foods and that these should be in addition to the currently permitted nutrient function claims (e.g. calcium is required for healthy bones and teeth).

There is also general recognition that health claims could be made for foods containing substances other than the traditionally recognised nutrients. A good example of such a case is where the cholesterol-lowering effects of a fat-based spread with the brand name Benecol are attributed to plant stanol esters, which are, at present, not recognised as nutrients.

The codes or agreements require that the claims are substantiated by appropriate scientific evidence. With the exception of the Belgian code, the others require a review and acceptance of the scientific evidence in support of the claim to be carried out by a panel of independent experts.

The most detailed requirements are given in the British code on health claims. This requires that the claim must be based on a systematic review of all the available scientific evidence relating to the validity of the claim, including published scientific literature. The conclusions of the review must be based on the totality of the evidence and not just that which supports the claim. The evidence must also be based on the most methodologically sound human studies and not just biochemical, cellular or animal studies, although other sources of information such as epidemiological evidence and animal, biochemical or cellular studies should be used to support the substantiation.

The evidence must be able to demonstrate that the food will contribute to a positive and significant physiological benefit when consumed by the target population as part of their normal diet. The claimed effect must be achievable with the consumption of a reasonable amount of the food on a regular basis or by the food making a reasonable contribution to the diet.

Expressed in the British and Dutch codes and implicit in the others is that the food as presented to the consumer must be demonstrated to produce the desired effects. The use of surrogate studies or reliance on bibliographical evidence only would not be acceptable.

It is also important that it can be demonstrated that the claimed effect is maintained over a reasonable period of time and is not just a short-term response to which the body later adjusts. The exceptions allowed are for health claims that are for situations that are only relevant for a short- or medium-term benefit. A good example is the requirement for folic acid pre-conceptually and for the first 12 weeks of pregnancy in the case of neural tube defects.

These stringent requirements for health claims resulted in considerable discussion between the development and marketing teams of the company as it became apparent that further studies would be required to support the substantiation. A cost–benefit appraisal had to be carried out by the marketing department to see if the cost of acquiring the extra data was likely to be returned from additional sales if the claim was made.

2.6 Packaging

The proposed packaging had not only to be tested for the barrier properties in terms of product stability but also checked for compliance with a number of laws.

The first group of legislation that had to be checked was that dealing with materials and articles in contact with food. Council Directive 89/109/EEC[25] as amended is the framework directive which lays down a general requirement that all materials that come into contact with food should not transfer their constituents to food in quantities that could endanger human health or make the food unacceptable to the consumer. The directive also restricts the use of vinyl chloride monomer in the manufacture of food-grade plastics and places controls on the use of regenerated cellulose film coming into contact with food.

Under the framework directive there are a number of more specific directives, including Commission Directive 97/48/EC[26] on plastic materials and articles in contact with food and directives on the methods of testing the migration of the constituents of plastics to foods.

As the inner surface of the packaging that came into contact with the product was a plastic, these directives were particularly relevant and certification of compliance to the directives had to be obtained from the supplier of the packaging.

Although not directly part of European food law, the requirements of the directive on packaging and packaging waste (94/62/EC) also had to be considered.[27]

Aspects of this directive have a direct relevance to the packaging of the product. The main ones to be considered were the requirements that the packaging used must be the minimal subject to the safety, hygiene and acceptance for the packed product and for the consumer. The packaging used must be recoverable through at least one of the following:

- material recycling
- incineration with energy recovery
- composting or biodegradation.

The directive also permits packaging to be reusable, but this was not appropriate for the product concept. Any noxious or hazardous substances in the packaging must be minimised in any emissions, ash or leachate from either incineration or landfill.

Within the directive there is also a very specific requirement for heavy metal limits in packaging or any of its components. These limits, which refer to the total concentration of cadmium, mercury, lead and hexavalent chromium, refer to packaging in general and not just to that which comes into contact with food. The heavy metal limits were 250 parts per million (ppm) by weight for any packaging used on or after 30 June 1999 and these reduce to 100ppm by weight on or after 30 June 2001. Again, assurances had to be obtained from the manufacturers of all the components of the packaging that their products complied with the directive, both in terms of recovery and the ability to meet the heavy metal limits.

Instructions also had to be given to the packaging designers to ensure that the requirements for minimalisation of the packaging were taken into consideration.

2.7 Labelling

Once the pack design had been agreed it was important that all the legal requirements could appear on the label in the appropriate manner. The list of compulsory requirements is given in Directive 79/112/EEC (as amended) and the main ones include the name of the product as a generic name, the list of ingredients, instructions for use, a statement of minimum durability, storage conditions and the name of the manufacturer, packer or seller established within the EU. The declaration of minimum durability, in this case a 'Best before end:' statement and the storage conditions, were based on the results of the product shelf-life trials.

In the case of the declaration of ingredients, the marketing department had a preference to exercise the option of declaring the additives by their generic names as given in the directives instead of using the 'E' numbers for the additives.

As the original development of the product had taken place in North America, many of the values in the nutrition labelling had to be adjusted to the European requirements given in Directive 90/496/EEC. Not only were the factors for calculating the energy content from the energy nutrients different between the two continents but there were also significant differences in the calculation of the activity of a number of vitamins. For example, the thiamin (vitamin B_1) level had been originally calculated on the basis of input of the salt, whereas in Europe the declaration is as the amount of the thiamin cation present. There was also a major discrepancy in the calculation of vitamin A activity in betacarotene.

The formulation was checked to ensure that the composition did not trigger any statutory warnings or statements such as those required in Directive 94/35/EC on sweeteners where the presence in a product of the intense sweetener aspartame or polyols require prescribed warning statements. The national requirements in this area also had to be taken into consideration. For example, in the UK there is a voluntary agreement between the British Department of Health and the food industry that products containing added vitamin A (as retinol) should carry a warning for pregnant women if the vitamin A content of the recommended daily intake of the product exceeds 800μg. The contribution of betacarotene to the vitamin A content is excluded from this requirement.

2.8 Manufacture

The manufacture of the product was a dry-blending process followed by the spraying into the mix of oil and lecithin. While it was envisaged that the production for the launch of the product would be carried out in North America, there was a requirement to find a suitable production facility in Europe.

As part of the evaluation of potential contract manufacturers, a technical, quality and hygiene audit was carried out on the main contenders. The hygiene part of the audit was designed to ensure that all the requirements of Directive 93/43/EEC[28] on food hygiene were in compliance. This included confirmation that a hazard analysis and critical control point assessment (HACCP) had been carried out by the company as required by the directive.

2.9 References

1 European Council Directive 90/496/EEC on nutrition labelling for foodstuffs. *O.J. of E.C.* L276/40 of 6 October 1990.
2 European Council Directive 89/398/EEC on foodstuffs for particular nutritional uses. *O.J. of E.C.* L186/27 of 30 June 1989.
3 Commission Directive 96/8/EC on foods intended for use in energy-restricted diets for weight control. *O.J. of E.C.* L55/22 of 6 March 1996.
4 European Council Regulation (EC) No. 1139/98 on compulsory labelling of certain foodstuffs produced from genetically modified organisms. *O.J. of E.C.* L159/4 of 3 June 1998 as amended by Commission Regulation (EC) No. 49/2000. *O.J. of E.C.* L6/13 of 11 January 2000.

5 European Council Directive 83/417/EEC relating to caseins and caseinates. *O.J. of E.C.* L237/25 of 26 August 1983.

6 European Council Directive 76/621/EEC on the maximum level of erucic acid in oils, fats and foodstuffs for human consumption. *O.J. of E.C.* L202/35 of 28 July 1976.

7 European Council Directive 80/891/EEC on method of analysis for determining the erucic acid content of fats and oils. *O.J. of E.C.* L254/35 of 27 September 1980.

8 European Parliament and Council Directive 95/2/EC on food additives other than colours and sweeteners. *O.J. of E.C.* L61/1 of 18 March 1995.

9 European Commission Regulation (EC) No. 50/2000 on the labelling of foodstuffs containing additives or flavourings that have been genetically modified. *O.J. of E.C.* L6/15 of 11 January 2000.

10 Ministry of Agriculture, Fisheries and Food (UK). Definition and Determination of Dietary Fibre. Letter and statement dated 1 May 1996.

11 Food Safety Information Bulletin, MAFF, UK. Definition of Dietary Fibre. Bulletin No. 109, June 1999.

12 European Commission DG III. 'Addition of vitamins and minerals to foods and food supplements – a discussion paper'. III/5934/97, 1997, Brussels.

13 Scientific Committee on Food of the European Commission. Opinion on substances for nutritional purposes which have been proposed for use in the manufacture of foods for particular nutritional uses. SCF/CS/ADD/NUT/20/ Final of 12 May 1999.

14 European Parliament and Council Regulation (EC) No. 258/97 concerning novel foods and novel food ingredients. *O.J. of E.C.* L43/1 of 14 February.

15 European Parliament and European Council Directive 94/36/EC on colours for use in foodstuffs. *O.J. of E.C.* L237/13 of 10 September 1994.

16 European Council Directive 88/388/EEC on flavourings used in foodstuffs and source materials used in their production. *O.J. of E.C.* L184/61 of 15 July 1988.

17 European Council Directive 79/112/EEC relating to the labelling, presentation and advertising of foodstuffs. *O.J. of E.C.* L33/1 of 8 February 1979.

18 European Council Directive 65/65/EEC relating to proprietary medicinal products. *O.J. of E.C.* 22 February 1965.

19 Federation of Swedish Food Industries *et al.* Health Claims in the Labelling and Marketing of Food Products. Food Industry's Rules (Self-Regulating Programme). Revised programme of 28 August 1996.

20 Federatie Voedingsindustrie/Fédération de l'Industrie Alimentaire (Belgium). Health Claims Code of Conduct, draft, 21 October 1998.

21 Voedingscentrum (Netherlands). Code of practice assessing the scientific evidence for health benefits stated in health claims on food and drink products. April 1998.

22 Joint Health Claims Initiative (United Kingdom). Code of Practice on Health Claims on Foods. Final text, 9 November 1998.

23 Joint 'Ministerio de Sonidad y Consumo' (Ministry of Health, Spain) and Federación de Industrias de Alimentación y Bebidas (Spanish Federation of Food and Drink Manufacturers) agreement on health claims on foods of 20 March 1998.

24 Conseil National de l'Alimentation (France). Allégations faisant un lien entre alimentation et santé. Avis No. 21, 30 June 1998, Paris.

25 European Council Directive 89/109/EEC relating to materials and articles intended to come into contact with foodstuffs. *O.J. of E.C.* L40/30 of 11 February 1989.

26 European Commission Directive 97/48/EC on plastic materials and articles in contact with food (*O.J. of E.C.* L222 of 12 August 1997) amending Council Directive 82/711/EEC. *O.J. of E.C.* L297/26 of 23 October 1982.

27 European Parliament and Council Directive 94/62/EC on packaging and packaging waste. *O.J. of E.C.* L365/10 of 31 December 1994.

28 European Council Directive 93/43/EEC on the hygiene of foodstuffs *O.J. of E.C.* L175/1 of 19 July 1993.

3

US legislation and functional health claims

M.K. Schmidl and T.P. Labuza, University of Minnesota

3.1 Introduction

With the enactment of the Orphan Drug Act (ODA) of 1988 (Pub. L. 100–290),[1] Nutrition Labeling and Education Act (NLEA) of 1990 (Pub. L. 101–535),[2] Dietary Supplement Health and Education Act (DSHEA) of 1994 (Pub. L. 103–417),[3] and the Food and Drug Administration Modernization Act (FDAMA) of 1997 (Pub. L. 105–115),[4] food laws and regulations have been substantially reformed,[5–8] opening up entirely new opportunities to promote both the health benefits of foods and to design so-called 'functional foods' and 'nutraceuticals' which can provide targeted nutritional, disease-preventing or health benefits to the consumer. These new legislative mandates and the regulations that follow helped to clarify a somewhat confusing situation. For example, in 1963, the US government seized a table sugar product, which was essentially sucrose fortified with 19 vitamins and minerals, on the basis that the addition of these nutrients were of no value since they were already available in the US diet. The courts (*US* v. *Dextra Brand Sugar* 231 F. Supp 561; 2/21/63) overturned the government action on the basis that it should not interfere with commerce and the product was neither misbranded nor adulterated. The company was responding to the consumer concern at that time that some products were considered to be empty calories (containing no vitamins or minerals); thus fortifying the sugar brought it into the 'healthy' food category.

In the US, any statements or claims on a packaged food are covered under the Federal Food, Drug and Cosmetic Act (FFDCA). These statements on the label are considered labeling, and as such, any false or misleading statements are considered to be 'misbranding'. In addition, any promotional material, such as a book, in close proximity to the food at point of sale has also been considered to be labeling and subject to the law under the FFDCA. In fact the federal government has seized products on this point of law and the Supreme Court has ruled this to be constitutionally correct (*US* v. *Kordel* 397 US 1; 1970). Section 403(a)(1) of the FFDCA declares as misbranding any false or misleading statements. In addition, Section 201(n) also makes a food misbranded if the label fails to reveal facts material to the product. The latter came into play prior to the requirement for nutrition labeling on all foods, when in 1974, the Food and Drug Administration (FDA), the agency responsible for administering the FFDCA, decided that if one made a nutrient claim on the label, then the label had to have a specific nutrient-based table containing information on calories, fat, protein, carbohydrates and eight vitamins and minerals, i.e. more encompassing than just saying 'contains a high amount of vitamin C.' In 1990, the US Congress enhanced this by passing NLEA, thus essentially requiring nutrition labeling for all processed foods on the basis that the specific label was material to the facts about any food, not just if specific content claim were made.

3.2 Definitions

Because laws and regulations have become extremely complex in the US, we will introduce the subject with the definition of a few key terms. 'Content claims' in labeling refer to such adjectival descriptors of food characteristics as 'low fat,' 'low sugar,' 'reduced calorie,' and 'healthy.' No mention of disease is involved. 'Health claims' prose is a bit of a misnomer because it involves label claims referring to specific diseases or conditions such as 'osteoporosis,' 'cardiovascular disease,' and 'hypertension.' Such claims are better categorized as disease-specific claims. 'Structure–function claims' refers to claims that may also be made on conventional food or dietary supplement labels if products qualify. No mention of disease or symptoms of disease may be stated, e.g. 'Calcium builds strong bones.'

When Congress (the House and Senate) votes to pass a new law (a Congressional Bill), it becomes a public law and is first denoted as Pub. L. xx–yy where Pub. L. is Public Law, xx denotes that number of the Congress (note each Congress is two years in length) and yy denotes the bill number in order of passage over the two-year period, thus FDAMA is PL 105–115 or the 115th bill passed by the 105th Congress in their two-year term. After the President (the Executive Branch of the three-part US government structure) signs the legislation, it becomes an Act; thus we have the Federal Food Drug and Cosmetic Act (FFDCA) of 1938 (21 USC 301–394) as amended (many times) and the Wholesome Meat Act of 1967 (21 USC 672). Once published, an Act officially becomes an official statute (e.g. the FFDCA is 52 Statute 1040 *et seq.*). Eventually statutes get published in the United States Code (USC), thus the FFDCA became 21 USC 301–394. Because Acts are broad and non-specific, the President of the USA is given the responsibility of the carrying out the Acts through promulgation (creation) of regulations as done by the various regulatory departments. These regulations give details and are more specific. As noted for foods, the main administrative organization within the Executive Branch is the Food and Drug Administration which is part of the Department of Health and Human Services. Within the FDA, the critical administrative branch related to food is the Center for Food Safety and Applied Nutrition (CFSAN). Meats are not legally foods and meat labeling is under the control of the Food Safety and Inspection Service (FSIS) of the United States Department of Agriculture (USDA). As required by the Administrative Procedure Act (APA) of 1946, all regulations proposed by the Executive Branch of the government must go through a public proposal process, instituted by publishing in the Federal Register (FR). The FR is published every working day of the year and provides an enormous array of notices by every administrative unit. It is imperative that anyone dealing with label claims keeps abreast of the proposed and finalized regulations as any changes can affect their business. The FR process allows all affected citizens and organizations to make public comment, and gives the agency a chance to respond.

Once due process is complete in a rather complex procedure of reproposals and a finalized regulation, the regulation has the power of law, unless reinterpreted by the courts (the third part of the US legislature–executive– judicial government design). The US Court's job is to resolve disputes based on US Constitutional issues, thus they must take into consideration the intent of Congress (legislature) and the concept of whether such regulation is arbitrary, capricious and not ripe for adjudication. The latter point means that although there might be a potential effect of the regulation on a party, unless someone can prove that actual harm has occurred or definitely will occur, the regulation stands as law. The seminal case of *Abbott Labs* v. *Gardner* (38 US 136; 1967) set the standard for the ripeness test. Thus if it were a misbranding issue due to a claim, the FDA would have to seize product because it felt the claim was illegal and then the regulation could be challenged. In addition, one might propose that the regulation precludes a claim that you want to make, and if you are going to print a label, prevention of the potential use of the label causes financial harm. Challenging regulations in court is not an uncommon way in which the regulation becomes better defined. Once a regulation is promulgated, it then gets published as an official regulation in an appropriate title (21 Code of Federal Regulations (CFR) for foods, 9 CFR for meats).

It should be noted that the court system has three tiers. The lowest courts are known as District Courts, with 94 courts spread over the whole USA, US possessions and territories. The next tier is the US Circuit Court of Appeals (CCA), of which there are 11 plus one for the District of Columbia, the latter of which hears cases arising out of conflict with regulations. The final court of appeal is the US Supreme Court. The Supreme Court (SC) gets close to 3,000 cases a year, but hears only 250–300 of them. These are designated by granting *certiorari* (agreement to hear the case). The rest are sent back to the Circuit Court for retrial or the SC states that they agree with the CCA decision. Very few food cases get to the US Supreme Court.

Another important aspect of the US system of law, i.e. legislature–executive–judicial, is that the courts have the final say (at least until Congress passes a new law) as to what a law means. In what may seem to be a trivial matter, but important to health and nutrition claims, the FFDCA defines food in the Section 201(f) as 'articles used for food and drink for man and animals and chewing gum.' This rather circular definition obviously has some limitations but served its purpose for almost 80 years until its definition was challenged in a US court case, *NutriLab, Inc.* v. *Schweiker*. The opinion was published October 5, 1982 and upheld by the Circuit Court of Appeals (713 F. 2nd. 335, 7th Circuit August 23, 1983). In essence, the Circuit Court said that the word 'food' means 'items consumed for taste, aroma or nutritive value.' It should be noted, based on agreements between US federal agencies, that a product with < 3% meat is a food (3% or more meat comes under the Wholesome Meat Act), if < 2% poultry it is a food (i.e. 2% or more of poultry in a food brings it under the Poultry Inspection Act) and if in a sandwich form, it is a food if it has < 16% meat. One can thus see why US food laws and regulations are so confusing to the international community.

3.3 Nutrient modification and specific nutrient claims

Nutrient modification claims (nutrient descriptors) have been developed for products for which there is a calorie, cholesterol, fatty acids, sugar, sodium or cholesterol reduction. These are claims used to attract the consumer and as such usually appear as a statement on the front panel of the food package. Because of the complexity of these rules, they will not be repeated here but a few examples are provided in part, e.g. the labeling of products for which the level of calories has been modified (21 CFR 101.60 *et seq.*; 58 FR 49020; September 18, 1993). A claim of 'free of calories' (or a trivial amount) can be made if there is less than 5 calories; a low-calorie food must be less than 40 calories for a serving size over 30 g (or > 50 g as prepared); and a reduced caloric claim requires it to be 25% lower than a reference value of a product in the same category. The 'free of' claim is one that is confusing to consumers because the product may not be entirely free of 'x'. An example is a commercial 'fat-free' butter substitute that has these words on the front label whereas the nutrition facts statement shows that it contains approximately 0.5 g fat which is the allowed upper limit for a fat-free claim and that it has 5 calories from fat (21 CFR 101.60(b)(1)(i)).

For specific nutrient claims, such as 'an excellent source of vitamin C,' 21 CFR 101.62 requires the product to have at least 20% of the RDI or DRV whereas when claiming the product as a good source, there must be between 10% and 19% of the value. The regulations also have preclusions that disallow the use of a content claim for one nutrient when other nutrients present in the food would make the product have less of a health benefit, e.g. one can claim a lite sodium product only if the sodium reduction is > 50% and the fat content is less than 3 g per serving (21 CFR 101.56). Importantly, the FDA revoked many standards of identity (formulas) for foods, including those for most dairy products, based on petitions from both industry and consumer organizations, such that terms like 'skim' now are consistent with the new labeling practices, i.e., lower fat milk now has to provide the percentage fat content on the front label panel.

USDA's final rules governing nutrition labeling of meat and poultry products (now 9 CFR part 317, 320 and 381) states that FSIS's nutrition labeling final regulations for meat and poultry products, as authorized by the Federal Meat Inspection Act, the Wholesome Meat Act and the Poultry Products Inspection Act, will parallel to the extent possible, FDA's nutrition labeling regulations promulgated under the Nutrition Labeling and Education Act. Consequently, USDA labeling in the marketplace is almost identical to FDA-labeled products. USDA's regulations provide for 'voluntary nutrition labeling on single-ingredient, raw meat and poultry products and by establishing mandatory nutrition labeling for all other meat and poultry products, with certain exceptions.' USDA accepted most of FDA's nutrient-content claim definitions but had a problem with lipids, simply because meat and poultry by nature contribute significantly to lipid intake. USDA therefore emphasized additional adjectival descriptors such as 'lean' and 'extra lean.' For example, 9 CFR 317.362 states: 'The term "lean" may be used on the label or in labeling of a meat product, provided that the product contains less than 10 grams fat, less than 4 grams saturated fat and less than 95 milligrams cholesterol per 100 grams and the Reference Amount Customarily Consumed (RACC) for individual foods and per 100 grams and labeled serving size for meat-type products.' It should be noted that FDA also has 'lean' claims (21 CFR 101.62 (e)(2)) for meal products or main dish products (such as a frozen dinner) which requires less than 10 g total fat, less than 4 g saturated fat and less than 95 mg of cholesterol in a serving. Extra lean claims require less than 5 g total fat, less than 2 g saturated fat and less than 95 mg cholesterol in a serving.

3.4 Disease-specific claims or disease-prevention (health) claims

Up until 1993, FDA regulations (21 CFR 101.9 (i)(1)) prevented any food label from bearing a disease-specific/disease-prevention or health-related claim. If it did, the FDA considered the product to be a drug, i.e. a drug is any article that 'is intended for use in the diagnosis, cure, mitigation, treatment or prevention of disease in man or other animals' (FFDCA Section 201 (g)). Thus in the case mentioned earlier, *NutriLab, Inc.* v. *Schweiker*, the government seized a NutriLab product, a starch blocker, because it was intended to affect the structure/function of the body in the prevention of a disease, obesity.

On January 6, 1993 and amended several times, FDA's final rules (21 CFR 101.14; 58 FR 44036; August 18, 1993, 59 FR 24232; May 10, 1994, 62 FR 15390; May 1, 1997) for disease-specific/disease-prevention claims were issued. Under these rules one may petition FDA to issue a regulation to approve a 'health claim,' but FDA will issue such a regulation only when it determines, based on the totality of publicly available scientific evidence, including evidence from well-designed studies conducted in a manner that is consistent with generally recognized scientific procedures and principles, that there is significant scientific agreement, among experts qualified by scientific training and experience to evaluate such claims, that the claim is supported by such evidence, i.e. that there is a national health risk and that the ingredient has been shown scientifically to reduce that risk (21 CFR 101.14(b)). In addition to this very high standard of scientific proof that FDA will require to issue such a regulation, an approved 'health claim' may be used in labeling for any product that meets the conditions set forth in the regulation, not just the petitioner's product.[9, 10] It should be noted that in 63 FR 14349 (April 25, 1998), FDA revised the food labeling definition of 'healthy' to permit processed fruits and vegetables and standardized enriched cereal grain products (to which iron, thiamin, niacin and riboflavin have been added, in the appropriate levels) that conform to bear this term.

The model health claims that appeared in 21 CFR 101.71 (*et seq.*) through December 2000 are as follows:

1.   Calcium and Osteoporosis: Regular exercise and a healthy diet with enough calcium helps teen and young adult white and Asian women maintain good bone health and may reduce their high risk of osteoporosis later in life (21 CFR 101.72; 58 FR 2665; January 6, 1993). In order to make the claim on the label the food must satisfy the following specific nutritional standards:
     • The food must be 'high' in calcium.
     • The calcium must be assimilable.
     • Dietary supplements must meet United States Pharmacopeia (USP) standards for disintegration and dissolution, or if no USP standard applies, appropriate assimilability under the conditions of use must be stated on the product label.
     • The food or supplement must not contain more phosphorus than calcium on a weight per weight basis.

2.   Dietary Lipids and Cancer: Development of cancer depends on many factors. A diet low in total fat may reduce the risk of some cancers (21 CFR 101.73; 58 FR 2787; January 6, 1993). In order to make the claim on the label the food must satisfy the following specific nutritional standards:
     • The food must meet the requirements for a 'low fat' food.
     • Fish and game meat may meet the requirements for 'extra lean' instead of 'low fat.'

3.   Sodium and Hypertension: Diets low in sodium may reduce the risk of high blood pressure, a disease associated with many factors (21 CFR 101.74; 58 FR 2820; January 6, 1993). In order to make the claim on the label the food must satisfy the following specific nutritional standard:
     • The food shall meet the requirements of a 'low sodium' food.

4. Dietary Saturated Fat and Cholesterol and Risk of Coronary Heart Disease: Development of heart disease depends upon many factors, but its risk may be reduced by diets low in saturated fat and cholesterol and healthy lifestyles (21 CFR 101.75; 58 FR 2739; January 6, 1993). In order to make the claim on the label the food must satisfy the following specific nutritional standards:
    * The food must meet the requirements for a 'low saturated fat,' 'low cholesterol' and 'low fat' food.
    * Fish and game meat may meet the requirements for 'extra lean' instead of 'low fat' food.

5. Fiber-Containing Grain Products, Fruits and Vegetables and Cancer: Low fat diets rich in fiber-containing grain products, fruits and vegetables may reduce the risk of some types of cancer, a disease associated with many factors (21 CFR 101.76; 58 FR 2537; January 6, 1993). In order to make the claim on the label the food must satisfy the following specific nutritional standards:
    * The food must meet the requirements for a 'low fat' food.
    * The food must meet the requirements for a 'good source' of dietary fiber without fortification.
    * Food must be, or contain, a grain product, fruit or vegetable.

6. Fruits, Vegetables and Grain Products that contain Fiber, particularly Soluble Fiber, and Risk of Coronary Heart Disease: Diets low in saturated fat and cholesterol and rich in fruits, vegetables and grain products that contain some types of dietary fiber, particularly soluble fiber, may reduce the risk of heart disease, a disease associated with many factors (21 CFR 101.77; 58 FR 2552; January 6, 1993). In order to make the claim on the label the food must satisfy the following specific nutritional standards:
    * The food must meet the requirements for a 'low saturated fat,' 'low cholesterol,' and 'low fat' food.
    * The food must contain at least 0.6 gram soluble fiber per reference amount customarily consumed without fortification. The content of soluble fiber must be declared on the nutrition information panel.
    * The food must be or contain a grain product, fruit or vegetable.

7. Fruits and Vegetables and Cancer: Low fat diets rich in fruits and vegetables (foods that are low in fat and may contain dietary fiber, vitamin A and vitamin C) may reduce the risk of some types of cancer, a disease associated with many factors. Broccoli is high in vitamins A and C and it is a good source of dietary fiber (21 CFR 101.78; 58 FR 2552; January 6, 1993). In order to make the claim on the label the food must satisfy the following specific nutritional standards:
    * The food must meet the requirements of a 'low fat' food.
    * The food must qualify as a 'good source' of vitamin A, vitamin C or dietary fiber without fortification.
    * The food must be or contain a fruit or vegetable.

8. Folate and Neural Tube Defects: Healthful diets with adequate folate may reduce a woman's risk of having a child with a brain or spinal cord birth defect (21 CFR 101.79; 61 FR 8752; April 15, 1996). In order to make the claim on the label the food must satisfy the following specific nutritional standards:
    - The food shall meet or exceed the requirements for a 'good source' of folate (i.e., provides 10 to 19 percent of the daily value per reference amount of food). ·
    - Dietary supplements shall meet the United States Pharmacopeia (USP) standards for disintegration and dissolution, except that if there are no applicable USP standards the folate in the dietary supplements shall be shown to be bioavailable under the conditions of use stated on the product label.
    - The food shall not contain more than 100 percent of the RDI for vitamin A as retinol or preformed vitamin A and vitamin D per serving or per unit.

9. Dietary Sugar Alcohol and Dental Caries: For packages with total surface area available for labeling of less than 15 square inches: 'Useful only in not promoting tooth decay.' For packages with total surface area available for labeling of 15 or more square inches: 'Frequent between meal consumption of foods high in sugars and starches promotes tooth decay. The sugar alcohols in (name of food) do not promote tooth decay' (21 CFR 101.80; 61 FR 43433). It should be noted that sugar free (sorbitol) chewing gum manufacturers had been using the claim 'Does not promote tooth decay' for almost 30 years with no interference from the FDA. The promulgation of this claim thus gave regulatory credence to this practice. In order to make the claim on the label the food must satisfy the following specific nutritional standards:
    - The sugar alcohol in the food must be xylitol, sorbitol, mannitol, maltitol, isomalt, lactitol, hydrogenated starch hydrolysates, hydrogenated glucose syrups, erythritol or a combination of these.
    - The food must contain less than 0.5 gram of sugar per reference amount customarily consumed and per labeled serving.
    - The sugar-alcohol containing food must not lower plaque pH below 5.7 by bacterial fermentation either during consumption or up to 30 minutes after consumption as measured by in vivo tests.

10. Soluble Fiber From Certain Foods and Risk of Coronary Heart Disease: Diets low in saturated fat and cholesterol that include soluble fiber from (name of whole oat or psyllium source and, if desired, the name of the food product) may reduce the risk of heart disease (21 CFR 101.81; 61 FR 296; January 4, 1996, 62 FR 15343; April 31, 1997, 63 FR 8103; February 18, 1998).[10] It should be noted that with respect to soluble fiber, 21 CFR 101.17 warns that the label should state that the consumer should consume adequate quantities of water if the fiber source is from psyllium. One should also note that the oat health claim was promulgated first and when

the psyllium claim was finalized, the two were combined, thus in effect there are actually 11 promulgated final health claim regulations found in the Federal Register. In order to make the claim on the label the food must satisfy the following specific nutritional standards:

- The food product must contain one or more of the whole oat foods: oat bran, rolled oats or whole oat flour, and the whole oat foods shall contain at least 0.75 grams of soluble fiber per reference amount customarily consumed of the food product; or psyllium husk (as defined in the regulations), and the pysllium food shall contain at least 1.7 g of soluble fiber per reference amount customarily consumed of the food product.
- The amount of soluble fiber must be declared in the nutrition label.
- The food must meet the requirements for a 'low saturated fat,' 'low cholesterol' or 'low fat' food.

11. Soy Protein and Risk of Coronary Heart Disease (see below).

None of the above health claims can be made under 21 CFR 101.14 (a) (5) if the product contains: >13 g total fat, >4 g saturated fat, >60 mg cholesterol or >480 mg sodium, per reference amount customarily consumed and per labeled serving size. For meal-type products, similar claims can be made but the above restrictions are >26 g total fat, >8 g saturated fat, >120 mg cholesterol and >960 mg sodium per labeled serving. For main dish products, these levels are >19.5 g fat, >6 g saturated fat, >90 mg cholesterol, or >720 mg sodium per labeled serving. It should be noted that the CFR for each claim contains all the FR notice references. For those interested in the scientific basis used to establish each claim they should obtain these FR notices. Very importantly, FDA also issued the so-called 'jelly bean' rule (21 CFR 101.14 (e) (6)) precluding adding an ingredient to a food so as to be able to make a health claim, if the original food contains less than 10% of the RDI or DRV for vitamins A and C, iron, calcium, protein, or dietary fiber before supplementing. The FDA has suggested this requirement is problematic and could be modified in the future to allow claims for some vitamin-fortified foods. This rule does not apply to dietary supplements. Finally, in 21 CFR 101.71, FDA specifically has stated that since there was no significant scientific agreement there can be no claims made (yet) for dietary fiber and cancer (58 FR 53296; 1993), dietary fiber and cardiovascular disease (58 FR 53298; 1993), antioxidants and cancer (58 FR 53302; 1993), zinc and immune function and omega 3-fatty acid and cardiovascular disease (58 FR 53304; 1993). Because the timetable was vague as to the time period in which FDA had to publish a final regulation on any health claim once it was first published, the dietary supplement industry sued (*Nutritional Health Alliance* v. *Shalala* 953 F. Supp. 526; S.D.N.Y. 1997). This forced FDA to promulgate 62 FR 12579 (March 17, 1997) and 62 FR 28230 (February 22, 1997) in which they agreed to a 270-day time period between initial FR proposal and final regulation with two possible 90-day extensions. Furthermore, several courts overturned parts of 21 CFR 101.71 dealing with the above ban on claims for dietary fiber and colorectal cancer (21 CFR 101.71(c)), the antioxidant vitamins and cancer, omega-3 fatty acids and coronary heart disease (21 CFR 101.71(e)) and a claim in (21 CFR 101.79(c)(a)(i)(g)) regarding a statement that the effectiveness of a specified amount of folate per serving from one particular source for reducing risk of neural tube defects was better than another source (61 FR 8752, 8760; 1996; *Pearson and Shaw* v. *Shalala*; 164 F. 3d 650; DC Cir. 1999; *National Council for Improved Health* v. *Shalala* (122 F. 3d 878; 10th Cir. 1997; *Nutritional Health Alliance* v. *Shalala* 144 F. 3d 220, 2d Cir 1998) Circuit 98-5043; US Appl. Lexis 464). The legal overturning of the regulations was directed towards dietary supplements but it appears it may also apply to conventional foods. The court said that fears that claims would be misleading could be addressed effectively through disclaimers, rather than through suppression of the claim, thus the courts in these cases found that both foods and dietary supplements could carry a disclaimer if a health claim is made. Allowing of the 'disclaimer' along with the health claim would therefore allow for non-violation of the First Amendment, allowing commercial free speech. The agency was directed to reconsider these health claims and provide guidance on what information is needed to meet the 'significant scientific agreement' standard for approval of health claims and not to do so would be in violation of the First Amendment related to commercial free speech (59 FR 395, 405, 422–23; 1994). Thus the courts said to FDA that the disclaimer could carry the burden as to the level of scientific support for the claim v. against the claim. The court was concerned, however, that this could lead to consumer confusion. The court also reiterated that if FDA denied a claim, it would be subject to review by the court. In addition, in an earlier case (*Pearson* v. *Shalala* 14 F. Supp 2d.10 D.C. 1998), the issue of improper procedures with respect to promulgation of the regulations under the APA were raised but the court felt that the time line to get approval was appropriate.

Other instances in which part of these regulations were challenged include (1) *National Council for Improved Health* v. *Shalala* (122 F. 3d 878; 884–85; 10th Cir. 1997) in which the case against the government was thrown out on the basis that there was no particular injury to the parties, and (2) *Nutritional Health Alliance* v. *Shalala* (144 F. 3d 220, 225–227; 953 F. Supp. 526 (S.D.N.Y.); 1997 2nd Cir 1998 cert. denied; U.S.L.W. 3113–3122, December 7, 1998) in which the case was thrown out on the basis of it being unripe for adjudication since the challengers did not try to go through the normal regulatory proposal procedure even though that could take up to 540 days as noted above. For a good review of the implication of commercial free speech on dietary supplement claims see Sidale.[11] These cases thus support the principle that one can have appropriate health claims and structure–function claims on both conventional foods and dietary supplements, if they qualify. Structure–function claims require a different type of wording but also must be truthful and not misleading and will be discussed later in this chapter. Note that in a Federal Trade Commission (FTC) action on advertising (*American Home Products Corp.* v. *FTC* 695 F. 2d 681, 684, 696–702; 3d Cir. 1983) the FTC required the advertiser of an unsubstantiated claim to have a disclaimer that said that the claim was open to substantial question.

On November 10, 1998 (63 FR 62977) the FDA also proposed allowing a health claim about the role that soy protein may have in reducing the risk of coronary heart disease (CHD) on the labels and labeling of food containing soy protein. This proposal is based on the agency's determination that soy protein, as part of a diet low in saturated fat and cholesterol, may reduce the risk of CHD. In proposing this health claim, FDA concluded that foods containing protein from the soybean as part of a diet low in saturated fat and cholesterol may reduce the risk of heart disease by lowering blood total cholesterol and LDL-cholesterol. The amino acid content in soy protein is different from that of animal protein and most other vegetable proteins, and appears to alter the synthesis and metabolism of cholesterol in the liver. Because soy protein occurs in or can be added to a wide variety of foods and beverages, it is possible to eat soy protein-containing products as many as four times a day (three meals and a snack), according to the FDA. Studies show that 25 g soy protein per day has a cholesterol-lowering effect. Therefore, for a food to qualify for the health claim, each serving of the food must contain at least 6.25 g soy protein, or one-fourth of the 25 g amount shown to have a cholesterol-lowering effect. This claim is different than the claim of 'maintains healthy cholesterol' on 'Take Control^{TM}' a Promise(r) margarine-like product being marketed as a conventional food as of May 1999. In this case, Unilever (through T.J. Lipton) used the self-declaration allowance to deem a soy lipid sterol as a Generally Recognized As Safe (GRAS) substance so it could be added to foods. Its mode of action is through the inhibition of cholesterol absorption in the gastrointestinal tract.*

An interesting sidebar related to claims came on February 5, 1999 when the Bureau of Alcohol, Tobacco and Firearms (BATF) approved statements for wine labels that referred to health effects of wine consumption. The statements were amended versions of those submitted over three years ago by the Coalition for Truth and Balance, an *ad hoc* group of 12 US wineries. Use of the labels are voluntary. The two BATF-approved statements are: 'The proud people who made this wine encourage you to consult your family doctor about the health effects of wine consumption' and 'To learn the health effects of wine consumption, send for the Federal Government's Dietary Guidelines for Americans, Center for Nutrition Policy and Promotion, USDA, 1120 20th Street, NW, Washington DC 20036 or visit its website.' As noted in their press release from BATF, under existing law, BATF can only deny labeling statements if they are false or misleading, and since these were not and, more importantly, they were not direct health claims, the statements were allowed after they had done a survey on wine drinkers. BATF does not intend to go through the FR public notice process for this action. They will, however, seek federal legislation to strengthen their authority over alcoholic beverages. According to the definition in the FFDCA, drink is food and thus should

---

* Since this chapter was written, the FDA proposal for a health claim on soy protein (63 FR 62977 November 10, 1998) was finalized on October 26, 1999 (64 FR 57700). This allows for a health claim related to soy protein and coronary heart disease. The regulation appears as 21 CFR 101.82 and requires at least 6.25 grams of soy protein per serving such that a person can acheive 25 grams per day (4 servings). All other restrictions on fat, sodium, calories, etc. apply.

be regulated by the FDA. However, since BATF already has inspectors in alcoholic beverage manufacturing facilities and the presence of alcohol inhibits pathogenic growth, FDA beginning in 1938 deferred all authority to them, although the FDA still could seize adulterated product. In 1974 FDA asked BATF to issue ingredient labeling requirements for alcoholic beverages. Since they refused, FDA terminated their memorandum of understanding with BATF in 1975 (40 FR 54536) and were going to pursue such practice. The alcoholic beverage industry sued to prevent this (*Brown Forman Distillers* v. *Mathews* 436 F supp 5, 1976; *Brown Forman Distillers* v. *Califono*, DC West KY, 1979) and won the action to prevent FDA from doing so. In 1980 BATF did propose labeling requirements (46 FR 40538) but withdrew the proposal in 1982 (48 FR 11884) after significant objection by the liquor industry.

It appears that most consumers find the new labels easier to understand, but considerable concern about label accuracy remains. In many cases, consumers are downright suspicious of health or other claims, particularly because of the plethora of often-conflicting health claims to which they are subjected in the media based on analysis of research studies showing opposing effects of various foods, ingredients or nutrients, e.g., the positive v. negative value of drinking coffee. Many believe that the label information is at the discretion of the manufacturer and that such information is not strictly regulated by FDA. At best, one can reasonably conclude that implementation of the NLEA has been only a modest success in terms of education, in spite of the enormous efforts devoted to its implementation.[12]

In some regards, FDA has been a bit overzealous in implementing the wording in the labeling for disease-specific claims. For example, consider the regulation for calcium and osteoporosis. Most manufacturers would simply like to claim that 'calcium helps prevent osteoporosis,' when their food product contains a reasonable amount of calcium. However, the FDA regulation provides several model label statements that they anticipate should be used. For example, one such model for foods exceptionally high in calcium that can be used for most calcium supplements states: 'Regular exercise and a healthy diet with enough calcium helps teen and young adult white and Asian women maintain good bone health and may reduce their high rate of osteoporosis later in life. Adequate calcium intake is important, but daily intakes above about 2,000 mg are not likely to provide any additional benefit.' Given the limited space on food labels, the statement is too long. In addition it ignores the large population of African American women who also might benefit from use of calcium and an Asian American group objected to it on the basis that it discriminated against Asian women. Thus, there are not a lot of disease-specific claims being made in the marketplace at present. For the most part, the American public seems nutritionally illiterate, and they will remain so until the schools make nutritional education an integral part of health and science education. The food label does not substitute for such education although it can be used as a means in the process. This brings up another interesting twist in the US legal system as was noted earlier. Since about the 1950s, the government seized food products if pamphlets, flyers, books, etc. were in close proximity to the product and such material contained disease-related claims specific to the product. The US targeted this mainly on supplement products (for example *US* v. *Kordel*

335–345; 69 S. Ct. 106; 1948; *US* v. *Kordel* 397 US 1; 90 S. Ct. 763; 1970). Since the last case mentioned, the FDA has had little action in this area although it remains as a Sword of Damocles on promotional material in close proximity to the product when held for sale. This promotional material was also considered in DSHEA, as will be seen.

3.5 The Food and Drug Administration Modernization Act 1997

The FDA Modernization Act amended the FFDCA to allow an alternative procedure for a nutrient content claim or a health claim that is the subject of a published authoritative statement by a scientific body of the US government with official responsibility for public health protection or research directly relating to human nutrition (such as the National Institutes of Health or the Centers for Disease Control and Prevention or the National Academy of Sciences). The person who wants to use the claim must give FDA at least 120 days' prior notice, including the exact claim to be used, a copy of the authoritative statement and a balanced representation of the scientific literature related to the claim. The FDAMA authorized FDA to exercise its discretion to allow use of the new nutrient content claim at the time that FDA publishes the FR proposal to permit use of the claim for public comment. This authority could also be used to remove an existing claim at the proposal stage.

With regard to this new method for health claims, the claim must be stated in a manner such that the claim is an accurate representation of the authoritative statement and in a manner that the claim enables the public to comprehend the information provided in the claim and to understand the relative significance of such information in the context of a total daily diet. FDA published the regulations pursuant to this as a guidance document in 63 FR 32102, June 11, 1998. This document is available in the Compliance Policy Guides Manual (CPGM). Because of concern by Congress for these rules, FDA on 1/21/99 (64 FR 3250) published a proposed regulation for this process which would comprise 21 CFR 101.90. The health claim may be made only if the food does not contain a nutrient in an amount that increases the risk to persons in the general population and/or the risk of a disease or health-related condition that is diet related, taking into account the significance of the food in the total daily diet. In addition, the health claim may not be false or misleading in any particular, which includes a prohibition on failure to reveal facts that are 'material in the light of' the claim. FDA will continue to be the final arbiter about whether such a health claim may be made because the claim may be made only until either (a) FDA issues a regulation prohibiting or modifying the claim or finding that the requirements to make the claim have not been met, or (b) a District Court of the US finds, in an enforcement proceeding, that the requirements to make the claim have not been met. In addition, FDA has the authority to make a proposed health claim regulation effective immediately upon the date of publication of the proposal.[4, 13] Finally FDAMA revised the requirement for referral statements. Previously, referral statements such as 'see side panel for nutrition information' on the front panel of a food label were made whenever a disease prevention claim or a nutrient descriptor claim was made for a food. Under FDAMA this will no longer be true. Such a referral statement will be required only if FDA makes a determination that the food contains a nutrient at a level that increases the risk of disease. This provision will significantly reduce label clutter, and significantly increase the incentive for useful nutrition information in labeling.

3.6 Medical foods

One type of food product that may bear a 'disease claim' is the medical food. A medical food is defined as a food that is specially formulated for the feeding of a patient who has a special medically determined nutrient requirement, the dietary management of which cannot be achieved by the modification of the normal diet alone and the food is labeled to be used under the supervision of a physician or under medical supervision (Orphan Drug Act 1988 (Pub. L. 100–290)).

The medical food's label and labeling may bear information about its usefulness for the dietary management of a disease or medical condition for which distinctive nutritional requirements, based on recognized scientific principles, are established by medical evaluation (21 CFR 101.9 (j) (8)).[1, 14, 15, 16] A food is subject to this exemption only if:

- It is a specially formulated and processed product (as opposed to a naturally occurring foodstuff used in its natural state) for the partial or exclusive feeding of a patient by means of oral intake or enteral feeding by tube.
- It is intended for the dietary management of a patient who, because of therapeutic or chronic medical needs, has limited or impaired capacity to ingest, digest, absorb, or metabolize ordinary foodstuffs or certain nutrients, or who has other special medically determined nutrient requirements, the dietary management of which cannot be achieved by the modification of the normal diet alone.
- It provides nutritional support specifically modified for the management of the unique nutrient needs that result from the specific disease or condition, as determined by medical evaluation.
- It is intended to be used under medical supervision.
- It is intended only for a patient receiving active and ongoing medical supervision wherein the patient requires medical care on a recurring basis for, among other things, instruction on the use of the medical food (21 CFR 101.9 (j) (8)).

If a food qualifies as a medical food, it is exempt from the pre-approval requirements that otherwise generally apply for FDA approval of health claims and nutrient content claims used in labeling. It also is not a drug even though it is used in the management of a disease (e.g. low phenylalanine products for those with phenylketonuria disease). A company that is responsible for a medical food must possess data that are sufficient to show that no claim made on the label or in other labeling is either false or misleading in any particular manner. However, there is no requirement to notify FDA that one is manufacturing or marketing a medical food or to obtain FDA approval or even notify FDA with respect to the use of medical food labeling claims. A medical food is not authorized to bear a claim to cure, mitigate, treat or prevent a disease – such a claim would create drug status for the product. Instead a medical food is permitted to make a claim to address a patient's special dietary needs that exist because of a disease. This type of claim is distinguished from a claim to treat the disease. The distinction should be kept in mind in developing any labeling claims for a medical food.[1, 15] Typical medical food products include foods useful in the treatment of:

- Genetic disorders, e.g., phenylketonuria, celiac disease, maple syrup urine disease.
- Stress conditions, e.g., surgery, chemotherapy, radiation therapy, burns.
- Cancer and HIV/AIDS patients.
- Neurological disorders, e.g., Alzheimer's disease.
- Gastrointestinal disorders, e.g., Crohn's disease, ulcerative colitis.

3.7 The Dietary Supplement Health and Education Act 1994

Beginning in the early 1950s, the FDA became increasingly concerned about what it felt were illegal label and formulation claims on vitamin and mineral products. In 1973, it promulgated an especially threatening regulation to the dietary supplement industry which resulted in a strong Congressional lobby effort to change the law (38 FR 2143, 2152, January 19, 1973 and 38 FR 20708; 38 FR 20730, September 2, 1973). In addition the industry had several portions of the regulations overturned in court, dealing with limits or levels of addition of ingredients (*National Nutritional Foods Association* v. *FDA*, 504 F. 2d 761, 2d Cir 1974 and *National Nutritional Foods Association* v. *Kennedy* 572 F. 2d 377; 2d. Cir. 1978). Because of this FDA was forced to withdraw 'all' of the above regulations (44 FR 16005, March 16, 1979). Congress also acted, upon the urging of Senator Proxmire of Wisconsin, by passing the Vitamin–Mineral Amendment of 1976 which prohibited FDA from imposing any limits on the level of safe vitamins and minerals in dietary supplements, from classifying them as drugs, and from limiting any combination thereof. This very hard hand slapping forced the issue and FDA discontinued going after dietary supplement manufacturers.

However, when NLEA was passed, FDA again began to stake their claim on these products. FDA published several regulations suggesting that NLEA applied (58 FR 33700, June 18, 1993; 58 FR 53296, October 14, 1993; 59 FR

395, January 4, 1994). During the period between 1992 and 1994, there again was extensive pressure on Congress by the industry to amend NLEA and the FFDCA to preclude any FDA action on dietary supplements which included vitamins, minerals, specific metabolic compounds and herbal supplements. On October 7, 1992, Congress passed an amendment to the FFDCA (Dietary Supplement Act 1992, Pub. L. 102–571; 106 Stat. 4491, 4500) to create a moratorium which inhibited the FDA from applying NLEA requirements on dietary supplements. Following passage of this Act, until passage of the Dietary Supplement Health and Education Act 1994, many US Senators and the House of Representatives claimed to be receiving more mail, more phone calls, and generally more constituent pressure on this subject than on anything else, including health-care reform, abortion or the budget deficit.[17]

Not surprisingly, given all this pressure, Congress eventually passed the Dietary Supplement Health and Education Act (DSHEA) 1994 (Pub. L. 102–571). The House of Representatives approved the measure by unanimous consent on October 7, 1994 and the Senate approved it, also by unanimous consent on October 8, 1994. The President signed it into law on October 25, 1994.[16] FDA has published over 25 Federal Register notices pursuant to this law, some of which have been finalized as regulations.

The new law, like virtually all legislation and the regulations pursuant to it (62 FR 49826; 62FR 49883; 62 FR 41886; 49859; 63 FR 23633), is a compromise. It does not include all of the restraints on FDA regulation of dietary supplements that the sponsors had originally wanted. Furthermore, it imposes some significantly new requirements for such products. Nevertheless, viewed as a whole, this legislation is a very favorable development for those who want to sell or consume a free range of dietary supplements including vitamins, minerals, herbs, other botanicals, amino acids and other similar dietary substances as mentioned earlier. The latter could be any compound in any metabolic pathway.

'Dietary supplements' are now defined by Sec 201(ff) of the FFDCA as amended by the DSHEA as products intended to be ingested in the form of a tablet, capsule, powder, softgel, gelcap or liquid droplet (or, if not in such form, are not represented for use as a conventional food or as a sole item of a meal or the diet) and which contains one or more of the following dietary ingredients: a vitamin, mineral, herb or other botanical, amino acid or other dietary substance for use to supplement the diet by increasing the total dietary intake, including a concentrate, metabolite, constituent, extract, or combination of any of the above.[3] Thus under Section 3(c) of DSHEA, a food containing an added supplemental ingredient can be sold as a dietary supplement as long as it does not claim it is a food and does state on the front panel that it is a dietary supplement. This thus supersedes the 1976 Vitamin Mineral Amendment which disallowed a food from the category (Section 411(c)(3) of the FFDCA). To further distinguish the product as a dietary supplement, a new type of panel was required called 'Supplement Facts'. Thus a chicken soup-like product with added echinacea can be sold as a dietary supplement if it states on the front panel of the label 'a hot liquid preparation with echinacea', suggesting that it is not a food but rather an item to supplement the diet, and the front panel also has the required words 'Dietary Supplement'. It should also be noted that FDA additionally promulgated several definitions in 62 FR 49868, September 23, 1997 including descriptors such as 'high potency' and the definitions for 'high in antioxidants,' claims that might be used on the front principal display panel.

While an unapproved health claim is generally not permitted on the label or other labeling of a food (including a dietary supplement) unless the claim meets the FDA approved health claims or FDAMA requirements previously discussed, for dietary supplement products only, there is an exception that permits four types of statements of nutritional support to be made on the label or in other labeling. These statements of nutritional support are as follows:

1. A statement that claims a benefit related to a classical nutrient deficiency disease and discloses the prevalence of such disease in the USA.
2. A statement that describes the role of a nutrient or dietary ingredient intended to affect the structure or function of the body in humans.
3. A statement that characterizes the documented mechanism by which a nutrient or dietary ingredient acts to maintain such structure or function.
4. A statement that describes general well-being from consumption of a nutrient or dietary ingredient.[3, 17, 18]

Any of the above four types of statements of nutritional support may be made in labeling for a dietary supplement without the approval of a health claim regulation under 21 CFR 101.71, if the manufacturer has substantiation that such statement is truthful and not misleading. In addition the labeling must carry a prominent disclaimer which states that: 'This statement has not been evaluated by the Food and Drug Administration. This product is not intended to diagnose, treat, cure or prevent any disease.' The manufacturer must notify the FDA no later than 30 days after the first marketing of the dietary supplement with a structure–function statement that such a statement is being made.[3, 16] Of further importance, FFDCA, Section 403 (b) *et seq.* made it clear that the FDA should not use the Kordel decision mentioned earlier to prevent separate published material from being sold. This new section thus allows publications to be in close proximity, but physically separated from the product. It also requires that such printed material should present a balanced view of the available scientific literature on the dietary supplement. The publication also cannot promote a particular manufacturer or brand of a dietary supplement and this cannot be subverted by applying a sticker to the publication or on the product. Most importantly, 403 (k) puts the burden on the FDA to establish proof that the material is false or misleading.

The new claims allowed for dietary supplements are generally referred to as 'structure–function' claims. Over 4,000 statements of nutritional support have now been filed with FDA by companies that have told the agency that they are using such a statement in labeling. FDA has responded to a few hundred, through a 'courtesy letter,' in those instances where the agency believes that the claims were improper 'disease' claims. The firm is told either to drop the claim or to contact the FDA Drug Center for more information. Obviously in these cases the FDA feels that the claims make the product a drug, and thus it is illegal since the product has not gone through the drug approval process and the product is both adulterated and misbranded.

To provide guidance to industry, in April 1998, FDA proposed a rule stating criteria to determine when a structure–function claim for a dietary supplement constitutes an impermissible disease claim (63 FR 23624).[19] The proposal generated more than 100,000 comments from manufacturers, trade associations, health-care professionals, consumers, Congress and other federal, state and local governmental agencies. The overwhelming majority of the respondents were highly critical of the proposal. The proposed rule first expands FDA's definition of disease to be 'any deviation from, impairment of, or interruption of the normal structure or function of any part, organ or system (or combination thereof) of the body that is manifested by a characteristic set of one or more signs or symptoms, including laboratory or clinical measurement that are characteristic of a disease.' FDA states in the preamble that the laboratory or clinical measurements that are characteristic of a disease include elevated cholesterol fraction, uric acid, blood sugar and glycosylated hemoglobin and that characteristic signs of disease include elevated blood pressure or intraocular pressure. The agency then proposed ten criteria for identifying disease claims that would be impermissible for a dietary supplement unless the products were to comply with drug requirements or with an applicable health claim regulation*:

1. *Claimed effect on a specific disease or class of diseases.* FDA's examples of such claims (disease claims) include: protection against the development of cancer; reduces the pain and stiffness associated with arthritis; decreases the effect of alcohol intoxication; alleviates constipation. Claims that FDA acknowledges would not be disease claims include: helps promote urinary tract health; helps maintain cardiovascular function and a healthy circulatory system; helps maintain intestinal flora; promotes relaxation.

2. *Claimed effect on signs or symptoms.* The second type of disease claim identified by FDA is a claim of an effect on signs or symptoms (presenting symptoms) that are recognizable to the health-care professional or consumers as being characteristic of a specific disease or of a number of different specific diseases. Examples of these claims are: improves urine flow in men over 50 years old; lowers cholesterol; reduces joint pain; relieves headache. Examples of claims that FDA acknowledges are not disease claims because the signs or symptoms are not by themselves sufficient to characterize a specific disease or diseases include: reduces stress and frustration; improves absentmindedness. FDA also states that if the context did not suggest treatment or prevention of a disease, a claim that a substance helps maintain normal function would not ordinarily be a

*FDA promulgated final regulations for structure functions claims in 65 FR 999-1050 on January 6, 2000. The summary document is extensive in describing the claims and does not preclude them from use on conventional foods. The regulation appears as 21 CFR 101.93.

disease claim. The agency gives as examples of these appropriate claims: helps maintain a healthy cholesterol level that is already within the normal range; helps maintain regularity. However, the agency was concerned that the only reason for maintaining normal function is to prevent a specific disease or diseases associated with abnormal function.

3.   *Claimed effect on a consequence of a natural state that presents a characteristic set of signs or symptoms.* These are claims about certain natural states (pregnancy, aging, menstrual cycle) that are not diseases but are sometimes associated with abnormalities that are characterized by a specific set of signs or symptoms that are recognizable to health-care professionals or consumers as constituting an abnormality of the body. FDA gives as examples of these abnormalities: toxemia of pregnancy; premenstrual syndrome; abnormalities associated with aging such as presbyopia; decreased sexual function; Alzheimer's disease; or hot flashes. Examples of claims that FDA acknowledges would not be disease claims are, for example: for men over 50 years old; to meet nutritional needs during pregnancy.

4.   *Claimed effect on disease through name of products, claims about ingredients in product, citation of publication, use of disease term, illustrations.* Examples of names of products that the FDA feels would constitute a disease claim include: Carpaltum (carpal tunnel syndrome); Raynaudin (Raynaud's phenomenon); Hepatacure (liver problems). Names that FDA states do not imply an effect on disease include: Cardiohealth; Heart Tabs. A claim that a dietary supplement contains an ingredient that has been regulated primarily by FDA as a drug and is well known to consumers for its use in preventing or treating a disease (e.g. aspirin, digoxin and laetrile) would be a disease claim. Citing a title of a publication or other reference if the title refers to a disease use would be a disease claim. Pictures, vignettes, symbols or other illustrations that suggest an effect on disease are also said by FDA to be disease claims. FDA gives the following as examples: electrocardiogram tracings; pictures of organs that suggest prevention or treatment of a disease state; the prescription symbol (Rx); or any reference to prescription use.

5.   *Claims that products belong to a class of products intended to diagnose, mitigate, treat, cure or prevent disease.* This category includes identifying a product as antibiotic, antimicrobial, laxative, antiseptic, analgesic, antidepressant, antiviral, vaccine or diuretic. In contrast, FDA states that acceptable identifiers would be: rejuvenative; revitalizer; adaptogen.

6.   *Claim that product is substitute for therapy product.* These include claims that a product has the same effect as that of a recognized drug or disease therapy, for example, Herbal Prozac. Prozac is an approved prescription drug used for depression.

7.   *Claim that product augments a particular therapy or drug action.* These are claims that a product should be used as an adjunct to a recognized drug or disease therapy in the treatment of disease. For example, a claim for use as part of your diet when taking insulin to help maintain a healthy blood sugar level.

8. *Claim that product has a role in body's response to disease or to a vector of disease.* These are claims that a product augments the body's own disease-fighting capabilities. Examples include: supports the body's antiviral capabilities; supports the body's ability to resist infection. This category also includes claims that a product is intended to affect the body's ability to kill or neutralize pathogenic microorganisms, or to mitigate the consequences of the action of pathogenic microorganisms on the body (i.e. the signs and symptoms of infection). In contrast, FDA states that an example of an acceptable claim in this area would be 'supports the immune system.'

9. *Claimed effect on adverse events associated with disease therapy.* These are claims that a product treats, prevents or mitigates adverse events that are associated with a medical therapy or procedure and manifested by a characteristic set of signs or symptoms. Examples of these disease claims identified by FDA are: reduces nausea associated with chemotherapy; helps avoid diarrhea associated with antibiotic use; to aid patients with reduced or compromised immune function such as patients undergoing chemotherapy. On the other hand FDA acknowledges that 'helps maintain healthy intestinal flora' would be an acceptable claim for a dietary supplement. Such a claim can be found on quite a number of fermented dairy-based dietary supplements which contain bifidobacteria.

10. *'Catch-all' provision.* FDA states that any claim that otherwise suggests an effect on a disease or diseases is also a disease claim.[19]

One month after the publication of the above proposed regulation on structure–function claims (May 20, 1999) FDA issued a notice to Pharmanex Inc. (Siam Valley, CA) that their dietary supplement product, Cholestin, was a drug and therefore misbranded. At that time, the product label stated that it could reduce both total cholesterol and LDL cholesterol by 10%. Cholestin is a fermented red yeast rice product that was imported from China where it was used to both color foods and in traditional Chinese medicine (TCM). The yeast fermentation produces a compound, mevinolin, exactly the same compound as a drug called Mevacor(r) (lovastatin). This was manufactured by Merck and approved in 1987 to inhibit cholesterol synthesis in the liver and thereby reduce cholesterol levels in the blood. In 1998, the FDA asked the Bureau of Customs to prevent (blocklist) the major ingredient at all ports of entry into the US, i.e. preventing Pharmanex from getting their raw material to manufacture their dietary supplement. Subsequently Pharmanex sued the US (*Pharmanex* v. *Shalala* case 2:97 CV 0262K DC Utah) to overturn that decision. On February 16, 1999 the DC agreed and overturned the FDA decision, declaring that Cholestin is a dietary supplement on the basis that DSHEA, 21 USC Section 321(ff)(3)(B)(I) declares that a dietary supplement does not include 'an article that is approved as a new drug under Section 355 ... which was not before such approval ... marketed as a dietary supplement or as a food.' Thus the courts ruled that this section only applies to new drugs and Cholestin is a dietary supplement which was used as such in China before passage of DSHEA. What this says is that a dietary supplement may contain a substance with drug-like activity, but if that substance was being used or marketed as a supplement by one party prior to DSHEA, the fact that it was also marketed as a drug by another party prior to that time does not make the supplement a drug. This case followed the standard set by *Fmali Herb, Inc.* v. *Heckler* (715 F. 2d 1383; D.C.N.C., September 15, 1983). Prior to Fmali, FDA held that foods, herbs, and botanicals not consumed in the US prior to passage of the 1958 Food Additives Amendment were either an unapproved food additive, or if not such, then the company introducing it had to either get a GRAS declaration or go through the food additive process. In 1973, FDA thus prevented a sassafras herb tea from being marketed because it contained safrole, an unapproved food additive that was a carcinogen (*US* v. *Select Natural Herb Tea* Civ #73-1370 RF; D.C. Cal; July 15, 1973). The Fmali case essentially overturned the blocklist that FDA instituted on a Korean herb (renshren-fenwang-jiang) on the basis that the Food Additives Amendment did not apply only to the US, i.e., if a product was consumed safely somewhere in the world prior to 1958, it can be imported into the US. It should also be noted that FDA instituted a new self-affirmation process for GRAS declaration (62 FR 18938; April 17, 1997) which has not been finalized. Thus some new, never before used herb would have to be declared GRAS before its use in food or it could be more easily introduced as a new dietary ingredient under DSHEA, as will be mentioned below. FDA has decided to appeal the Pharmanex decision to the Circuit Court. This certainly makes the decision of what is a drug versus a dietary supplement in the US market up for further legal interpretation.

As a final note to this section, the current laws and regulations and their interpretation have created a watershed for new products. It is not clear from DSHEA or the relevant regulations as to what data the manufacturer must have in order to substantiate the claim on the label (21 CFR 101.9(c)). The current feeling is that claims are being made based on single research articles or fairly uncontrolled in house clinical studies, perhaps bringing us to the climate in the 1950s. In addition, under DSHEA a manufacturer of a dietary supplement may use any ingredient in the product as long as they notify the FDA 75 days prior to its use (62 FR 49886 now in 21 CFR 190.6). Moreover these ingredients are exempted from the GRAS or the food additive definition, including the Delaney Clause (Section 409 (c) (3)(a)) which in itself prevents use of potential carcinogens as ingredients (Section 201 (s)(6)). Furthermore, DSHEA requires that the burden of proof on safety exists with the FDA (see Section 402 (f)(1)(D)); i.e., the manufacturers are not required to prove safety before introduction into the marketplace. Thus, ingredients that are not approved for use as a food additive (see Section 409 of the FFDCA) can be added to a dietary supplement as long as the manufacturer has some data in their files as to its safety and toxicity. For example, the compound stevioside, a sweetener extracted from the leaves of chrysanthemum species, though petitioned for, has not been approved for use in foods, but is now found in several dietary supplements in the US market. Thus based on the Fmali case discussed above, the leaves of the stevia plant could be imported and used in a dietary supplement, but using the effective compound in a purified form (stevioside) would be illegal since the compound has neither GRAS nor an approved food additive status unless petitioned for (e.g., the soy oil sterol mentioned earlier). It is also likely that stevioside could be declared as a new dietary supplement ingredient under 21 CFR 190.6 and be used in supplements.

3.8 The controversy over labeling

There is some controversy, as mentioned earlier, over whether the labeling of a food other than a dietary supplement may include a structure/function claim. The FDCA recognized that a food may be intended to affect the structure or any function of the body. Accordingly, it has long been felt that a food may make a label claim or other labeling representation about its dietary impact on the structure or function of the human body, provided that the particular claim used does not also suggest that the food will cure, mitigate, treat, or prevent disease (which would give it drug status) and provide further that the claim does not trigger some other requirement for FDA preclearance. In practice, FDA generally has tolerated a few claims of this type over the years, without asserting that the claim creates drug status or is a health claim. For example, claims that calcium helps build strong bones, protein helps build strong muscles and bread builds strong bodies in twelve ways have been made in food labeling and have been tolerated by FDA as appropriate claims about the impact of a food on the structure or function of the body. As noted before, the same was true about certain sorbitol-containing chewing gums that claimed 'does not promote tooth decay.' This latter claim was legitimatized when FDA allowed this as one of the ten approved health claims.

To make the situation even more confusing, on December 7, 1998 the US Supreme Court declined to review a US 2nd Circuit Court of Appeals decision on the FDA prohibition of the 'health claims' on dietary supplements (*Nutritional Health Alliance* v. *Shalala* 953 F. Supp 526; S.D.N.Y.; 1997). The court basically upheld the practice that although such a claim is within the Constitutional allowance of commercial free speech, if the FDA felt there was not significant scientific agreement of the benefit, for a product in particular, then it can deny the use of the claim.

In principle, these structure–function claims can be extended to other truthful and non-misleading statements. For example, it would appear to be potentially defensible to claim that a substance in a food helps maintain a normal, healthy cardiovascular system without triggering either drug status or requirements for approval of a health claim. However, there is some uncertainty about how far this type of structure–function claim can be pushed before FDA will assert either drug status or an unapproved health claim status.

A preamble statement on FDA's final labeling rules on dietary supplements, in the Federal Register of September 23, 1997 (62 FR 49860) stated:

> FDA points out that the claim that cranberry juice cocktail prevents the reoccurrence of urinary tract infections is a claim that brings the product within the 'drug' definition whether it appears on a conventional food or on a dietary supplement because it is a claim that the product will prevent disease. However, a claim that cranberry products help to maintain urinary tract health may be permissible on both cranberry products in conventional food form and dietary supplement form if it is truthful, not misleading and derives from the nutritional value of cranberries. If the claim derives from the nutritive value of cranberries, the claim would describe an effect of a food on the structure or function of the body and thus fall under one exception to the definition for the term drug. The claim is not a health claim because no disease is mentioned explicitly or implicitly.[20]

FDA's statements in this regard may not be entirely consistent with governing law, regulations or the court's varied interpretations. There is at least some basis for concluding that a food can have other uses, as acknowledged by the courts with respect to prunes and coffee in *Nutrilab, Inc.* v. *Schweiker*. The major food trade associations are in favor of an interpretation that would treat conventional food in the same regulatory manner as dietary supplements in this respect. This then brings up the vision that the grocery store will eventually supplant the medical care system and the pharmacy.

3.9 Advertising and the Federal Trade Commission

Information and claims about a food in the print or electronic media are considered to be advertising, while information on the food label is labeling. This was resolved in 1938 by the Wheeler-Lea Act (52 Stat 111) and reaffirmed in 1966 with the Fair Packaging and Labeling Act (Pub. L. 89–755; 80 Stat 1296) which excluded food labeling from being considered advertising. The prior sections covered the laws and regulations with respect to labeling which is under the aegis of misbranding under the FFDCA or the Wholesome Meat Act. Advertising is covered under the Federal Trade Commission Act (15 USC 52–56) passed in 1914 and amended many times. The Act created a stand-alone commission, the FTC, to deal with unfair and deceptive practices in advertising, thus control of advertising goes beyond mere 'truth,' it also includes 'unfairness.' There are no requirements for preclearance of advertising claims by the FTC. Instead, the FTC maintains that an advertiser should be in possession of a reasonable basis of substantiation for an advertising claim from the time that the claim is first made (no allowance to claim now and then substantiate later). Under its current policies and practices, the FTC would assert that an advertiser should be in possession of competent and reliable scientific evidence to substantiate a claim of health-related benefit. Competent and reliable scientific evidence means tests, analyses, research studies, or other evidence based on the expertise of professionals in the relevant area, that have been conducted and evaluated in an objective manner by persons qualified to do so, using procedures generally accepted in the profession to yield accurate and reliable results. This is exactly the question the courts made in several of the FDA cases discussed earlier, i.e. what level of science constitutes substantiation? The FTC maintains that an advertiser should possess substantiation for all objective claims that it makes, whether explicit or implicit. The FTC sometimes alleges that an objective claim has been made implicitly and should have been substantiated, although the surprised advertiser does not believe that the alleged claim was made at all.[20, 21, 22]

Insofar as a company repeats, in advertising, particular claims that are appropriate under FDA's rules for use in labeling, the company is likely to be in compliance with the FTC's standards for advertising. In particular, the FTC has stated that it would not likely question the use in advertising of a health claim or a nutrient content claim covered by an FDA regulation.[23] In addition, if a company has sufficient data to substantiate other types of health-related claims for FDA purposes, the data are likely to satisfy the FTC. Occasionally, it may be possible to include in advertising a claim that is not necessarily appropriate for use in labeling. For example, a company may have sufficient data to substantiate a health claim but the claim has not been approved by FDA for use in labeling. Because there are no requirements for FTC preclearance of health claims used in advertising, the company could use the claim in advertising if the claim can be adequately substantiated. The FTC has recently published a guidance document for industry with respect to advertising dietary supplements, which reaffirm the above principles.[24]

One key difference in FTC actions is the 'cease and desist' principle (FTC Act Section 6 (f)). In a rather complicated process, if the FTC finds fault with a company and the company agrees to this fault, the company can agree to cease and desist from using the same advertisement in the future. This action and acceptance then becomes no admission of guilt. FTC cease and desist decisions are published in the Federal Register. Several interesting cases include: *FTC* v. *ITT Continental Baking* (36 FR 18521; 1971) for advertising of a thin sliced bread useful for weight reduction; *FTC* v. *TJ Lipton* (38 FR 18366; 1973) for advertising of gelatin as nutritious; and more recently *FTC* v. *Body Gold* (62 FR 11201; March 11, 1997) for advertising of a dietary supplement based on chromium for weight loss.

3.10 Future trends

Although the complex set of US laws may seem unduly restrictive, there is clearly a trend towards allowing more information to be available to the consumer, on some basis of substantiation. As demand from the consumer rises and is recognized by the US Congress, FDA will undoubtedly have to adapt its regulatory policies to accommodate unique foods. The market then will only continue to increase in dollar value and size.

3.11 Further reading

For additional reading on interpretation of the Food Drug and Cosmetic Act that relates to health claims and dietary supplements, see the following:

HUTT, P.B. and HUTT II, P.B. 'A history of government regulation of adulteration and misbranding of food.' *Food Drug Cosmetic Law Journal*, 39: 2–73, 1984.

HUTT, P.B. 'Government regulation of health claims in food labeling and advertizing.' *Food Drug Cosmetic Law Journal*, 41(3): 52–63, 1986.

HUTT, P.B. and MERRILL, R.A. *Food and Drug Law: Cases and Materials*, 2nd edn, Mineola Press, Long Island NY, 1991.

3.12 References

1   US Congress. 100th Congress. Orphan Drug Amendments of 1988. Pub. L. 100–290. Amendment of Section 526(a)(1) of the Federal Food, Drug and Cosmetic Act, 21 U.S.C. 360bb(ax1). Library of Congress, Washington, DC, 1988.

2   US Congress. 101st Congress. Nutrition Labeling and Education Act of 1990. Pub. L. 101–535. Amendment of Section 403 of the Federal Food, Drug and Cosmetic Act, 21 U.S.C. 343. Library of Congress, Washington, DC, 1990.

3   US Congress. 103rd Congress. Dietary Supplement Health and Education Act of 1994. Pub. L. 103–417. 108 Stat/4325-4335, Library of Congress, Washington, DC, 1994.

4   US Congress. 105th Congress. Food and Drug Administration Moderniza- tion Act of 1997. Pub. L. 105–115. 111 Stat. 2296, Library of Congress, Washington, DC, 1997.

5   FDA. 'Food labeling regulations implementing the Nutrition Labeling and Education Act of 1990, final rule, opportunity for comments.' Fed. Register 58 2066-2963, 1993.

6   FDA. 'Food labeling; mandatory status of nutrition labeling and nutrient content revisions; format for nutrition label.' Fed. Register 58 2079, 1993.

7   FDA. 'Food labeling; establishment of date of application.' Fed. Register 58 2070, 1993.

8   FDA. 'Food labeling; serving sizes Final rule.' Fed. Register 58 2070, 1993.

9   FDA. 'Labeling: General requirements for health claims for food. Proposed rule.' Fed. Reg. 56:60537-60689, 1991.

10 FDA. 'Authorized health claims.' 21 Code of Federal Regulations, 1999,

Part 101.72(e)–101.81.

11 SIDALE, M. 'Dietary supplements and commercial free speech.' *Food and Drug Law Journal*, 48: 441–55, 1993.

12 OWE, S. 'Functional foods: Consumers are ready, are we?' Society for Nutrition Education symposium, Montreal, Quebec, July 26, 1997.

13 HUTT, P.B. 'A guide to the FDA Modernization Act of 1997.' *Food Technology*, 52(5): 54, 1998.

14 HATTAN, D.G. and MACKEY, D. 'A review of medical foods: Enterally administered formulations used in the treatment of disease and disorders.' *Food Drug Cosmetic Law J.*, 44: 479–501, 1989.

15 SCHMIDL, M.K. and LABUZA, T.P. 'Medical food. A scientific status summary by the Institute of Food Technologists Expert Panel on Food Safety and Nutrition.' *Food Technology*, 46: 87–96, 1992.

16 MUELLER, C. and NESTLE, M. 'Regulation of medical foods: toward a rational policy.' *Nutrition in Clinical Practice*, 10: 8–15, 1995.

17 MCNAMARA, S.H. 'Dietary supplement legislation enhances opportunities to market nutraceutical-type products.' *Journal of Nutraceuticals, Functional & Medical Foods*, 1: 47–59, 1997.

18 NESHEIM, M.C. 'The regulation of dietary supplement.' *Nutrition Today*, 33(2): 62–8, 1998.

19 FDA. 'Regulations on statements made for dietary supplements concerning the effect of the product on the structure or function of the body; proposed rule and dietary supplements: Comments on report of the commission on dietary supplement labels.' Fed. Reg. 63:23624-23632, 1998.

20 FDA. 'Food labeling regulation, amendments; food regulation uniform compliance date; and new dietary ingredient premarket notification; final rules.' Fed. Reg. 62: 49826-49868, 1997.

21 Federal Trade Commission Act. Part 5, 12, 1984.

22 *Consolidated Book Publishers Inc.* v. *Federal Trade Commission*, 53 F. 2d 942, cert. denied, 286 US. 553, 1931.

23 FTC. 'Food advertising enforcement policy statement.' 59 Fed Reg 28388, 1994.

24 FTC. 'Business guide for dietary supplement industry released by FTC staff.' FTC File No 974506, Washington, DC, 1998.

Part II

Functional foods and health

4

Colonic functional foods

R.A. Rastall (University of Reading), R. Fuller (Russett House, Reading), H.R. Gaskins (University of Illinois, Champaign, Urbana), and G.R. Gibson (University of Reading)

4.1 Introduction

The microbiota of the human gastrointestinal tract plays a key role in nutrition and health.[1, 2] Through the process of fermentation, gut bacteria metabolise various substrates (principally dietary components) to form end products such as short chain fatty acids and gases. This anaerobic metabolism is thought to contribute positively towards host daily energy requirements. The human large intestine is the body's most metabolically active organ, a fact attributable to the resident microflora and its activities. Usually, the human host lives in harmony with the complex gut microbiota. However, under certain circumstances like antimicrobial intake, stress, poor diet and living conditions, the microflora 'balance' may be upset. Moreover, the normal fermentative process may produce undesirable metabolites like ammonia, phenolic compounds, toxins, etc. The gut flora is also susceptible to contamination from transient pathogens, which further upset the normal community structure. These factors can have consequences that may onset gut disorder, which can be manifest through both acute and chronic means. As such, the large intestine is a prime focus for functional foods that serve to fortify normal gut function, and help to prevent dysfunction.

It is clear that the colonic microbiota is susceptible to manipulation through dietary mechanisms that target specific bacterial groups.[3] There is current interest in the use of dietary components that help to maintain, or even improve, the normal gut microflora composition and activities. This is a critical aspect of functional food science, which targets benign, or even beneficial, gut bacteria.

One much-used approach is *probiotics*. Here, live microbial additions are made to appropriate food vehicles like yoghurts or other fermented milks.[4–6]

The micro-organisms used in this respect are usually lactic acid bacteria such as lactobacilli and/or bifidobacteria. It is proposed that probiotics exert certain advantageous properties in the gastrointestinal ecosystem. These are thought to include improved resistance to pathogens, reduced blood lipids, positive immuno-modulatory properties and better protection from chronic gut disorder.[7,8] To be effective, probiotics should remain viable and stable, be able to survive in the intestinal ecosystem and the host animal should gain beneficially from harbouring the probiotic.[9]

Prebiotics serve a similar purpose to probiotics in that they aim to improve the gut microflora community structure. A prebiotic is a non-digestible food ingredient that beneficially affects the host by selectively stimulating the growth and/or activity of one or a limited number of bacteria in the colon, that may improve the host health.[10–12] As such, the approach advocates the targeting of selected indigenous bacteria through non-viable food ingredients. A further aspect is the development of *synbiotics,* which combine and therefore exploit the two concepts and seek to enhance probiotic survival by using a selective metabolic adjunct.[10]

4.2 What are colonic functional foods?

A complex, resident gastrointestinal microflora is present in humans. While the transit of residual foodstuffs through the stomach and small intestine is probably too rapid for the microflora to exert a significant impact, this slows markedly in the colon.[13] As such, colonic micro-organisms have ample opportunity to degrade available substrates, of which around 70g/d may be derived from the diet. These can be recognised as 'colonic foods', metabolism of which occurs through the anaerobic metabolic process known as fermentation. Table 4.1 shows approximate levels of colonic foods in the typical Western diet.

Fermentation by gut bacteria consists of a series of energy yielding reactions that do not use oxygen in the respiratory chains. The electron acceptors may be

Table 4.1 Type of substrates available for bacterial growth in the human large intestine

Substrate	Estimated quantity (g/d)
Resistant starch	8–40
Non-starch polysaccharides	8–18
Unabsorbed sugars	2–10
Oligosaccharides	2–8
Chitins, amino sugars, synthetic carbohydrates, food additives	?
Dietary protein	3–9
Mucins	?
Bacterial recycling	?
Sloughed epithelial cells	?

organic (e.g. some products of the fermentation) or inorganic (e.g. sulphate, nitrate). As carbohydrates form the principal precursors for fermentation, ATP is usually formed through substrate level phosphorylation by saccharolytic micro-organisms. Principal sources of carbon and energy for bacteria growing in the human large intestine are resistant starches, plant cell wall polysaccharides and host mucopolysaccharides, together with various proteins, peptides and low molecular weight carbohydrates that escape digestion and absorption in the upper part of the gastrointestinal tract (Table 4.1). A wide range of bacterial endo- and exo-glycosidases, proteases and amino-peptidases degrade these complex polymers, forming smaller oligomers and their component sugars and amino acids. Intestinal bacteria are then able to ferment these intermediates to other metabolites (discussed in section 4.3). The hydrolysis and metabolism of carbohydrates in the large gut is influenced by a variety of physical, chemical, biological and environmental factors (Table 4.2). Of these, it is probably the nature and amount of available substrate that has most significance, making diet the principal and easiest mechanism by which the fermentation profile may be influenced.

4.3 How are colonic foods metabolised?

Bacteria resident in the large gut depend upon a supply of fermentable substrate for their growth and activities. Principally, this is provided by the diet, although there is also a contribution from endogenous sources like mucins and chondroitin sulphate.[2] Any foodstuff that resists digestion in the upper gastrointestinal tract (stomach, small intestine) can serve as a colonic food in that it feeds the resident microbiota. Dependent on the type of fermentation that occurs, this may have positive or negative implications for host health.

In terms of end products, a variety of different metabolites arise in the large bowel, some of which exist transiently. The principal products of carbohydrate fermentation are short chain fatty acids (SCFA) and gases. The majority of these end products (95–99%) are absorbed into the blood stream.[14] Major SCFA produced are acetate, propionate and butyrate. It is thought that acetate is cleared in peripheral tissues such as muscle. Propionate is largely broken down in the

Table 4.2 Factors affecting colonisation and growth of bacteria in the gut

Physicochemical	Microbial
Amount and type of substrate	Competition between species for colonisation sites and nutrients
pH of gut contents	Inhibition through metabolic end products, e.g. acids, peroxides
Redox potential	Specific inhibitory substances, e.g. bacteriocins Bile salts Immunological events

liver, whereas butyrate acts as the primary source of fuel for colonocytes. The systemic metabolism of SCFA in the liver is thought to contribute about 7–8% of host daily energy requirements[14] – which in itself confirms the significant role of gut micro-organisms in human nutritional processes. Other organic acids such as succinate and pyruvate act as 'electron sink' products whose further bacterial metabolism, to SCFA, serve to increase fermentation efficiency in the large gut.

Gases are also derived by bacterial action in the large intestine. Principally, these are hydrogen, carbon dioxide, methane and hydrogen sulphide.[15] While gas formation is usually considered to be the terminal stage of food digestion, it remains an enigmatic process through the 'balance' of H_2 generation/ metabolism. A number of possible fates occur for intestinal H_2 in that it may be excreted or further metabolised by gut bacteria. In the latter case, sulphate reducers (producing H_2S), methanogens (expiring CH_4) and acetogens (excreting acetate) may all be involved. Microbial competition for the availability of these gases is of much scientific interest from both the ecological and clinical perspectives. Studies on gut microbial diversity are leading to the description of new bacteriological interactions, as well as improved recognition of how hydrogenoptrophic organisms interact. Medically, H_2 and its fate have been, at least tenuously but usually scientifically, linked with pneumatosis cystoides intestinalis, ulcerative colitis and bowel cancer.[15]

Predominant end products of protein fermentation are SCFA, including branched chain forms, as well as phenolic compounds, ammonia and some amines.[16] These metabolites have been associated with various clinical states such as tumourigenesis, schizophrenia, migraine.[17] In very general terms, the metabolites of a saccharolytic metabolism in the gut are benign, whereas those that arise from proteolysis can be detrimental.[18] As such, there can be positive or negative outcomes associated with gut bacterial fermentation. As dietary residues form the principal substrates for this metabolic process, careful consideration of foodstuffs may allow a more benevolent microbiological function. This necessitates a clear understanding of microbial composition and activities. Future baseline studies that use a molecular approach towards bacteria characterisation will have clear relevance in this respect.[19]

Hitherto, our knowledge of gut flora composition has been derived from studies where the microbiota has been determined through the use of 'selective' agars followed by phenotypic identification. While this gives an unrealistic measure of the full diversity, the general picture has been agreed. It is accepted that the 'normal' colonic flora contains around 400–500 different microbial species. The main numerically important group seem to be the bacteroides, with substantial contributions also from bifidobacteria, clostridia, fusobacteria, eubacteria, lactobacilli, coliforms, peptococci, peptostreptococci, anaerobic streptococci, methanogens, sulphate reducers and acetogens.[1, 2, 13]

Numerically, the large gut bacterial population can be as high as 10^{12} per gram of faecal material. As there is usually 100–200 g of contents in the typical adult colon, this makes the hindgut the most heavily colonised, and metabolically active, area of the human body. As such, the conventional function of the large gut as being largely an organ for the storage and excretion of waste material, as well as offering some absorptive capacity, has been replaced with the realisation that it has an authentic and important role in nutrition.

The normal flora of the human colon contains components that can be considered to be pathogenic in nature as a result of their proteolytic activities. Moreover, the organ is the site of infection for transient pathogens, such as various parasites, viruses and bacteria.[20] Major food-borne bacterial pathogens include campylobacters, salmonellae, *Listeria* and certain strains of *Escherichia coli*, such as the verocytoxin producing *E. coli* (VTEC) O157, responsible for various outbreaks including the notorious Wishaw episode (in 1996) involving 21 fatalities.

It is also hypothesised that certain components of the gut flora may be involved in the aetiology and/or maintenance of more severe gut diseases such as inflammatory bowel disease (ulcerative colitis, Crohn's disease), colon cancer and pseudomembranous colitis.[20] It has also recently been demonstrated that the important stomach pathogen *H. pylori* can be isolated from faeces.[21] This bacterium has been implicated in type B gastritis, the formation of gastric and duodenal ulcers and stomach cancer. However, the pathological role (if any) of *H. pylori* carriage in the colon has not been determined. As will be discussed later, a number of resident bacteria may be of some benefit to host health.[10] Generally, the various components of the large intestinal microbiota may be considered as exerting pathogenic effects or they may have potential health-promoting values. Examples include lactobacilli and bifidobacteria, both of which are present in the human colon in significant numbers.[2] Probiotics, prebiotics and synbiotics are all approaches to the improvement of host health by the fortification of selected bacteria in the gut. Because of the huge impact that food has on hindgut interactions, the way in which this 'balance' may be controlled is through appropriate use of diet.

4.4 Probiotics

The most tried and tested manner in which the gut microbiota composition may be influenced is through the use of live microbial dietary additions, as probiotics. In fact, the concept dates back as far as pre-biblical ages. The first records of ingestion of live bacteria by humans are over 2,000 years old.[22] However, at the beginning of this century probiotics were first put onto a scientific basis by the work of Metchnikoff at the Pasteur Institute in Paris.[23] Metchnikoff hypothesised that the normal gut microflora could exert adverse effects on the host and that consumption of 'soured milks' reversed this effect. Metchnikoff refined the treatment by using pure cultures of what is now called *Lactobacillus delbrueckii* subsp. *bulgaricus* which, with *Streptococcus salivarius* subsp. *thermophilus*, is used to ferment milk in the production of traditional yoghurt. A formal probiotic definition is a live microbial feed supplement which beneficially affects the host animal by improving its intestinal microbial balance.[4, 7] This has recently been modified by a European working party on gastrointestinal function foods to 'a live microbial food ingredient that is beneficial to health'.[3] This implies that health outcomes should be defined and proven, which is not an easy task. Most research has been directed towards the use of intestinal isolates of bacteria as probiotics. Over the years, many species of micro-organisms have been used. They consist not only of lactic acid bacteria (lactobacilli, streptococci, enterococci, lactococci, bifidobacteria) but also *Bacillus* spp. and fungi such as *Saccharomyces* spp. and *Aspergillus* spp.

Main positive effects associated with probiotics include cholesterol and/or triglyceride reduction, anti-tumour properties, protection against gastroenteritis, improved lactose tolerance and stimulation of the immune system through non-pathogenic means.[8] Over half the world's population is unable to utilise lactose effectively. The basis for improved digestibility of lactose in probiotics may involve β-galactosidase activity of the bacteria or a stimulation of the host's mucosal β-galactosidase activity. Various claims have been made for beneficial effects of probiotics against infectious diarrhoea conditions. The manner in which probiotics improve colonisation resistance may be due to the production of strong acids/other anti-microbial compounds, immune stimulation, metabolism of toxins and/or occupation of potential colonisation sites. Bacterial enzymes, which convert pre-carcinogens to carcinogens, are produced in the gut but their involvement in the pathogenesis of cancer is unclear. However, some probiotics (*in vitro*) are effective at decreasing the activities of such enzymes. Studies to show that probiotic supplementation can affect plasma cholesterol concentrations, and consequently the incidence of coronary heart disease, have given very equivocal data.[24]

Probiotic use in animals may take the form of powders, tablets, sprays and pastes. In humans, the most commonly used vector involves fermented milk products and 'over the counter' freeze-dried preparations of lactic acid bacteria in capsules. Recently, the market has expanded to include other foods such as flavoured drinks and pharmaceutical preparations such as tablets. Selection criteria for efficacious probiotics are listed in Table 4.3.

One of the most problematic areas is survival of the live micro-organism after ingestion. Many of the purported health-promoting aspects of probiotics rely on good culture viability. The rather variable nature of much probiotic research

Table 4.3   Selection criteria for probiotics

- Must exert a beneficial effect on the consumer
- Non-pathogenic and non-toxic
- Contain a large number of viable cells
- Survive in the gastrointestinal tract
- Good sensory properties
- Preferably be isolated from the same species as the intended use

may, at least partly, be explained by poor culture survival *in vivo*. It is possible that certain commercially used probiotic strains (e.g. *Lactobacillus acidophilus*, *Lactobacillus casei*, *Bifidobacterium infantis*, *Bifidobacterium bifidum*) may survive well when exposed to gastric acid or certain small intestinal secretions. However, as mentioned earlier, the large intestine is occupied by a very diverse and metabolically active microbiota. In this case (and if, as is usual, the colon is the target organ), the survival of the probiotic is questionable, particularly as the live feed addition may have been compromised in the upper gastrointestinal tract.

A major problem with establishing the survivability of a probiotic is the need to specifically detect the added organism against the background of the indigenous microflora. This can now be overcome, however, by the use of molecular biological techniques.

A strain-specific oligonucleotide probe can be constructed, given appropriate sequence information on the probiotic micro-organism. Certain diagnostic regions of 16S rRNA genes are targeted and the oligonucleotide probes can be fluorescently labelled. Such probes can be used to reliably quantify probiotic populations using direct (*in situ*) fluorescent microscopy (FISH).[25] Another approach that is still being developed is the use of genetic fingerprinting of the micro-organisms that grow on culture plates. DNA is isolated from colonies growing on agar plates and subjected to PCR-based AFLP (amplified fragment length polymorphism) analysis.[26] The resolution of AFLP is at least an order of magnitude greater than other commonly used fingerprinting methods and facilitates clear differentiation of the probiotic from any indigenous strains of the same species. Molecular methods such as these are an essential strategy, as in the past, studies have failed to address the problem of distinguishing between added (probiotic) and indigenous strains.

4.5 Prebiotics

Prebiotics allow the selective growth of certain indigenous gut bacteria. Thus, the prebiotic approach involves administration of a non-viable food component and considers that many potentially health-promoting micro-organisms such as bifidobacteria and lactobacilli are already resident in the human colon. To be an effective prebiotic a colonic food must:[10]

- neither be hydrolysed nor absorbed in the upper part of the gastrointestinal tract;
- have a selective fermentation such that the composition of the large intestinal microbiota is altered towards a healthier composition.

A good prebiotic would utilise the gut bacterial fermentation and physiology in a very tailored manner. While the obvious way in which this can be achieved is through stimulation of the indigenous beneficial flora, there is further potential for enhanced functionality. This may be through anti-infective as well as attenuative properties.[12] These aspects are under investigation. Future research will identify multi-functional prebiotics.

4.5.1 Commercially available prebiotics

The prebiotic activity of fructose-containing oligosaccharides (FOSs) has been confirmed.[27–31] As such, these prebiotics are the European market leaders. This is because these carbohydrates have a specific colonic fermentation directed towards bifidobacteria, which are purported to have a number of health-promoting properties.[1, 10] Bifidobacteria are able to breakdown and utilise fructo-oligosaccharides due to their possession of the β-fructofuranosidase enzyme, providing a competitive advantage in a mixed culture environment like the human gut.[32] FOSs have proven prebiotic effects in human trials.[12]

Galacto-oligosaccharides (GOSs) are another class of prebiotics that are manufactured and marketed in Europe as well as Japan. These consist of a lactose core with one or more galactosyl residues linked via $\beta 1 \rightarrow 3$, $\beta 1 \rightarrow 4$ and $\beta 1 \rightarrow 6$ linkages.[33] They have found application in infant formula foods as they are naturally present (albeit in very low quantities) in human milk.

A different class of galacto-oligosaccharides, used as prebiotics in Japan, are those isolated from soybean whey. These soybean oligosaccharides (SOSs) are built up of galactosyl residues linked $\alpha 1 \rightarrow 6$ to a sucrose core.[33]

Gluco-oligosaccharides can also act as prebiotics. Isomalto-oligosaccharides (IMOs) are comprised of glucosyl residues linked by $\alpha 1 \rightarrow 6$ bonds.[33] Strictly speaking, these oligosaccharides are only partially prebiotic since they are metabolised by humans. They are, however, very slowly metabolised and the bulk of isomalto-oligosaccharide added to a food passes through to the colon.

Xylo-oligosaccharides (XOSs) are also used as prebiotics in Japan. These consist of xylosyl residues linked by $\beta 1 \rightarrow 4$ linkages[33] and are much more acid stable than other prebiotics. For this reason, they have found application in soft drinks which tend to be acidic.

An interesting prebiotic oligosaccharide is lactosucrose (LS). This is a hybrid molecule between sucrose and lactose: $Gal\beta 1 \rightarrow 4Glc\alpha 1 \leftrightarrow 2\alpha Fru$.[33] This non-reducing oligosaccharide is a very promising prebiotic with rapidly developing applications in Japan.

Dietary fibres (e.g. from wheat, maize, rice, soya) have always been considered to have a beneficial effect on gut function and colonic bacteria, but this is a generalised stimulatory effect and such polysaccharides are not *selectively* fermented in the colon.

4.5.2 Commercial manufacture of prebiotics

Currently, most oligosaccharides are produced using enyzmatic reactions, either by building up the desired oligosaccharide from readily available sugars by transglycosylation or by the hydrolysis of large polysaccharides.[34] Major exceptions are lactulose, which is produced by the alkali catalysed isomerisation of lactose, soybean oligosaccharides which are directly extracted from soybean whey by the Calpis Food Industry Co. (Tokyo) and inulin, which is extracted from chicory by several companies in Europe, of which Orafti (Tienen, Belgium) is the most significant.

4.5.3 Future aspects

Some future developments for prebiotic research are given below. At the present time we do not know enough about the structure–function relationships among oligosaccharides to realise all of this potential. In addition, we will need innovations in the manufacturing technology in order to produce more sophisticated oligosaccharides at prices that the food industry can afford. Research in this area is currently in progress.

Incorporation into a wider range of food vehicles

The advantage of prebiotics is that they do not rely on culture viability in a given product. As such, any food normally containing carbohydrates is potentially receptive to the approach. The food technologist is thus faced with less of a challenge in terms of efficacy of use and consumer acceptance, and can exert more creativity in the design of novel products. Cereals, biscuits, infant formula feeds, weaning foods, confectionery, cakes, savoury products, spreads and pastes are all amenable to incorporation of prebiotics.

Multiple biological properties

Bifidobacteria are known to inhibit the growth of various pathogens *in vitro*. This occurs due to several mechanisms and can be dubbed the '*Bifidobacterium* barrier' (Fig. 4.1):

- Production of SCFA results in a hostile environment for pathogens such as *E. coli*.
- Bifidobacteria produce anti-microbial agents active against Gram negative and Gram positive pathogens.[35]

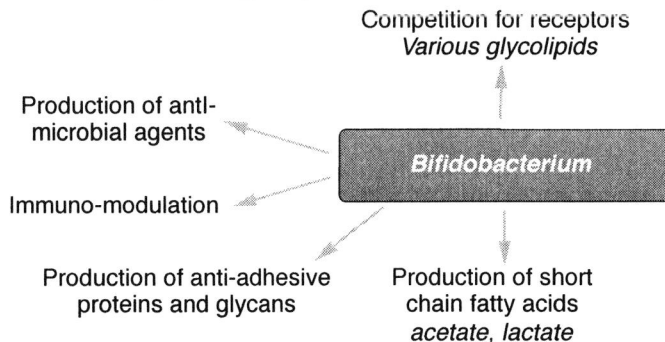

Competition for receptors
Various glycolipids

Production of anti-microbial agents

Immuno-modulation

Bifidobacterium

Production of anti-adhesive proteins and glycans

Production of short chain fatty acids
acetate, lactate

Fig. 4.1 The bifidobacterium barrier. The diagram indicates different mechanisms whereby bifidobacteria may inhibit pathogen persistence in the gut.

- Bifidobacteria bind to various cell-surface glycolipids, occupying receptor sites for pathogens.[36, 37]
- Bifidobacteria are reported to produce anti-adhesive glycans and proteins, inhibiting the binding of pathogens to their cellular receptors.[36]

Recently, the fact that oligosaccharides act as cellular receptors for pathogens has led to the development of therapeutic oligosaccharide-based agents directed against gastrointestinal (GI) pathogens.[38] These are complex (and expensive) drugs. There is, however, potential in using soluble oligosaccharides as 'decoy oligosaccharides' in food. The idea is that invading pathogens would bind to the soluble oligosaccharide as well as the cellular receptor, thus inhibiting colonisation. Until an economic manufacturing technology for such oligosaccharides is developed (under way at the present time) the value of this approach cannot be determined. Of particular interest in this regard would be oligosaccharides such as manno-oligosaccharides. These are receptors for type 1 fimbriated pathogens such as *E. coli*, *Salmonella* sp., *Shigella* sp., etc. Such oligosaccharides can be manufactured using enzymatic techniques,[39, 40] and their potential as anti-adhesive prebiotics is currently under investigation.

Low dosage forms
The intake doses of FOSs which have elicited a bifidogenic effect in human studies range from 4 to 40 g/d.[12] However, it is important that the minimal operative dose is used, such that unwanted side-effects like flatulence are reduced. The target organisms for prebiotic use are not gas producers. As such, if distension difficulties arise after prebiotic ingestion, it is due to a non-selective metabolism which, most likely, would arise from too high a dosage. Low dosage forms will depend upon highly selective fermentation by the target organisms. The food industry would find it useful to have different prebiotics that have a range of minimum active doses. This would maximise flexibility with respect to the type of food vehicle that could be developed.

Persistence through the colon
Most prebiotics are metabolised in the proximal (right side) colon, making this a very saccharolytic region of the gut. In contrast, the distal (left side) colon is much more proteolytic, with relatively high levels of the pro-carcinogens and toxins discussed above. A very desirable property in a prebiotic would be the ability to induce a saccharolytic metabolism throughout the length of the colon. This may be achievable by producing prebiotics with an appropriate molecular weight distribution such that low molecular weight molecules were metabolised in the left side and high molecular weight molecules were more slowly metabolised and reached the right side. This is represented diagrammatically in Fig. 4.2.

Physiological advantages
Other physiological properties could be identified that would be desirable in a prebiotic. These would include, for instance, non-carcinogenic properties, i.e.

Transverse colon

Proximal colon
~ saccharolytic

Distal colon
~ proteolytic

May be achieved with a mixture of low
and high molecular weight prebiotics

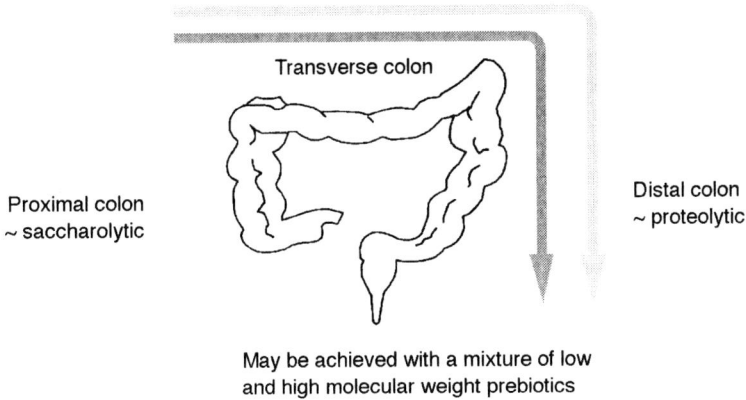

Fig. 4.2 A schematic representation of persistent prebiotics. Most prebiotics are predominantly metabolised in the saccharolytic area of the right colon. However, most gut disorders are of distal origin. It is therefore more desirable that prebiotic fermentation occurs in the left side; this may be achieved through the action of slowly metabolised or persistent forms.

not being amenable to fermentation by oral bacteria to produce acid. An ideal prebiotic would also have a low calorific value. The definition of a prebiotic given above states that it should not be metabolisable by humans, and therefore have no calorific value. This is not always achieved in practice, for instance the isomalto-oligosaccharides are partially metabolisable by humans and have some calorific value.

Useful technological properties
If prebiotics are to make a significant impact on human health they must be incorporated into a wide range of foods. If this is to be realised, they must also be useful food ingredients as well as possessing useful biological (prebiotic) activity. It is possible to identify desirable technological properties in a prebiotic. Ideally they would be available with a range of viscosities, and a range of sweetness. They would also have good preservative and drying characteristics.

4.6 Synbiotics

A synbiotic is a marriage of the concepts of probiotics and prebiotics. A synbiotic consists of a live microbial food additive together with a prebiotic oligosaccharide. The advantages are that a commercial probiotic with known benefits can be used and the prebiotic aids the establishment of the organism in the complex colonic environment. There is thus great flexibility in the choice of probiotic micro-organisms and oligosaccharide and the best combination for a specific desired outcome can be determined.

The survival of the probiotic part of a synbiotic can be determined *in vitro* using a model of the human gut.[41] The system has been validated against gut contents from sudden death victims and gives a very close analogy to bacterial activities and composition in different areas of the hindgut. The system consists of three vessels, of increasing size, aligned in series such that a sequential feeding of growth medium occurs. The vessels are pH regulated to reflect *in vivo* differences. As such, vessel 1 has a high availability of substrate, bacteria grow quickly and it is operated at an acidic pH, similar to events in the proximal colon. In contrast, the final vessel resembles the neutral pH, slow bacterial growth rate and low substrate availability that is characteristic of distal regions. After inoculation with faeces, an equilibration period is followed by identification of the bacterial profiles that have developed in response to their imposed conditions. Survival experiments with and without different prebiotics can then be carried out.

Determining the survival of a synbiotic suffers from the same problems of identification against the indigenous background flora as probiotics discussed above. Much the best way of achieving this is to use molecular markers as described above. If the survivability is determined in the *in vitro* gut model system, then an alternative approach can be considered. This is to incorporate detectable marker genes into the target species. At the present time the best such marker gene is the green fluorescent protein (GFP) from the jellyfish *Aequorea victoria*. The protein emits green light when excited with blue light and has the advantage that no exogenous substrates or cofactors are required. Epifluorescent microscopy is then used to demonstrate GFP expression.

4.7 Health aspects of functional colonic foods

There needs to be a clear distinction between functional and health claims that are levelled against colonic foods. It is our contention that targeting of the human colon with probiotics, prebiotics or synbiotics and/or manipulation of the gut flora composition are functional aspects of intestinal microbiology. The desirability of identifying concomitant health advantages is obvious.

4.7.1 Colonic cancer

In humans, the colon is the second most frequent site for carcinonoma formation. It is thought that tumours arise 100 times more often in the colon compared to the small intestine. This has led to speculation that the hindgut microflora are involved in colonic cancer onset. Some large intestinal bacteria are able to produce carcinogenic, or tumour-promoting, compounds during their metabolism.[42] Dietary strategies that lead to a reduction in the accumulation of such products, and hence their effects, are worthy of attention. Two approaches are possible.

First, some bacterial metabolites may offer a protective role in tumourogenesis. For example, butyrate, which is a common fermentation end product, has received attention as a stimulator of apoptosis and as a preferred fuel for the healthy gut mucosa.[43] In this case, it would be desirable to increase overall butyrate levels in the large gut and the prebiotic approach offers such potential.[44] The fermentation of resistant starches forms relatively high quantities of butyric acid. However, it is important that careful consideration is given to the nature of the bacteria stimulated by prebiotics; starches, for instance, are well fermented by clostridia, which may also be pathogenic. Less specifically, the overall carbohydrate load in the large intestine has relevance, as an increased bulk of gut organisms may have the effect of aiding excretion of toxic materials from the bowel.

Second, it may be possible to 'subvert' certain entities of the microbiota such that their metabolism favours more benign end products. The shift away from a proteolytic fermentation by clostridia and/or bacteroides to a saccharolytic one is an obvious example. Another is the direct inhibitory effect that lactic acid bacteria may have on bacteria that produce pro-carcinogenic faecal enzymes such as azoreductase, nitroreductase and β-glucuronidase.

Similarly, dietary lipids may enter the colon in reasonable amounts and it is accepted that the faecal stream contains lipid-derived carcinogens, which are formed by bacterial activities. These include diacylglycerol, which is thought mainly to be produced by the activities of certain clostridia.[45] In conjunction with bile salts, an intake of some lipids (e.g. phosphatidylcholine) gives rise to the formation of diacylglyercol at physiologically significant quantities. The result of an accumulation of this metabolite may be the activation of protein kinase C, which is thought to be a potent stimulator of mucosal cell proliferation; it may be possible to advocate certain prebiotics that reduce *in situ* levels of this tumour promoter.

4.7.2 Immunological effects

The immunomodulatory capabilities of lactic acid bacteria have received much attention.[46] It is thought that such bacteria act as *adjuvants*, able to stimulate both non-specific host defence mechanisms and some cells involved in the specific response.[47] The result is often an increased phagocytic activity and/or elevated immune molecules such as secretory IgA, which may affect pathogens such as salmonellae. Most attention in this respect has been diverted towards the intake of probiotics[48] and interactions between cell wall components and immune cells. It is also hypothesised that the immune stimulation may exert effects against tumour cells.[8] It is more difficult to envisage specific effects through the prebiotic approach, where the target organ is very heavily colonised with a wide variety of bacteria.

4.7.3 Systemic effects on blood lipids

It is thought that elevated cholesterol levels in the blood represent a significant risk factor for coronary heart disease. In this context, there is some evidence that lactic acid bacteria may be of use for reducing total and low density lipoprotein (LDL) cholesterol levels. The mechanisms whereby lactic acid micro-organisms are able to reduce blood lipid concentrations have not been definitively proven.[24] However, the following aspects are identifiable:

- The formation of certain bacterial end products of fermentation (e.g. acetate and propionate possible in combination with L-lactate) may affect systemic lipid and cholesterol levels.
- Lactic acid bacteria may be able to directly assimilate cholesterol. This has been hypothesised from some *in vitro* experiments, but is a source of contention in that the data are conflicting.
- Deconjugation of bile salts may increase their faecal excretion, although this would mainly be a small intestinal effect and therefore not a target for the prebiotic concept.
- Lactic acid bacteria may interfere with cholesterol absorption from the intestine.

4.7.4 Effects on pathogens

The lactic microflora of the human gastrointestinal tract is thought to play a significant role in improved colonisation resistance.[49] There are a number of possible mechanisms in operation:

- Metabolic end products such as acids excreted by these micro-organisms may lower the gut pH, in a microniche, to levels below those at which pathogens are able compete effectively.
- Competitive effects from occupation of normal colonisation sites.
- Direct antagonism through natural anti-microbial excretion.
- Competition for nutrients.

The outbreak of *E. coli* O157 in Lanarkshire, Scotland, at the end of 1996 resulted in 21 fatalities and was one of the world's most serious food poisoning incidents ever. The deaths have highlighted the continuing concern of bacterial gastroenteritis to consumers, the food industry, researchers and the medical profession. In recent laboratory tests we have also shown that some bifidobacteria exert powerful antagonistic effects towards *E. coli* O157. The inhibition was variable in species of bifidobacteria, with *Bifidobacterium infantis* and *B. longum* exerting the greatest effect on *E. coli*. The possibility exists therefore that increased levels of bifidobacteria (and consideration of the species type) in the large gut may, along with other factors such as immune status, offer improved protection.

Above the age of about 55 years, faecal bifidobacterial counts are known to show a marked decrease in comparison to those of younger persons.[50] It may be of some relevance that the UK fatalities during the *E. coli* outbreak all involved the elderly, while hundreds of people in different age groups reported the infection. A potential correlation exists with reduced pathogen resistance, decreased numbers of bifidobacteria in the elderly and the production of natural resistance factors. In essence, the natural gut flora may have been compromised through reduced bifidobacterial numbers and have a diminished ability to deal with pathogens. If prebiotics are used to increase bifidobacteria or lactobacilli towards being the numerically predominant genus in the colon, an improved colonisation resistance ought to result, but has not been proven. Moreover, oligosaccharides themselves may act as anti-infective agent through the occupation of bacterial ligands for pathogen colonisation/receptor sites.[38]

The prebiotic concept may be extrapolated further by considering an attenuation of virulence in certain food-borne pathogens. For example, the plant derived carbohydrate cellobiose is able to repress the pathogenicity of *Listeria monocytogenes* through down regulation of its virulence factors.[51] As such, this organism is avirulent in its natural habitat of soil, where it is exposed to rotting vegetation and therefore cellobiose. In the human body, an absence of cellobiose may allow the virulence factors to be expressed, and it is possible that further incorporation of this disaccharide to foods susceptible to *Listeria* contamination could reduce this virulence.

4.8 Host–microbe interaction

4.8.1 Therapeutic use of probiotic organisms

Interest in the administration of beneficial organisms to compete with 'toxin-producing' bacteria in the intestine has persisted since Metchnikoff's writings concerning the benefits of drinking fermented milk at the beginning of the twentieth century.[23, 52] The premise is that when the microbial balance is shifted in favour of pathogenic bacteria, such as in times of stress, antibiotic compromise, or dietary changes, the intake of probiotic organisms has the potential to re-establish microbial equilibrium, and if given routinely, may prevent pathogenic invasion.

There is increasing evidence that probiotics increase host immunity to a range of intestinal pathogens including *E. coli*, *Salmonella* and *Shigella*,[53] and may prevent antibiotic-induced pseudomembranous colitis by *C. difficile*.[54] Some *Lactobacillus* strains can also activate macrophages[55, 56] and enhance natural killer cell activity in mice.[57] The findings of Perdigon and co-workers,[55] which demonstrate that both *Lactobacillus casei* and *L. bulgaricus* given perorally enhanced peritoneal macrophage function in mice, is particularly illustrative, because a marked difference in macrophage phagocytic activity was observed in response to the two microbial species; phagocytic activity was enhanced by peroral administration of *L. casei*, a resident gut bacterial species, but not by *L. bulgaricus*, a species that does not survive in the intestinal tract. This finding offers an impressive example of the ability of non-pathogenic, indigenous microbial species to enhance the immunological function of the host. The use of organisms generally recognised as safe (GRAS) and which provide the host with resistance to pathogenic colonisation and enhance immunological function is therefore a therapeutic alternative which merits further experimentation and elucidation. Most knowledge on the contributions of normal gut bacteria to the structure and functions of the intestinal immune system is derived from a substantial literature on germ-free rodents.

4.8.2 Characteristics of germ-free mice

Animals living under sterile, germ-free (GF) conditions have immunologically relevant physical characteristics which make them distinguishable from conventional (CV) animals, which harbour a normal population of autochthonous bacteria. The caecum, for example, is much larger in GF than in CV mice as a result of water retention.[58] On the other hand, many immunologically relevant organs, such as the small intestine and mesenteric lymph nodes, are smaller and weigh less in GF animals.[59] This decreased size may be the result of lower water content and leukocyte populations in the mucosal and submucosal layers.[59, 60] In addition to decreased size, the lymph nodes, spleen and other lymphoid tissues have few germinal centres,[60–62] sites within lymph nodes and other lymphoid tissues where antigen presentation occurs, leading to B cell proliferation and the differentiation of antibody-secreting plasma cells. Those germinal centres that are present in GF animals are suspected to result from (a) basal activity, (b) antigens in the diet, or (c) a response to endogenous viruses which are present even in GF colonies.[61, 63] The thymus, though following a pattern of growth and regression similar to that observed in CV animals, grows at a slower rate in GF animals and never reaches the sizes attained in CV mice.[64] The smaller thymus in GF animals can be expected to affect long-term immunity adversely, as there will be fewer T helper (TH) cells to activate B cells, resulting in an absence of memory cells. A parallel can be drawn between this condition in the GF mouse and the elderly, where decreased immune function can be partially attributed to the paucity of T cells which results from the involution of the thymus with age. Cell-mediated immunity has not been well characterised in GF mice. However, evidence does exist for delayed type hypersensitivity and normal allograft responses in GF mice.[64–66] Regarding humoral immunity, GF mice have low levels of immunoglobulins[67–69] and little or no detectable IgA.[70] GF mice do respond to antigen with antibodies, but at lower concentrations than CV mice.[71, 72] GF mice are also five times more resistant to LPS-induced lethality than CV mice.[73] It has been demonstrated that transfer of T cells from CV to GF mice lowered this resistance, which led to the hypothesis that Gram-negative bacteria in the gut contribute towards production of a T cell population which regulates B cell responses to lipopolysaccharides (LPS).[74] Substantial differences have been demonstrated between GF and CV animals regarding the numbers and function of macrophages, which are among the cell types most responsive to microbial alterations. For example, relative to CV animals, macrophages from axenic animals (a) are fewer in number,[75] (b) are less active metabolically,[76] (c) are less capable of antigen degradation,[77, 78] (d) are less responsive to chemotactic stimuli,[79-81] and (e) have diminished tumoricidal capabilities,[82-83] and (f) have decreased microbicidal activity toward certain pathogens such as *Listeria* spp. and *E. coli*.[66] It is of note that macrophages are identified as being responsive to micro-ecological changes in early GF work and in our recent attempts to identify host components that are responsive to the intestinal microbiota.

The physiological differences between GF and CV animals invite speculation of the role played by the conventional microbiota in the development of immunity in the host. The existence of GF animals, which can be associated with members of the normal microbiota, can therefore serve as valuable tools for understanding interactions between the host and specific members of the autochthonous microbiota, as well as interactions between different members of the microbiota. A detailed description of microbial–host and microbe–microbe interactions using a differential model will allow more precise characterisation of host responses to foreign inflammatory or immunogenic agents and the ability of probiotic organisms to provide protection to the host.

4.8.3 Characterisation of microbial populations in CV mice

The constituent members and the relative proportions of the species making up the autochthonous microbiota can vary according to animal species and strain, the age of the individual, diet, the external environment and stress. The microbiota in all regions consists of obligate anaerobes, but significant populations of micro-aerophilic and facultative anaerobes are also present.[84] Gram-positive genera (lactobacilli) generally dominate the regions proximal to the stomach; Gram-negative and Gram-positive microbiota (*Bacteroides*, fusiforms) tend to inhabit the more distal regions. It should be noted, however, that bacteria that inhabit the more proximal regions are eventually passed down to the more distal areas. Moreover, characterisation of compartmental populations of microbes in CV mice is therefore an indication of those species that are found in those compartments at the highest numbers, but not necessarily the species that have highest affinity for the local environment. Given the difficulties with assigning particular species to specific localities of the GI tract, a complete microbial 'census' of the various GI compartments is lacking.

4.8.4 Reassociation of GF mice with members of the autochthonous microflora

The eventual outcome of microbial association of GF mice is subject to various factors; GF mice have physiological characteristics, such as different oxygen tensions and degrees of proteolytic activity, which account for differences between GF and CV mice in microbial adhesion potentials along the intestinal epithelium.[85, 86] When only one microbe is introduced to a GF animal, it will attain numbers far higher than those seen in CV animals and will generally colonise both the small and large intestines, perhaps due to retarded peristalsis in GF animals.[84] The order of introduction can also determine the dominant species that persist. Furthermore, competition between introduced species may produce unexpected alterations in microbial composition.[87]

4.8.5 Immunological changes in GF mice upon introduction of autochthonous bacteria

Upon introduction of the complete repertoire of autochthonous microbiota, GF animals develop a physiology comparable to that observed in CV animals: within two days the caecum becomes smaller and thicker-walled, with more solid contents than GF animals; the spleen, lymph nodes, and Peyer's patches develop germinal centres and begin to grow, reaching CV dimensions within a week of association; the lamina propria is thickened and becomes more cellular; and serum immunoglobulin concentrations increase.[88, 89] Coliforms, which colonise the host immediately following exposure, are believed to be responsible for these changes, whereas strict anaerobes are not observed until much later.[90] Differential host responses to specific bacterial species has led Dubos et al.[91] to suggest that, among the bacteria normally found in the host intestine, some are truely symbiotic and constitute the autochthonous microbiota, while other microbial types present in the gut gain access to the host due to their presence in the environment but do not establish a symbiotic relationship with the host. Many subsequent studies have shown that the host reaction to individual species is dependent on the microbial species, with some species provoking a strong immunological response, and others producing little, if any, noticeable change on the host.[88, 89, 92–97] A representative study is that of Carter and Pollard,[88] where GF mice were monoassociated with either *Lactobacillus casei, Clostridium difficile,* or *Bacteroides fragilis* var. *vulgatus*. Upon sacrifice, antibody titres against the microbial strains utilised in the experiments could not be demonstrated in the mice remaining germ-free. The *L. casei*-associated mice were similar to the GF controls, with thin-walled, watery caeca, small Peyer's patches with sparse, small germinal centre zones, and with mesenteric lymph nodes and spleen resembling GF mice. The *B. vulgatus*-monoassociated mice developed caeca characteristic of CV mice, but the Peyer's patches neither increased in size nor develped germinal zones. After two weeks, small germinal zones had developed in the MLN, as well as weak antibody response to *B. vulgatus*. The *C. difficile*-associated mice developed CV characteristics within 2–5 weeks, as opposed to the two days required for CV animals.

Although the monoassociation of gnotobiotic animals with native microbial strains appears to have no effect on the host immune system, as seen in the Carter and Pollard study,[88] this may be an artefact of using a GF model with only one microbial species. Indeed, studies performed by Moreau et al.[95] indicated that, although many autochthonous strains are non-immunogenic when monoassociated with GF animals, when two or more strains are associated with the animals they do induce an increase in IgA+ plasma cells.

4.9 Conclusion

Functional foods probably first arose through the necessity to supplement the diet with vitamins. Certainly the first generation of functional foods involved the addition of trace minerals to appropriate foodstuffs, with cereals being a popular vehicle for use. It is the case that most current thinking and product development is centred towards gastrointestinal activity and microbial interactions specifically. Probiotics have a long history of use in humans, but have never realised their full potential. This is probably because of some poor science that has been associated with the concept. Often trials have been carried out in a very subjective manner. Today, the concept of gut flora modulation is enjoying new popularity and it is imperative that well-conducted human studies are used to test and validate probiotics, prebiotics and synbiotics. These should have rigorous control and include appropriate placebo. New advances in molecular biology allow a highly sophisticated tracking of the microbiota changes in response to dietary intervention. Similarly, this chapter has reviewed the use of certain animal models for probiotic use. Here, many hypotheses have arisen on immunological status. Again, these need to be confirmed in humans. It is implicit that any effects seen through the use of functional foods identify a plausible mechanism of effect.

It is important that diet fulfils all the nutritional requirements of humans; however, an added bonus may be the health-enhancing effects. While the population ages and pharmaceutical expenses increase, the route of using diet for the prophylactic management of disorder is an attractive concept – especially when the human gut is considered.

4.10 References

1 GIBSON, G.R. and ROBERFROID, M.B. (eds) *Colonic Microbiota*, Nutrition and Health. Kluwer Academic Publishers, Dordrecht, 1999.
2 CUMMINGS, J.H. and MACFARLANE, G.T. 'The control and consequences of bacterial fermentation in the human colon', *J Appl Bacteriol*, 1991, **70**, 443–59.
3 SALMINEN, S., BOU8LEY, C., BOUTRON-RUAULT, M.-C., CUMMINGS, J.H., FRANCK, A., GIBSON, G.R., ISOLAURI, E., MOREAU, M.-C., ROBERFROID, M. and ROWLAND, I.R. 'Functional food science and gastrointestinal physiology and function', *Brit J Nutrition*, 1998, **80**, S147–71.
4 FULLER, R. 'Probiotics in man and animals', *J Appl Bacteriol*, 1989, **66**, 365–78.
5 TANNOCK, G.W. (ed.) *Probiotics: A Critical Review*, Horizon Scientific Press, Wymondham, 1999.
6 FULLER, R. and GIBSON, G.R. 'Modification of the intestinal microflora using probiotics and prebiotics', *Scan J Gastroenterol*, 1997, **32**, 28–31.

7   FULLER, R. (ed.) *Probiotics: The Scientific Basis*, London, Chapman & Hall, 1992.

8   FULLER, R. (ed.) *Probiotics 2: Applications and Practical Aspects*, London, Chapman & Hall, 1997.

9   LEE, Y.-K., NOMOTO, K., SALMINEN, S. and GORBACH, S.L., *Handbook of Probiotics*, New York, John Wiley, 1999.

10 GIBSON, G.R. and ROBERFROID, M.B., 'Dietary modulation of the human colonic microbiota: introducing the concept of prebiotics', *J Nutr*, 1995, **125**, 1401–12.

11 GIBSON, G.R. and COLLINS, M.D., 'Concept of balanced colonic microbiota, prebiotics and synbiotics'. In *Probiotics, Other Nutritional Factors and Intestinal Microflora*, L.A. Hanson and R.H. Yolken (eds), Nestlé Nutrition Workshop Series, vol. 42, pp. 139–56, Nestec Ltd. Vevey/Lippincott-Raven Publishers, Philadelphia, 1999.

12 GIBSON, G.R., BERRY OTTAWAY, P. and RASTALL, R.A., *Prebiotics: New Developments in Functional Foods*, Oxford, Chandos Limited, 2000.

13 MACFARLANE, G.T., GIBSON, G.R. and CUMMINGS, J.H., 'Comparison of fermentation reactions in different regions of the colon', *J Appl Bacteriol*, 1992, **72**, 57–64.

14 CUMMINGS, J.H. 'Short chain fatty acids'. In *Human Colonic Bacteria: Role in Nutrition, Physiology and Pathology*, G.R. Gibson and G.T. Macfarlane (eds) pp. 101–30, CRC Press, Boca Raton, 1995.

15 LEVITT, M.D., GIBSON, G.R. and CHRISTL, S.U. 'Gas metabolism in the large intestine'. In *Human Colonic Bacteria: Role in Nutrition, Physiology and Pathology*, G.R. Gibson and G.T. Macfarlane (eds), pp. 131–54, CRC Press, Boca Raton, 1995.

16 MACFARLANE, G.T., GIBSON, G.R., BEATTY, E.A. and CUMMINGS, J.H. 'Estimation of short chain fatty acid production from protein by human intestinal bacteria, based on branched chain fatty acid measurements', *FEMS Microbiol Ecol*, 1992, **101**, 81–8.

17 MACFARLANE, G.T., CUMMINGS, J.H. and ALLISON, C. 'Protein degradation by human intestinal bacteria', *J Gen Microbiol*, 1986, **132**, 1647–56.

18 MACFARLANE, G.T., GIBSON, R., DRASAR, B.S., CUMMINGS, J.H. 'Metabolic significance of the gut microflora', *Gastrointestinal and Oesophageal Pathology*, R. Whitehead (ed.), pp. 249–74, Edinburgh, Churchill Livingstone, 1995.

19 COLLINS, M.D. and GIBSON, G.R. 'Probiotics, prebiotics and synbiotics: Dietary approaches for the modulation of microbial ecology', *American J Clinical Nutrition*, 1999, **69**, 1052–7.

20 GIBSON, G.R. and MACFARLANE, G.T. 'Intestinal bacteria and disease', *Human Health: The Contribution of Microorganisms*, S.A.W. Gibson (ed.), pp. 53–62, London, Springer-Verlag, 1994.

21 KELLY, S.M., PITCHER, M.C.L., FARMERY, S.M. and GIBSON, G.R. 'Isolation of *Helicobacter pylori* from feces of patients with dyspepsia in the United Kingdom', *Gastroenterol*, 1994, **107**, 1671–4.

22 SHORTT, C. 'Living it up for dinner', *Chemistry and Industry*, 1998, **8**, 300–3.

23 METCHNIKOFF, E. *Prolongation of life*, New York, G.P. Putnam, 1908.

24 DELZENNE, N. and WILLIAMS, C.M. 'Actions of non-digestible carbohydrates on blood lipids in humans and animals'. In *Colonic Microbiota, Nutrition and Health*, G.R. Gibson and M.B. Roberfroid (eds), pp. 213–31, Dordrecht, Kluwer Academic Publishers, 1999.

25 LANGENDIJK, P.S., SCHUT, F., JANSEN, G.J., RAANGS, G.C., KAMPHUIS, G.R., WILKINSON, M.H.F. and WELLING, G.W. 'Quantitative fluorescence in situ hybridisation of *Bifidobacterium* spp. with genus-specific 16S rRNA-targeted probes and its application in fecal samples', *Appl Environ Microbiol*, 1995, **61**, 3069–75.

26 MCCARTNEY, A.L., WENZHI, W. and TANNOCK, G.W. 'Molecular analysis of the composition of the bifidobacterial and lactobacillus microflora of humans', *Appl Environ Microbiol*, 1996, **62**, 4608–13.

27 MCCARTNEY, A.L. and GIBSON, G.R. 'The application of prebiotics in human health and nutrition'. In Proceeding Lactic 97, *Which Strains? For Which Products?*, Adria Normandie, pp. 59–73, 1998.

28 WANG, G. and GIBSON, G.R. 'Effects of the in vitro fermentation of oligofructose and inulin by bacteria growing in the human large intestine', *J Appl Bacteriol*, 1993, **75**, 373–80.

29 WILLIAMS, C.H., WITHERLY, S.A. and BUDDINGTON, R.K. 'Influence of dietary neosugar on selected bacterial groups of the human faecal microbiota', *Microb Ecol Health and Disease*, 1994, **7**, 91–7.

30 KLEESSEN, B., SYKURA, B., ZUNFT, H.-J. and BLAUT, M. 'Effects of inulin and lactose on fecal microflora, microbial activity and bowel habit in elderly constipated persons', *Am J Clin Nutr*, 1997, **65**, 1397–1402.

31 GIBSON, G.R., BEATTY, E.R., WANG, X. and CUMMINGS, J.H. 'Selective stimulation of bifidobacteria in the human colon by oligofructose and inulin', *Gastroenterol*, 1995, **108**, 975–82.

32 IMAMURA, L., HISAMITSU, K. and KOBASHI, K. 'Purification and characterization of β-fructofuranosidase from *Bifidobacterium infantis*', *Biol Pharm Bull*, 1994, **17** 596–602.

33 PLAYNE, M.J. and CRITTENDEN, R. 'Commercially available oligosaccharides', *Bull Int Dairy Foundation*, 1996, **313**, 10–22.

34 NAKAKUKI, T. (ed.) 'Oligosaccharides. Production, properties and applications', *Japanese Technology Reviews*, 1993, **3**, 107–17, Yverdon, Gordon & Breach.

35 GIBSON, G.R. and WANG, X. 'Regulatory effects of bifidobacteria on the growth of other colonic bacteria', *J Appl Bacteriol*, 1994, **77**, 412–20.

36 FUJIWARA, S., HASHIBARA, H., HIROTA, T. and FORSTNER, J.F. 'Proteinaceous factor(s) in culture supernatant fluids of bifidobacteria which prevents the binding of enterotoxigenic *Escherichia coli* to gangliotetraosylceramide', *Appl Environ Microbiol*, 1987, **63**, 506–12.

37 UMESAKI, Y. 'Intestinal glycolipids and their possible role in microbial colonisation of mice', *Bifid Microflora*, 1989, **8**, 13–22.

38 ZOPF, D. and ROTH, S. 'Oligosaccharide anti-infective agents', *The Lancet*, 1996, **347**, 1017–21.

39 RASTALL, R.A. and BUCKE, C. 'Enzymatic synthesis of oligosaccharides', *Biotech Gen Eng Rev*, 1992, **10**, 253–81.

40 SUWASONO, S. and RASTALL, R.A. 'A highly regioselective synthesis of mannobiose and mannotriose by reverse hydrolysis using specific α1,2-mannosidase from *Aspergillus phoenicis*', *Biotech Lett*, 1996, **18**, 851–6.

41 MACFARLANE, G.T., MACFARLANE, S. and GIBSON, G.R. 'Validation of a three-stage compound continuous culture system for investigating the effect of retention time on the ecology and metabolism of bacteria in the human colonic microbiot', *Microbial Ecol*, 1998, **35**, 180–7.

42 ROWLAND, I.R. (ed.) *Role of the Gut Flora in Toxicity and Cancer*, London, Academic Press, 1988.

43 KIM, Y.S., TSAO, D., MORITA, A. and BELLA, A. 'Effect of sodium butyrate and three human colorectal adenocarcinoma cell lines in culture', *Falk Symposium*, 1982, **31**, 317–23.

44 OLANO-MARTIN, E., MOUNTZOURIS, K.C., GIBSON, G.R. and RASTALL, R.A. 'Development of prebiotics based on dextran and oligodextran', *Bri J Nutr*, in press.

45 MOROTOMI, M., GUILLEM, J.G., LOGERFO, P. and WEINSTEN, I.B. 'Production of diacylglycerol, an activator of protein kinase C by human intestinal microflora', *Cancer Res*, 1990, **50**, 3595–9.

46 PERDIGON, G. and ALVAREZ, S. 'Probiotics and the immune stat'. In *Probiotics: The Scientific Basis*, R. Fuller (ed.), pp. 146–80, London, Chapman & Hall, 1992.

47 ISOLAURI, E., JUNTUNEN, M., RAUTANEN, T., SILLANAUKEE, P. and KOIVULA, T.A. 'Human Lactobacillus strain (Lactobacillus GG) promotes recovery from acute diarrhoea in children', *Pediatrics*, 1991, **88**, 90–7.

48 NAIDU, A.S., BIDLACK, W.R. and CLEMENS, R.A. 'Probiotic spectra of lactic acid bacteria', *Crit Rev Food Sci Nutr*, 1999, **38**, 13–126.

49 GIBSON, G.R., SAAVEDRA, J.M., MACFARLANE, S. and MACFARLANE, G.T. 'Gastrointestinal microbial disease'. In *Probiotics 2: Application and Practical Aspects*, R. Fuller (ed.), pp. 10–39, Andover, Chapman & Hall, 1997.

50 MITSUOKA, T. 'Bifidobacteria and their role in human health', *J Ind Microbiol*, 1990, **6**, 263–8.

51 PARK, S.F. and KROLL, R.G. 'Expression of listeriolysin and phosphatidyli-nositol-specific phospholipase C is repressed by the plant-derived molecule cellobiose in *Listeria monocytogenes*', *Molec Microbiol*, 1993, **8**, 653–61.

52 METCHNIKOFF, E. *The Nature of Man: Studies in Optimistic Philosophy*, Trans. P. Charles Mitchell XVI (ed.), New York, G.P. Putnam, 1903.

53 DALY, C. 'Lactic acid bacteria and milk fermentation', *J Chem Technol Biotechnol*, 1991, **51**, 544–8.

54 ABBAS, Z. and JAFRI, W. 'Yoghurt (dahi): A probiotic and therapeutic view', *J Pak Med Assoc*, 1992, **42**, 221–4.

55 PERDIGON, G., NADER DE MACIAS, E.,. ALVAREZ, S., OLIVER, G. and PESCE DE RUIZ HOLGADO, A.A. 'Effect of perorally administered lactobacilli on macrophage activation in mice', *Infect Immun*, 1986, **53**, 404–10.

56 SATO, K., SAITO, H. and TOMIOKA, H. 'Enhancement of host resistance against *Listeria* infection by *Lactobacillus casei*: Activation of liver macrophages and peritoneal macrophages by *Lactobacillus casei*', *Microbiol Immunol*, 1988, **32**, 689–98.

57 KATO, I., YOKOKURA, T. and MUTAI, M. 'Augmentation of mouse natural killer cell activity by *Lactobacillus casei* and its surface antigens', *Microbiol Immunol*, 1984, **27**, 209–17.

58 WALKER, R. 'Some observations on the phenomenon of caecal enlargement in the rat', *Chemical Toxicology of Foods*, C.L. Galli, R. Paoletti and G. Vettorazzi (eds), pp. 339–48, Amsterdam, Elsevier, 1978.

59 GORDON, H.A. 'Morphological and physiological characterization of germ-free life', *Ann N Y Acad Sci*, 1959, **78**, 208–20.

60 GORDON, H.A. and WOSTMANN, B.S. 'Morphological studies on the germfree albino rat', *Anat Rec*, 1960, **137**, 65.

61 POLLARD, M. 'Germinal centers in germfree animals'. In *Germinal Centers in Immune Response*, H. Cottier, R. Odartchenko, C. Schindler and C. Congdon (eds), pp. 343–6, New York, Springer-Verlag, 1967.

62 THORBECKE, G.J. 'Some histological and functional aspects of lymphoid tissue in germfree animals, I. Morphological studies', *Ann N Y Acad Sci*, 1959, **78**, 237–46.

63 POLLARD, M. 'Host responses to neoplastic diseases', *Proc Inst Med Chicago*, 1967, **26**, 9.

64 BEALMEAR, P.M. 'Host defense mechanisms in gnotobiotic animals'. In *Immunologic Defects in Laboratory Animals*, E. Gershwin and B. Marchant (eds), vol. 2, pp. 261–350, New York, Plenum Press, 1980.

65 SCOTT, M.T., MACDONALD, T.T. and CARTER P.B. '*C. parvum* in germfree mice', *Cancer Immunol Immunother*, 1978, **4**, 135.

66 MACDONALD, T.T. and CARTER, P.B. 'Contact sensitivity in the germ-free mouse', *J Reticuloendothelial Soc*, 1978, **24**, 287.

67 WOSTMANN, B.S. 'Recent studies on the serum proteins of germfree animals', *Ann N Y Acad Sci*, 1961, **94**, 272–83.

68 SELL, S. 'γ-Globulin metabolism in germfree guinea pigs', *J Immunol*, 1964, **92**, 559–64.

69 SELL, S. 'Immunoglobulins of the germfree guinea pig', *J Immunol*, 1964, **93**, 122–31.

70 ASOFSKY, R. and HYLTON, M.B. 'Some characteristics of a secretory immunoglobulin (IgA) in germfree and conventional mice', *Symposium on Gnotobiotic Research*, p. 6, Madison, Wisconsin, 1967.

71 OLSON, G.B. and WOSTMANN, B.S. 'Cellular and humoral immune response of germfree mice stimulated with 7S HGG or *Salmonella typhimurium*', *J Immunol*, 1966, **97**, 275–86.

72 OLSON, G.B. and WOSTMANN, B.S. 'Lymphocytopoiesis, plasmacytopoiesis

and cellular proliferation in nonantigenically stimulated germfree mice', *J Immunol*, 1966, **97**, 267–74.

73 KIYONO, H., MCGHEE, J.R. and MICHALEK, S.M. 'Lipopolysaccharide regulation of the immune response: Comparison of responses to LPS in germfree, *Escherichia coli*-monoassociated and conventional mice', *J Immunol*, 1980, **124**, 36–41.

74 MCGHEE, F.R., KYONO, H., MICHALEK, S.M., BABB, J.L., ROSENSTREICH, D.L. and MERGENHAGEN, S.E. 'Lipopolysaccharide (LPS) regulation of the immune response: T lymphocytes from normal mice suppress mitogenic and immunogenic responses to LPS', *J Immunol*, 1980, **124**, 1603–11.

75 WOOLVERTON, C.J., HOLT, L.C., MITCHELL, D. and SARTOR, R.B. 'Identification and characterization of rat intestinal lamina propria cells: consequences of microbial colonization', *Vet Immunol Immunopathol*, 1992, **34**, 127–38.

76 HEISE, E.R. and MYRVIK, Q.N. 'Levels of lysosomal hydrolases in alveolar and peritoneal macrophages from conventional and germ-free rats', *Fed Proc*, 1966, **25**, 439 (abstract).

77 BAUER, H., PARONETTO, F., BURNS, W.A. and EINHEBER, A. 'The enhancing effect of the microbial flora on macrophage function and the immune response: a study in germfree mice', *J Exp Med*, 1966, **123**, 1013–24.

78 HOROWITZ, R.E., BAUER, H., PARONETTO, F., ABRAMS, G.D., WATKINS, K.C. and POPPER, H. 'The response of the lymphatic system to bacterial antigen: studies in germfree mice', *Am J Path*, 1964, **44**, 747–56.

79 ABRAMS, G. and BISHOP, J.E. 'Normal flora and leukocyte mobilization', *Arch Path*, 1965, **79**, 213–17.

80 JUNGI, T.W. and MCGREGOR, D.D. 'Impaired chemotactic responsiveness of macrophages from gnotobiotic rats', *Infect Immun*, 1978, **19**, 553–61.

81 MORLAND, B., SMIEVOLL, A.I. and MIDTVEDT, T. 'Comparison of peritoneal macrophages from germfree and conventional mice', *Infect Immun*, 1979, **26**, 1129–36.

82 MELTZER, M.S. 'Tumoricidal responses in vitro of peritoneal macrophages from conventionally housed and germ-free nude mice', *Cell Immunol*, 1976, **22**, 176–81.

83 JOHNSON, W.I. and BALISH, E. 'Macrophage function in germ-free, athymic (nu/nu), and conventional-flora (nu/+) mice', *J Reticuloendothelial Soc*, 1980, **28**, 55–6.

84 TANNOCK, G.W. 'Influences of the normal microbiota on the animal host', In *Gastrointestinal Microbiology*, R.I. Mackie, B.A. White and R.E. Isaacson (eds), vol. 2, pp. 537–87, New York, Chapman and Hall, 1997.

85 DUCLUZEAU, R. and RAIBAUD, P. *Ecologie microbienne du tube digestif*, Paris, Masson, 1979.

86 NORIN, K.E., MIDTVEDT, T. and GUSTAFSSON, B.E. 'Influence of intestinal microflora on the tryptic activity during lactation in rats', *Lab Anim*, 1986, **20**, 234–7.

87 LEE, A. 'Neglected niches the microbial ecology of the gastrointestinal tract'. In *Advances in Microbial Ecology*, K.C. Marshall (ed.), vol. 8, pp. 115–62,

New York, Plenum Press, 1984.

88 CARTER, P.B. and POLLARD, M. 'Host responses to "normal" microbial flora in germfree mice', *J Reticuloendothel Soc*, 1971, **9**, 580–7.

89 WAGNER, M. 'Serological aspects of germfree life', *Ann N Y Acad Sci*, 1959, **78**, 261–71.

90 MAYHEW, J.W. and POLLARD, M. unpublished observations reported in P.B. Carter and M. Pollard, 'Host responses to "normal" microbial flora in germfree mice', *J Reticuloendothel Soc*, 1971, **9**, 580–7.

91 DUBOS, R., SCHAEDLER, W., COSTELLO, R. and HOET, P. 'Indigenous, normal, and autochthonous flora of the gastrointestinal tract', *J Exp Med*, 1965, **122**, 67–75.

92 CARTER, P.B. and POLLARD, M. 'Studies with *Lactobacillus casei* in gnotobiotic mice'. In *Germfree Research: Biological Effect of Gnotobiotic Environments*, J.B. Heneghan (ed.), pp. 379–83, New York, Academic Press, 1973.

93 BALISH, E., YALE, C.E. and HONG, R. 'Serum proteins of gnotobiotic rats', *Infect Immun*, 1972, **6**, 112–18.

94 FOO, M.C. and LEE, A. 'Immunological tolerance of mice to members of the autochthonous intestinal microflora', *Infec Immun*, 1972, **6**, 525–32.

95 MOREAU, M.C., DUCLUZEAU, R., GUY-GRAND, D. and MULLER, M.C. 'Increase in the population of duodenal immunoglobulin A plasmocytes in axenic mice associated with different living or dead bacterial strains of intestinal organs', *Infec Immun*, 1978, **21**, 532–9.

96 MORISHITA, Y. and MITSUOKA, T. 'Antibody responses in germ-free chickens to bacteria isolated from various sources', *Japan J Microbiol*, 1973, **17**, 181–7.

97 WELLS, C.L. and BALISH, E. 'Modulation of the rat's immune status', *Can J Microbiol*, 1980, **26**, 1192–8.

5

Coronary heart disease

J.A. Lovegrove and K.G. Jackson, University of Reading

5.1 Introduction

Coronary heart disease (CHD) is one of the major causes of death in adults in the Western world. Although there has been a trend over the past 15 years towards a reduction in the rates of CHD in the major industrialised nations (including USA, Australia and the UK) due to better health screening, drug treatment, smoking and dietary advice, there has been an alarming increase in CHD in Eastern Europe.

CHD is a condition in which the main coronary arteries supplying the heart are no longer able to supply sufficient blood and oxygen to the heart muscle (myocardium). The main cause of the reduced flow is an accumulation of plaques, mainly in the intima of arteries, a disease known as atherosclerosis. This is a slow but progressive disease which usually begins in childhood, but does not usually manifest itself until later life. Depending on the rate of the narrowing of the arteries and its ultimate severity, four syndromes may occur during the progression of CHD. These include angina pectoris, unstable angina pectoris, myocardial infarction and sudden death. Angina pectoris literally means a 'strangling sensation in the chest' and is often provoked by physical activity or stress. This pain, which often radiates from the chest to the left arm and neck, is caused by reduced blood flow in the coronary artery but this pain fades quite quickly when the patient is rested. Unstable angina pectoris occurs as the condition worsens and pain is experienced not only during physical activity but also during rest. This type of angina is thought to involve rupture or fissuring of a fixed lesion which, when untreated, leads to an acute myocardial infarction. The condition is responsible for a large proportion of deaths from CHD and occurs as a result of prolonged occlusion of the coronary artery leading to death of some of the heart muscle. Disturbances to the contraction of the heart can lead to disruption in the electrical contraction of heart muscle and the heart may go into an uncoordinated rhythm (ventricular fibrillation) or may completely stop. Sudden death from a severe myocardial infarction occurs within one hour of the attack and is generally associated with advanced atherosclerosis.

A number of risk factors known to predispose an individual to CHD have been categorised into those that are not modifiable, such as age, sex, race and family history, and those that are modifiable, such as hyperlipidaemia (high levels of lipids (fat) in the blood), hypertension (high blood pressure), obesity, cigarette smoking and lack of exercise. Epidemiological studies examining CHD risks in different populations have observed a positive correlation between an individual's fasting cholesterol level (i.e. cholesterol level before eating a meal), especially elevated levels of low density lipoprotein (LDL) cholesterol and development of CHD.[1] Low levels of high density lipoprotein (HDL) cholesterol have been shown to be another risk factor for CHD since an inverse relationship exists with CHD development. This lipoprotein is involved in reverse cholesterol transport, carrying cholesterol from cells to the liver for removal from the body and a low level of HDL cholesterol reflects an impairment in this process.

A recently recognised risk factor for CHD is an elevated level of triacylglycerol (TAG; major fat in the blood) in both the fasted and fed (postprandial) state and the strength of this association has been demonstrated in a number of observation studies.[2] The atherogenic lipoprotein phenotype (ALP) is a newly recognised condition that describes a collection of abnormalities of both classical and newly defined risk factors which predisposes an apparently healthy individual to an increased CHD risk.[3] The lipid abnormalities of the ALP are discussed in more detail in section 5.3.3. The development of techniques by which to characterise the LDL subclass of individuals with CHD and those without CHD has enabled the prevalence of those with ALP to be identified in the population. Heritability studies have revealed that 50% of the variability in expression is due to genetic factors, with the remainder being associated with environmental influences such as diet, smoking and a sedentary lifestyle.

Individuals with CHD and those with a high risk of developing the condition are treated in a number of ways to help lower their LDL cholesterol and TAG concentrations while elevating their HDL cholesterol. Many lines of evidence suggest that adverse dietary habits are a contributory factor in CHD and so the first line of treatment for individuals with moderately raised cholesterol (5.5–7.0 mmol/l) and/or TAG (1.5–3.0 mmol/l) levels is to modify their diet. This is implemented by reducing the percentage of dietary energy derived from fat to approximately 30%, with a reduction of saturated fatty acids (SFAs) to 10% of the dietary energy derived from fat. Candidate fats for the replacement of a large proportion of SFAs include polyunsaturated fatty acids (PUFAs) of the *n*-6 (linoleic) series and monounsaturated fatty acids (MUFAs). Although both PUFAs (*n*-6 series) and MUFAs have been shown to decrease total cholesterol and LDL cholesterol levels, MUFAs have also been shown to maintain or increase HDL cholesterol concentrations when they are used to substitute SFAs compared with n-6 PUFAs. PUFAs of the n-3 series (eicosapentaenoic acid (EPA) and docosahexaenoic acid (DHA)) have been shown to reduce plasma TAG levels in both the fed and fasted states and reduce thrombosis when added to the diet, but they do not usually reduce total and LDL cholesterol levels.

Individuals with cholesterol levels above 8.0 mmol/l and/or TAG levels above 3.0 mmol/l require not only dietary modification but also lipid-lowering drugs to help reduce their disorder. Drugs that are available are effective in a number of ways, including the following:

- reduced synthesis of very low density lipoprotein (VLDL) and LDL (e.g. nicotinic acid)
- enhanced VLDL clearance (e.g. benzafibrate)
- enhanced LDL clearance (e.g. cholestyramine) and hydroxy-methyl-glutaryl CoA (HMG-CoA) reductase inhibition (e.g. simvasatin).

A recently available drug, fenofibrate, has been shown not only to reduce cholesterol and TAG levels, but also increases HDL cholesterol concentrations and is able to shift the LDL class profile away from the more atherogenic small dense LDL. These drugs are more aggressive and although they cause greater reductions in lipid levels compared with dietary modification, they are often associated with unpleasant side-effects. Therefore this supports the need for effective dietary strategies that can reduce circulating lipid levels in both the fed and fasted state and which offer long-term efficacy comparable with most effective drug treatments. One dietary strategy that has been proposed to benefit the lipid profile involves the supplementation of the diet with prebiotics, probiotics and synbiotics which are mechanisms to improve the health of the host by supplementation and/or fortification of certain health promoting gut bacteria.

A *prebiotic* is a non-viable component of the diet that reaches the colon in an intact form and which is selectively fermented by colon bacteria such as bifidobacteria and lactobacilli. The term 'prebiotic' refers to non-digestible oligosaccharides derived from plants and also synthetically produced oligo-saccharides. Animal studies have shown that dietary supplementation with prebiotics markedly reduced circulating TAG and, to a lesser extent, cholesterol concentrations. The generation of short chain fatty acids (SCFAs) during fermentation of the prebiotic by the gut microflora has been proposed to be one of the mechanisms responsible for their lipid-lowering effects via inhibition of enzymes involved in *de novo* lipogenesis. Of the human studies conducted to date, there has been inconsistent findings with respect to changes in lipid levels, although on the whole there have been favourable outcomes.

A *probiotic* is a live microbial feed supplement which beneficially affects the host animal by improving its intestinal microbial balance and is generally fermented milk products containing lactic acid bacteria such as bifidobacteria and/or lactobacilli. The putative health benefits of probiotics include improved resistance to gastrointestinal infections, reduction in total cholesterol and TAG levels and stimulation of the immune system.[4] A number of mechanisms have been proposed to explain their putative lipid-lowering capacity and these include a 'milk factor' which has been thought to inhibit HMG-CoA reductase and the assimilation of cholesterol by certain bacteria.

A combination of a prebiotic and a probiotic, termed a *synbiotic*, is receiving attention at present since this association is thought to improve the survival of the probiotic bacteria in the colon. However, further well-controlled nutrition trials are required to investigate the mechanisms of action and effects of prebiotics, probiotics and synbiotics.

Manufacturers in the USA and Europe are starting to explore the commercial opportunities for foods that contain health-promoting food ingredients (probiotics, prebiotics and synbiotics). Issues considered important to the continuing development of the growing market include safety, consumer education, price and appropriate health claims. Until recently, most of the food products marketed were probiotics incorporated into dairy products. However, with the increasing interest in prebiotics, a more diverse food market has been opened up since prebiotics can be incorporated into many long-life foods ranging from bread to ice-cream. Although there is increasing interest in the use of prebiotics, probiotics and synbiotics as supplements to the diet, there is a need to ensure that claims for these products are based on carefully conducted human trials, which exploit up-to-date methodologies

5.2 Coronary heart disease and risk factors

Diseases of the circulatory system account for an appreciable proportion of total morbidity and mortality in adults throughout the world. In 1990, CHD accounted for 27% of all deaths in the UK and stroke for 12%. The rates of mortality due to CHD throughout the world vary. For example, in one study among men aged 40–59 years, initially free of CHD, the annual incidence rate (occurrence of new cases) varied from 15 per 100,000 in Japan to 198 per 100,000 in Finland.[5] In addition to different rates of disease of the circulatory system between countries, the conditions assume varying degrees of importance in developing and affluent countries. Rheumatic heart disease is common in developing countries, whereas CHD has assumed almost epidemic proportions in affluent societies.

Fig. 5.1 shows trends in CHD standardised mortality rates for the USA, Australia and the UK. Rates in the majority of countries are reducing, but the decline in CHD mortality in the UK began later than in the USA and Australia.[6] However, in Eastern Europe, rates of CHD are increasing dramatically, which is in contrast to many other parts of the world. Improved surgical procedures, more extensive use of cholesterol-lowering drugs and other medication, a reduction in smoking and increased health screening are in part responsible for this downturn. In addition, changes in diet, and especially in the type of fat consumed, may also have had a beneficial impact on disease incidence.

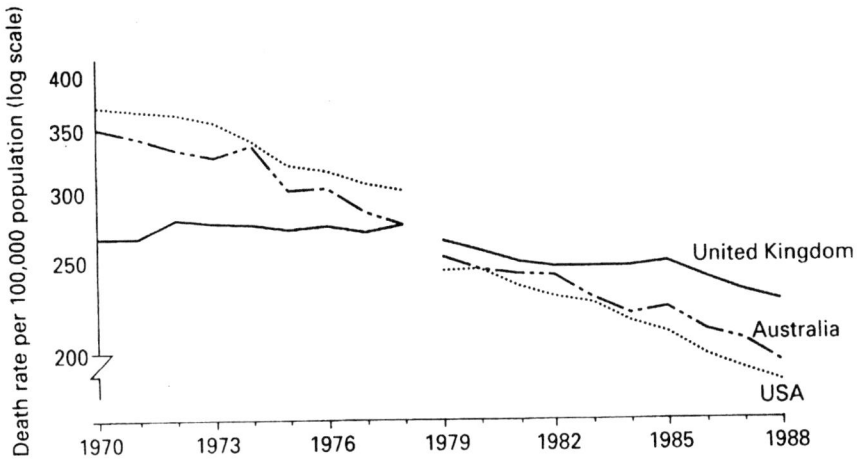

Fig. 5.1   Comparisons in the mortality from CHD in the UK, USA and Australia (1970–88). Data between the years 1978 and 1979 were by a change in classification from ICD8 to ICD9 (adapted from WHO, 1989).

5.2.1 Pathology of CHD development

The underlying basis for clinical cardiovascular disease is a combination of atherosclerosis and thrombosis. Atherosclerosis is a condition in which the arterial lining is thickened in places by raised plaques as a result of excessive accumulation of modified lipids, and of the proliferation and migration of smooth muscle cells from deeper layers of the arterial wall. The atherosclerotic plaque usually develops at a point of minor injury in the arterial wall. Tissue macrophages (a type of white blood cell) are attracted to this point of damage and engulf and accumulate LDL particles from the blood. Recent studies have shown that LDL particles that have become oxidised are more likely to be taken up and cause cholesterol accumulation in macrophages. The cholesterol-loaded macrophages are transformed into lipid-laden foam cells, which remain in the arterial wall. At a later stage, the plaque becomes sclerosed and calcified (hence the term 'hardening of the arteries').

Formation of an atherosclerotic plaque can occlude one or more of the arteries, mainly the coronary and cerebral arteries, resulting in CHD or a stroke, respectively. In addition, a superimposed thrombus or clot may further occlude the artery. An example of an artery that has atherosclerotic lesions and has been completely occluded by a thrombus is shown in Fig. 5.2. Blood clot formation is in part determined by a release of eicosanoids from platelets and the vessel walls. PUFAs released from platelet membranes are metabolised into thromboxane (an eicosanoid) which stimulates platelet aggregation and vasoconstriction. Simultaneously, the vessel walls also release PUFAs which are converted to prostacyclins (antagonistic eicosanoids), which inhibit platelet aggregation and cause vasodilation. The balance between production of thromboxane and prostacyclin, and the relative

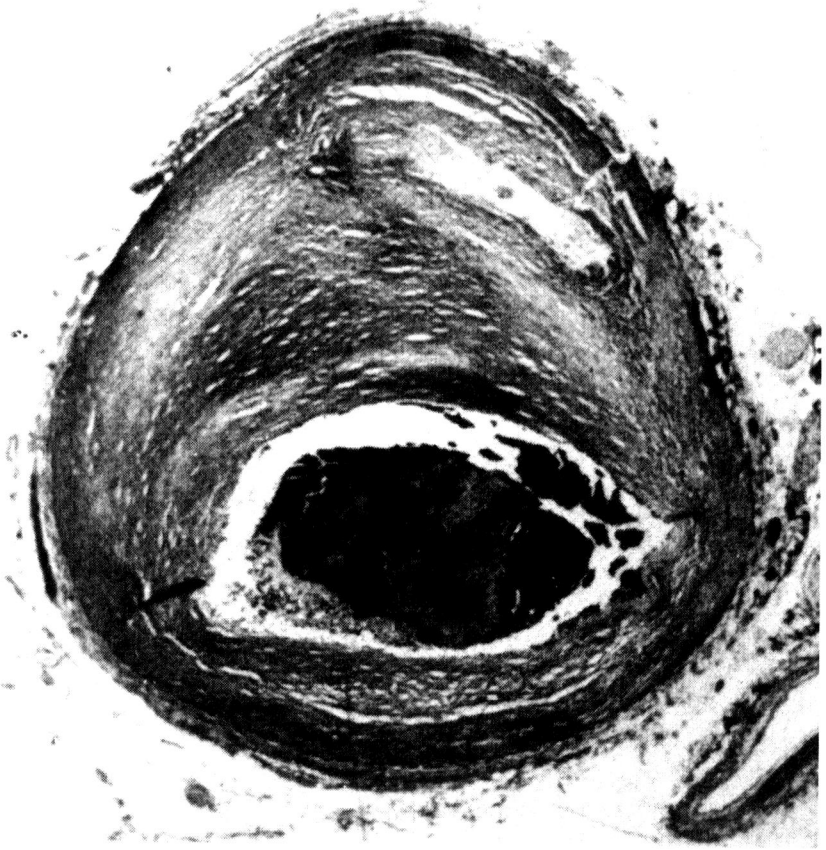

Fig. 5.2 Atherosclerotic plaque and thrombus completely occluding a coronary artery.

potencies of these two eicosanoids, will determine the extent of the blood clot formed.

Two major clinical conditions are associated with these processes: angina pectoris and coronary thrombosis or myocardial infarction. Angina pectoris is characterised by pain and discomfort in the chest, which is brought on by exertion and stress. It results from a reduction or temporary block in the blood flow through the coronary artery to the heart and seldom lasts for more than 15 minutes. A coronary thrombosis results from prolonged total occlusion of the artery, which causes infarct or death of some of the heart muscle and is associated with prolonged and usually excruciating central chest pain.

A variety of cells and lipids are involved in arterial thrombus, including lipoproteins, cholesterol, TAG, platelets, monocytes, endothelial cells, fibroblasts and smooth muscle cells. Nutrition may influence the development of CHD by modifying one or more of these factors and this will be discussed in more detail in section 5.4. For the purposes of this chapter the disease of the circulatory system that will be addressed is CHD, with little discussion of other CVD such as strokes.

5.2.2 Risk factors for the development of CHD

CHD is a multifaceted condition which has no single cause. The term 'risk factor' is used extensively, and often very loosely, to describe features of lifestyle and behaviour, as well as physical activity and biochemical attributes, which predict the likelihood of developing disease. Potential risk factors are continually being refined as research into the aetiology of CHD progresses. The known risk factors for development of CHD can be categorised into those that cannot be modified, those that can be changed, those associated with disease states and those related to geographic distribution, as shown in Table 5.1.

Some risk factors have a greater influence on CHD development than others. It has been demonstrated that there is a strong and consistent relationship between total plasma cholesterol and CHD risk.[7] The positive association is largely confined to the LDL fraction, which transports about 70% of cholesterol in the blood. In a large prospective study published in 1986, a fivefold difference in CHD mortality, over a range of plasma cholesterol levels, was observed in the US population.[7] In a recent cholesterol-lowering drug trial in a healthy population, a reduction of 20% and 26% in total and LDL cholesterol respectively was associated with a 31% reduction in the five-year incidence of myocardial infarction and CHD death.[8] It is this relationship between the plasma cholesterol levels and its link with CHD that forms the basis of most dietary guidelines, which recommend reductions in total fat and SFA intakes.

Table 5.1 Risk factors for the development of coronary heart disease

Unmodifiable	Being male
	Increasing age
	Genetic traits (including lipid metabolism abnormalities)
	Body build
	Ethnic origin
Modifiable	Cigarette smoking
	Some hyperlipidaemias (increased plasma cholesterol and triacylglycerol)
	Low levels of high density lipoprotein (HDL)
	Obesity
	Hypertension
	Low physical activity
	Increased thrombosis (ability to clot)
	Stress
	Alcohol consumption
Diseases	Diabetes (glucose intolerance)
Geographic	Climate and season: cold weather
	Soft drinking water

Table 5.2   Relative risk and yield of cases in the top fifth of the ranked distribution of risk factors in the men from the British Regional Heart Study after five years of follow-up. (Adapted from Shaper *et al.*, 1986.)

Factor	Relative risk	Yield in top fifth (%)
Age	4.7	34
Total cholesterol	3.1	31
Systolic BP	3.0	36
Diastolic BP	3.1	34
Body Mass Index (BMI)	1.8	28
'Smoking years'	5.1	38

If an individual presented with any one, or a combination, of risk factors it is not inevitable that that person will suffer from CHD. The ability to predict the occurrence of a myocardial infarct in individuals is fraught with complications. An obese, middle-aged man who suffers from diabetes, consumes a high-fat diet, smokes 40 cigarettes a day and has a stressful job, may never suffer from CHD; whereas a slim, physically active non-smoker who consumes a low-fat diet may die from a myocardial infarct prematurely. Despite this anomaly, individuals and populations are deemed at increasing risk of CHD according to the severity and number of identified risk factors. Table 5.2 shows the relative risk and yield of cases.[9]

The purpose of relative risk scores is in prediction, as it clearly contains items that cannot be modified. However, for the purpose of intervention, one must go beyond the items used to predict risk and consider issues such as diet, body weight, physical activity and stress (factors not used in the scoring system), as well as blood pressure and cigarette smoking, which are taken into account. General population dietary recommendations have been provided by a number of bodies which are aimed at reducing the incidence and severity of CHD within the population. Those specifically related to dietary factors are discussed in detail in section 5.4.

5.3 Relevant lipid particles

5.3.1 Plasma lipoprotein metabolism
Plasma lipoproteins are macromolecules representing complexes of lipids such as TAG, cholesterol and phospholipids, as well as one or more specific proteins referred to as apoproteins. They are involved in the transport of water-insoluble nutrients throughout the blood stream from their site of absorption or synthesis, to peripheral tissue. For the correct targeting of lipoproteins to sites of metabolism, the lipoproteins rely heavily on apoproteins associated with their surface coat.

The liver and intestine are the primary sites of lipoprotein synthesis and the two major transported lipid components, TAG and cholesterol, follow two separate fates. TAGs are shuttled primarily to adipose tissue for storage, and to muscle, where the fatty acids are oxidised for energy. Cholesterol, in contrast, is continuously shuttled among the liver, intestine and extrahepatic tissues by HDL.[10] Human lipoproteins are divided into five major classes according to their flotation density (Table 5.3). The density of the particles is inversely related to their sizes, reflecting the relative amounts of low density, non-polar lipid and high density surface protein present. The two largest lipoproteins contain mainly TAG within their core structures. These are chylomicrons (CMs), secreted by the enterocytes (cells of the small intestine), and VLDL, secreted by the hepatocytes (liver cells). Intermediate density lipoprotein (IDL) contains appreciable amounts of both TAG and cholesterol esters in their core. The two smallest classes, LDL and HDL, contain cholesterol esters in their core structures and the mature forms of these particles are not secreted directly from the liver but are produced by metabolic processes within the circulation. LDLs are produced as end products of the metabolism of VLDL, whereas components of HDL are secreted with CMs and VLDL. The lipid metabolic pathways can be divided into the exogenous and endogenous cycles, which are responsible for the transport of dietary and hepatically derived lipid respectively.[11]

Exogenous pathway
Following the digestion of dietary fat in the small intestine, long chain fatty acids are absorbed by the enterocyte. The nascent CM particle consists of a core of TAG (84–9% of the mass), cholesterol ester (3–5%) and surface free cholesterol (1–2%) and on the surface, phospholipids (7–9%) and apoproteins (1.5–2.5%).[12] Following secretion, the TAG component of the CM particle is hydrolysed by lipoprotein lipase (LPL) bound to the luminal surface of the endothelial cells in adipose tissue and muscle. Approximately 70–90% of the TAG is removed to produce a cholesterol ester-rich lipoprotein particle termed a CM remnant.[13] As the core of the CM remnant particle becomes smaller, surface materials, phospholipids, cholesterol and apolipoproteins are transferred to HDL to maintain stability of the particle. Uptake of these particles probably requires interaction with hepatic lipase (HL) which is situated on the surface of the liver. HL further hydrolyses the TAG and phospholipid components of the CM remnant before uptake by a receptor-mediated process in the liver.[14] The remnants are endocytosed and catabolised in lysosomes from which cholesterol can enter metabolic pathways in hepatocytes, including excretion into the bile (Fig. 5.3).

Endogenous pathway
VLDL provides a pathway for the transport of TAG from the liver to the peripheral circulation. Two subclasses of VLDL are released from the liver, $VLDL_1$ (large TAG-rich lipoprotein) and $VLDL_2$ (smaller, denser particles). LPL in the capillary bed extracts TAG from the secreted $VLDL_1$ but less efficiently when compared to CMs.[15] LDL receptors on the surface of the liver recognise the $VLDL_2$ particles and mediate the endocytosis of a fraction of these particles. Prolonged residency of some VLDL particles in the plasma results in

Table 5.3 Structure and function of lipoproteins (adapted from Erkelens, 1989)

Lipoprotein	Structural apolipoproteins	Apolipoproteins attached	Function
CM	B-48	A-I, A-IV, C-I, C-II and C-III	Carries exogenous TAG from gut to adipose tissue, muscle and liver
CM remnant	B-48	C-I, C-II, C-III	Carries exogenous cholesterol to the liver and periphery
VLDL (VLDL$_1$ and VLDL$_2$)	B-100	C-I, C-II, C-III and E	Carries endogenous TAG to the periphery
IDL	B-100	E	Carries endogenous cholesterol to the periphery
LDL	B-100	-	Carries cholesterol to the liver and periphery
HDL$_2$ and HDL$_3$	A-I and A-II	C-I, C-II, C-III, E, LCAT and CETP	Reverse cholesterol transport

Note:
Abbreviations: CM, chylomicron; VLDL, very low density lipoprotein; IDL, intermediate density lipoprotein; LDL, low density lipoprotein; HDL, high density lipoprotein; LCAT, lecithin cholesterol acyltransferase; CETP, cholesterol ester transfer protein.

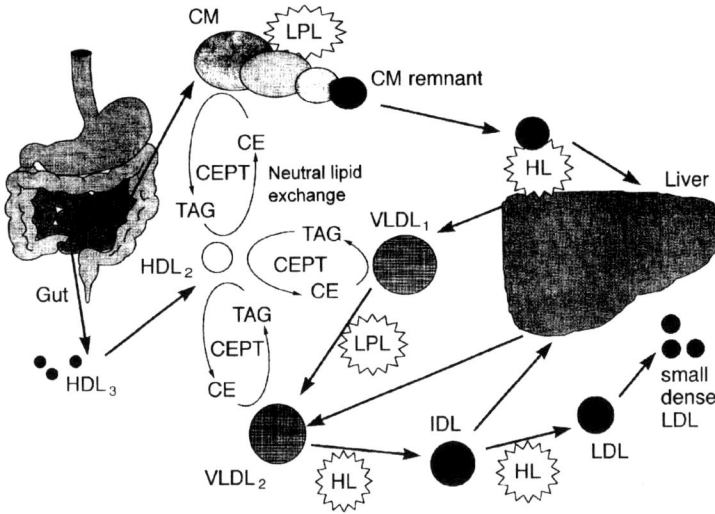

Fig. 5.3   Simplified overview of lipoprotein metabolism showing the inter-relationships between the exogenous and endogenous pathways.

further metabolism by LPL, and to some extent HL, to form the higher density IDL. HL, on the surface of hepatocytes, further hydrolyses IDL with eventual formation of LDL.[16] LDL is a heterogeneous population consisting of larger LDL species (LDL-I and LDL-II subclass) and smaller denser LDL particles (LDL-III). LDL can be taken up by LDL receptors present on the surface of hepatocytes and on extrahepatic cells.

Reverse cholesterol transport

A function of HDL is to trigger the flux of cholesterol from peripheral cells and from membranes undergoing turnover to the liver for excretion. The process of reverse cholesterol transport is mediated by an enzyme, lecithin cholesterol acyltransferase (LCAT), bound to species of HDL particles. It acts by trapping cholesterol into the core of the nascent HDL following interaction of this particle with a cell surface protein. The cholesterol is transferred to HDL_3, which in turn is converted to HDL_2. This particle can follow one of two pathways (direct or indirect) to deliver cholesterol to the liver.[17] In the direct pathway, the HDL_2 is removed via receptor-mediated endocytosis by the LDL receptor or via selective uptake of cholesterol ester from the HDL particle by the liver. The cholesterol ester transfer protein (CETP) is involved in the indirect pathway and transfers cholesterol ester to lower density lipoproteins (CMs and VLDL), in return for TAG, and is followed by their uptake by the liver (neutral lipid exchange) (Fig. 5.3).

The balance between the forward (exogenous and endogenous pathways) and the reverse pathway, which is tightly regulated by the secretion rates of the lipoproteins, determines the concentration of cholesterol in the plasma.

5.3.2 Classical lipid risk factors in coronary heart disease

Many epidemiological studies have shown a positive correlation between fasting total cholesterol levels, especially LDL cholesterol levels and CHD mortality.[1] Accumulation of LDL in the plasma leads to a deposition of cholesterol in the arterial wall, a process that involves oxidative modification of the LDL particles. The oxidised LDL is taken up by macrophages which eventually become foam cells and forms the basis of the early atherosclerotic plaque. It has been estimated that every 1% increase in LDL cholesterol level leads to a 2–3% increase in CHD risk.[18] The role of cholesterol lowering as a public health strategy in the primary prevention of CHD was unequivocally supported by the findings of the West Scotland Heart Study.[8] This lipid-lowering trial involved 6,595 middle-aged men with moderately raised cholesterol levels (5.8–8.0 mmol/l) but without any history of CHD. The study showed a 22% reduction in overall mortality and a 33% reduction in cardiovascular mortality in men receiving the active drug (prevastatin) compared with a placebo, in a five-year follow-up. Total cholesterol levels were reduced by 20%, with LDL cholesterol levels being reduced by 26% on the active drug treatment.

HDL cholesterol levels may influence the relationship between total cholesterol levels and CHD risk. A strong inverse relationship between fasting plasma HDL levels and the risk of development of CHD has been reported.[18] On average, HDL cholesterol levels are higher in women than in men. Factors that may lead to reduced HDL cholesterol levels include smoking, low physical activity and diabetes mellitus; whereas those that increase levels include moderate alcohol consumption. The Münster Heart Study, carried out between 1979 and 1991, investigated cardiovascular risk factors, stroke and mortality in people at work. Examination of fasting lipid parameters at the beginning of the study and with a follow-up six to seven years later demonstrated that HDL cholesterol concentrations were significantly lower in the group with major coronary events compared to the group that was free of such coronary events. Low HDL levels reflect a compromised pathway for the excretion of cholesterol and have been associated with a fivefold increase in risk of CHD compared to normal HDL values.[19]

5.3.3 Newly recognised risk factors

Elevated fasting and post-prandial TAG levels

Almost all of the epidemiological evidence for CHD risk has been determined from fasting lipoprotein concentrations, obtained following a 12-hour overnight fast. However, individuals spend a large proportion of the day in the post-prandial state when the lipid transport system is challenged by fat-containing meals. The magnitude and duration of post-prandial TAG concentrations following a fat load has been correlated with the risk of development of CHD. This has been shown in patients with CHD who show a more pronounced and prolonged TAG response following a meal compared with matched people without CHD, even though both groups showed similar fasting TAG concentrations.[2] The strength of the association between TAG levels and CHD has been demonstrated in a number of observational studies.[20] In the Framingham study, individuals were segregated according to their HDL cholesterol levels (classical risk factor) and it was observed that the group with the highest TAG and lowest HDL cholesterol concentrations had the greatest risk for CHD.[21] This also agreed with the observation by O'Meara et al.,[22] where the highest magnitude of lipaemia was found in individuals who had high fasting TAG compared with lower fasting TAG concentrations. Although univariate analysis has demonstrated the association between TAG concentrations and CHD risk, multivariate analysis, including other lipid parameters and especially HDL cholesterol levels, has abolished this statistical significance. However, this statistical correlation is a controversial issue since an inverse relationship exists between the levels of TAG and HDL cholesterol levels due to their metabolic interrelationships. Recent findings from the Münster Heart Study have demonstrated, using multivariate analysis, that total cholesterol, LDL cholesterol, HDL cholesterol and log-transformed values of TAG showed a significant age-adjusted association with the presence of major coronary events. This correlation with TAGs remained after adjustment for LDL and HDL cholesterol levels.[19] Therefore, a single measurement of these lipid parameters in an individual may provide insufficient information and so underestimate any association between these variables.

Elevated levels of chylomicrons and chylomicron remnants
The development of specific methods to differentiate between the exogenous and endogenous TAG-rich lipoproteins, CMs and VLDL, in post-prandial samples has enabled the atherogenicity of these lipoproteins to be investigated. A recent finding by Karpe et al.[23] has provided evidence that a delayed uptake of small CM remnants is associated with the progression of atherosclerosis. The abnormal clearance of CMs and CM remnants after a fat load have been implicated directly and/or indirectly with the presence of CHD. This may reflect the ability of CM remnants to infiltrate the arterial wall directly. The mechanism whereby CM remnants provide the building blocks of arterial lesions are thought to occur by one of two processes. First, the CM remnants may bind and penetrate the arterial surfaces (just in the same way as plasma LDL), therefore the rate of atherogenesis should be proportional to the plasma remnant concentrations. Second, CMs may be absorbed and then degraded to remnants on the arterial surface.[24] In each instance, the reaction leading to the endocytosis of remnants by smooth muscle cells may take place at sites where local injury has removed the endothelium.

The magnitude of post-prandial lipaemia is dependent on a number of factors including rates of clearance by peripheral tissue and receptor-mediated uptake of the remnants by the liver. Defects in any of these processes will cause an accumulation of CMs and their remnants which in turn can influence endogenous lipoproteins known to be atherogenic. In particular the transfer of TAG from CMs to LDL and HDL and a reciprocal transfer of cholesterol esters to the CMs by CETP may increase the atherogenic lipid profile. This is known as neutral lipid exchange. The transfer of cholesterol ester to CMs and VLDL makes them resistant to lipase action which impedes the normal metabolism of these TAG-rich lipoproteins. The cholesterol ester-enriched CM remnants are then able to be taken up by the macrophages in the arterial lesion. LDL and HDL, on the other hand, become suitable substrates for LPL and HL, causing a reduction in the size of these particles. This results in the development of an atherogenic lipoprotein profile in which the TAG-rich lipoproteins become cholesterol ester-enriched, LDL size is reduced and HDL cholesterol levels are reduced. The small dense nature of the LDL makes it unrecognisable by the LDL receptors in the liver and so makes it a favourable candidate for uptake by scavenger receptors present on macrophages in the arterial lesion.[25]

Elevated levels of small dense LDL (LDL-III)
It has long been established that elevated circulating LDL cholesterol levels represent a major risk factor for the development of CHD. Recently, with the use of density gradient ultracentrifugation techniques, LDL has been separated into three major subclasses. These are subdivided as light large LDL (LDL-I), intermediate size LDL (LDL-II) and small dense LDL (LDL-III).[26] In healthy normolipidemic males, a preponderance of LDL-II are seen, with only a small percentage of LDL-III being present.

A number of case control and cross-sectional studies has examined the relationship between LDL subclass and risk of CHD.[27] In studies in men with CHD, or those who had survived a myocardial infarction, it was demonstrated that small dense LDL-III was more common in the men with CHD than without. In 1988, Austin et al.[26] proposed that a preponderance of LDL-III in young men was associated with a threefold increase in CHD. However, more recently, a greater relative risk of CHD associated with raised LDL-III has been proposed.[28] The increased atherogenicity of small dense LDL-III is thought to be due to the increased residency of these particles in the circulation due to their slow uptake by the LDL receptor in the liver and peripheral tissues. This allows time for the small dense LDL to infiltrate into the intima of the arterial wall where it is thought that these particles are retained by extracellular matrix components before oxidation of the LDL particles occur. The modified small dense LDL-III is then taken up by the scavenger receptor on macrophages leading to the subsequent formation of foam cells.[29]

Atherogenic lipoprotein phenotype
The ALP is a collection of lipid abnormalities which confers an increased risk of CHD upon normal, healthy individuals. It has been proposed that 30–35% of middle-aged men in the Western world may be affected.[3] In the fasting state, this phenotype is characterised by a moderately raised TAG concentration (1.5 to 2.3 mmol/l), low HDL concentration (less than 1 mmol/l) and a predominance of small dense LDL-III (greater than 35% of LDL mass) and HDL particles. It is important to note that total cholesterol levels are usually in the normal range or

are only moderately raised. The atherogenic nature of the ALP may arise from the impairment of the removal of TAG-rich lipoproteins (CMs and VLDL) leading to the conversion of small, atherogenic cholesterol enriched remnants, LDL and HDL by neutral lipid exchange. It is generally considered that this collection of lipid abnormalities is closely associated with the insulin resistance syndrome.[30]

5.4 Diet and coronary heart disease: the evidence

There is a substantial, diverse and generally consistent body of evidence linking diet with cardiovascular disease. The evidence is most extensive for the relationship between CHD and dietary fat. Diet is believed to influence the risk of CHD through its effects on certain risk factors described in Table 5.1, for example blood lipids, blood pressure and probably also through thrombogenic mechanisms. More recently, evidence suggests a protective role for dietary antioxidants such as vitamins E and C and carotenes, possibly through a mechanism that prevents the oxidation of LDL cholesterol particles.

5.4.1 Dietary lipids and CHD risk

Epidemiological and clinical evidence clearly shows that the likelihood of death from CHD is directly related to the circulating level of total cholesterol (and more specifically LDL cholesterol). More recent evidence suggests that an exaggerated postprandial TAG response to fat-containing meals is also a significant risk factor for CHD.[2] Numerous studies have shown that the kinds and amounts of fat in the diet significantly influence plasma cholesterol levels. In the Seven Countries Study, mean concentrations of cholesterol of each group were highly correlated with percentage energy derived from SFAs, and even more strikingly related to a formula that also took into account the intake of PUFAs (see Fig. 5.4).[5]

Since this research, numerous other studies have supported the relationship between dietary intake of saturates and the raised plasma cholesterol levels. However, not all SFAs are equally potent in raising plasma cholesterol. Palmitic acid (16:0), the principal SFA in most diets, and myristic (14:0) are the most effective at elevating cholesterol; whereas stearic (18:0), lauric acid (12:0) and medium chain fatty acids (8:0 and 10:0) have little effect on plasma cholesterol levels.[31] The cholesterol response to a particular SFA may depend in part on the TAG structure,[32] and in part on LDL receptor activity.[33] The mechanism that is responsible for the increase in plasma cholesterol due to SFAs is at present unclear, but a reduction in the LDL receptor activity is one possibility. It has been recommended that the average contribution of SFAs to dietary energy be reduced to no more than 10%.[34] The current UK dietary intake is shown in Table 5.4. A considerable reduction from current levels of intake of dietary SFAs (average 33%) would be required to meet this recommendation.[35]

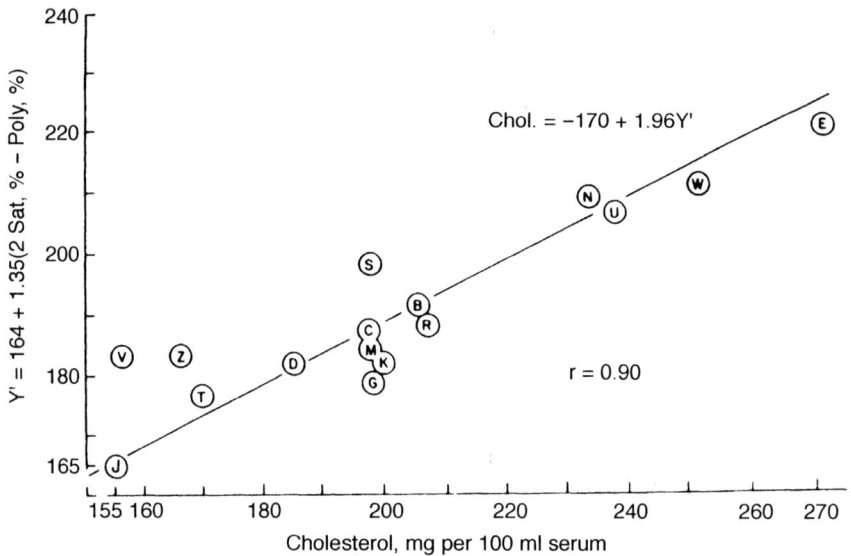

Fig. 5.4   Relationship of mean serum cholesterol concentration of the cohorts of Seven Countries Study to fat composition of the diet expressed in the multiple regression equation, including intakes of saturated and polyunsaturated fatty acids (A = Zregnjamin, B = Belgrade, C = Crevalcore, D = Dalmatia, E = East Finland, G = Corfu, J = Ushibuka, K = Crete, M = Montegiorgio, N = Zutphen, R = Rome, S = Slavonia, T = Tanushimara, U = USA, V = Velika Kisna, W = West Finland). (Adapted from Key, 1980.)

Table 5.4   Dietary intakes of selected nutrients for men and women aged 16–64 years. (Adapted from Gregory *et al.* 1990.)

Nutrients	Men	% total energy	Women	% total energy
Total energy (KJ)	10462		7174	
Fat (g)	102	37.6	74	39.2
SFA (g)	42	15.4	31	16.5
MUFA (g)	31	11.6	22	11.8
n-3 PUFA (g)	1.9	0.7	1.3	0.7
n-6 PUFA (g)	13.8	5.1	9.6	5.1
trans FA (g)	5.6	2.0	4.0	2.1
P:S ratio	0.40		0.38	
Cholesterol (mg)	390		280	
Carbohydrate (g)	272	41.6	193	43.0
Alcohol (g)	25	6.9	6.9	2.8
Fibre (g)	24.9		18.6	

The effect of the ingestion of different fatty acids on plasma cholesterol levels is varied and is summarised in Table 5.5. Substitution of SFAs by MUFAs or *n*-6 PUFAs significantly reduces LDL cholesterol levels although *n*-6 PUFA are more effective in this respect. There has been doubt as to whether MUFAs

Table 5.5 Effects of fatty acids on plasma lipoprotein concentrations

Fatty acid	Total cholesterol	LDL cholesterol	HDL cholesterol	Triacylglycerol
Saturated FA	Increase	Increase	Neutral	Neutral
n-6 PUFA	Decrease	Decrease	Decrease	NA
n-3 PUFA	Unchanged	Unchanged*	Increase	Decrease
Trans FA	Increase	Increase	Decrease	NA
MUFA	Decrease	Decrease	Neutral	Neutral
Cholesterol	Increase	Increase	NA	NA

Notes:
FA – fatty acid. PUFA – polyunsaturated fatty acid. MUFA – monounsaturated fatty acid. NA – not available. * May increase in hyperlipidaemics.

are effective in cholesterol-lowering or whether the observed decrease in plasma cholesterol was simply due to a replacement of SFAs. Some studies have suggested that the effect of oleic acid (cis 18:1) (the major MUFA in the diet) and linoleic acid (18:2) (major n-6 PUFA in the diet) on LDL cholesterol are similar, and that the greater effect of linoleic acid on total cholesterol is through reduction of HDL cholesterol.[36] In addition to this it has been reported that PUFAs incorporated into lipoproteins can increase their susceptibility to oxidation if there is insufficient antioxidant protection. Despite the beneficial lowering of LDL cholesterol associated with increased dietary PUFA, it has been proposed that the decreased levels of beneficial HDL cholesterol and greater susceptibility of lipoproteins containing n-6 PUFA to oxidation, result in pro-atherogenic effects of diets in which n-6 PUFA provide greater than 10% energy.[37] Substitution of saturates by oleic acid would avoid this and therefore MUFAs have theoretical advantages over PUFAs. It has long been recognised that, in Mediterranean populations, there is a significantly lower risk of CHD.[5] Their diet traditionally contains high amounts of olive oil in addition to fruit and vegetables compared to the UK diet. It has been speculated that a higher intake of MUFAs could contribute to the lower rate of CHD within this population. However, it could also be due to the higher antioxidants found in the fruit, vegetables and within virgin olive oil itself, in addition to other dietary and lifestyle factors. Research into the reasons for this link between the Mediterranean lifestyle and CHD risk is necessary to explain this observation fully.

As regards CHD, trans fatty acids appear to act similarly to SFA in their effects on blood cholesterol except that trans FA decreased HDL whereas SFA have little effect on HDL. In a trial conducted to compare the effects of different fatty acids, elaidic (trans 18:1), the principal trans fatty acid found in the diet, was found to decrease HDL and increase LDL levels significantly.[38] Some epidemiological evidence also supports these findings. Hydrogenated fats are a major dietary source of trans FA and are abundant in vegetable margarines and processed foods. However, due to the reported link between CHD risk and trans fatty acids, the level of these fatty acids has been substantially reduced in many margarines and manufactured foods.

The weight of evidence supports the view that raising cholesterol content of the diet increases plasma cholesterol, primarily LDL cholesterol, although there is considerable inter-individual response. Studies in humans over the past 25 years have indicated a threshold for an effect at an intake of about 95 mg/4300 KJ with a ceiling at about 450 mg/4300 KJ. Excess cholesterol is either not absorbed or suppresses endogenous production. As daily intake (Table 5.4) is at the lower end of this range, it is recommended that current dietary cholesterol intakes, measured per unit of dietary energy, should not rise.[34]

In contrast to dietary SFAs, MUFAs, *n*-6 PUFAs and *trans* fatty acids whose effects on cardiac health primarily reside in their ability to modify plasma LDL and HDL cholesterol levels, the benefits of an increased intake of *n*-3 PUFA lie in their ability to reduce thrombosis and decrease plasma TAG levels. The low incidence of CHD in Greenland Eskimos and Japanese fishermen, despite a high fat intake (fat providing 80% of dietary energy), has been attributed to their intake of marine foods high in EPA (20:5, *n*-3) and DHA (22:6, *n*-3).[39] In the DART trial, individuals who had suffered a previous myocardial infarction were advised to consume 1–2 portions of fatty fish per week. After a two-year follow-up period, a 29% reduction in mortality from CHD was reported in those advised to consume the fatty fish.[40]

Evidence has shown that fasting TAG levels and post-prandial (following a meal) TAG levels are a significant risk factor for CHD.[2] The mechanism is not fully understood but is believed to be associated with the TAG-rich lipoprotein particle (CM and VLDL) remnants which are potentially atherogenic. High

Table 5.6 Recommended daily intakes of dietary fat and fatty acids of the EEC and UK and the average daily consumption of these nutrients (% dietary energy)

	Total fat	SFA	PUFA	MUFA	Trans FA
Recommendations					
European	20-30[1]	10[1]	0.5[2] (*n*-3)	NR	NR
(EEC, 1992)			2.0[2] (*n*-6)		
UK	<35	<10	0.2g/day (*n*-3)	NR	2
(DH, 1994)			5.0 (*n*-6)		
Current intake					
UK (1990)	39	16	5 (*n*-6)	12	2
USA (1985)	37	13	7 (*n*-6)	13	-
France (1985–7)	36	15	6 (*n*-6)	13	-
Germany (1988)	40	15	6 (*n*-6)	12	-
Netherlands (1988)	40	16	7 (*n*-6)	15	-

Notes:
1. Ultimate goal.
2. Population reference intake.
NR – no recommendations.

levels of these remnants can contribute towards an increased risk of neutral lipid exchange (see section 5.3) which will in turn lead to an accumulation of small dense, more easily oxidised LDL-III, and a decreased circulation of beneficial HDL particles. Supplementation studies with *n*-3 PUFA have observed a significant reduction in blood TAG levels.[41] The proposed mechanism for this decrease in TAG is a reduction in the level of VLDL synthesis by the liver and an increased clearance of TAG-rich particles from the blood by the enzyme LPL (the enzyme that hydrolyses TAG within VLDL and CMs).

Fatty acids from the *n*-3 PUFA series also have a beneficial effect on thrombogenesis (blood clot formation). The utilisation of *n*-3 PUFAs instead of *n*-6 PUFAs in the production of eicosanoids (substances involved with the formation of blood clotting) can significantly reduce the rate of blood clot formation and thus reduce the risk of myocardial infarction. In addition, *n*-3 PUFA ingestion may result in the reduction in cardiac arrhythmias.[42] Sudden cardiac death is a serious problem in Western countries and no drug treatment, to date, has had any significant effect on incidence. Epidemiological studies have shown a reduced incidence of sudden death with *n*-3 PUFA intake, and animal and limited human evidence also suggests an anti-arrhythmic effect.[43]

At the present time most of the national and international guidelines for population intakes of dietary fat are based on the known adverse effects of SFAs in raising blood cholesterol levels with some consideration given to possible benefits of *n*-3 PUFAs on thrombosis. Table 5.6 shows the dietary guidelines of the European Community[44] and those of the UK Committee of Medical Aspects of Food Policy.[34] These recommendations are aimed at both the food industry and the general population. Due to high SFA intake compared with those recommended, which reflect consumer resistance to these recommendations, future recommendations may take greater account of the benefits of substituting SFAs with MUFAs, and the overall significance to human health of the absolute and relative amounts of *n*-6: *n*-3 PUFAs.

5.4.2 Carbohydrate intake and CHD risk

Recommendations for reductions in total fat in the diet have important implications for dietary carbohydrate intake. There is little variation in the proportion of energy derived from dietary protein; therefore there is a reciprocal relationship between the contributions of dietary fat and carbohydrate to energy. The metabolic effects of exchanging carbohydrate for fat depend mainly on the degree of substitution. Diets where about 60% of food energy is derived from carbohydrate are associated with lower HDL levels and higher TAG levels, and despite lower LDL levels have been suggested to be associated with a higher risk of CHD.[45, 46] However, a smaller increase in dietary carbohydrate levels to accommodate a reduction in dietary fat to 30% of energy has been reported to result in a small rise in TAG levels and no fall in HDL levels,[46] resulting in an overall positive benefit in CHD risk.

5.4.3 Non-starch polysaccharides and CHD risk

Four prospective studies have shown an inverse relationship between dietary 'fibre' intake and CHD. The studies have varied in the source of 'fibre' that was found to be effective. Morris et al.[47] found that cereal fibre was inversely related to cases of CHD, whereas others found that vegetable sources of fibre were associated with decreased risk.[48] On the contrary, a two-year intervention study in men who had suffered a previous heart attack, found no effect of increasing cereal 'fibre' intake on subsequent risk of mortality from cardiovascular disease.[40] The effect of a number of soluble NSPs which are selectively digested by the colonic gut microflora (classed as prebiotics) on the blood levels of cholesterol and especially LDL cholesterol will be discussed in detail in section 5.6.

5.4.4 Antioxidant nutrients and CHD risk

The cells of the body are under constant attack by activated oxygen species, which are produced naturally in the body. The protection of cells from the detrimental effects of these species is due to defence mechanisms, component parts of which are, or are derived from, the micronutrients called 'antioxidants'. These include the essential trace elements selenium, zinc and magnesium, and vitamin C and the various forms of vitamin E (the tocopherols and the tocotrienols). In addition, betacarotene, and other carotenoids, such as lutein and lycopene (present in large amounts in tomatoes) and flavonoids, present in red wine, tea and onions, probably also play a role.

There is a large body of evidence supporting a protective effect of the antioxidant vitamins E and C.[49] There are, however, inconsistencies in the amount of these antioxidants associated with reduced risk of CHD; this is especially the case for vitamin E. One explanation for these discrepancies is that vitamin E may be a marker for a diet that contains other dietary constituents (such as carotenoids and flavonoids) which have antioxidant potential. When vitamin E is taken in isolation as a supplement, higher levels might be necessary to achieve the same effect as diets that contain combinations of antioxidants. No specific recommendations on the levels of antioxidant intake have been given but a diet rich in vegetable and fruit and containing nuts and seeds is recommended.[50] The beneficial effects of red wine and olive oil on CHD risk could in part be attributed to antioxidants such as flavonoids and polyphenols contained within these foods.

5.4.5 Sodium and potassium and CHD risk

Sodium intake appears to be an important determinant of blood pressure in the population as a whole, at least in part by influencing the rise in blood pressure with age.[51, 52] A diet lower in common salt and higher in potassium would be expected to result in lower blood pressure and a smaller rise in blood pressure with age. Salt is the predominant source of sodium in the diet, with manufactured foods contributing to 65–85% of the total salt ingested. Blood pressure is an important risk factor for the development of CHD and strokes. It has been recommended that the population should reduce its salt intake by 3 g/day by reducing salt at the table and also the consumption of processed foods. Moreover, higher potassium levels within the diet are believed to reduce the blood pressure and foods such as fruit and vegetables, which contain this mineral, should be taken in higher amounts.

5.4.6 Alcohol and CHD risk

The debate surrounding the benefits of alcohol consumption and, more specifically, red wine consumption and the risk of CHD is one that has been running for many years. There is evidence that high consumption of alcohol is related to increased mortality, especially from CHD. However, alcohol consumption appears to be associated with relatively low risk of CHD across a variety of study populations. The benefit that is associated with alcohol consumption is almost entirely due to the increased levels of HDL cholesterol which is associated with reduced CHD risk.[53] However, other factors such as lower platelet activity, reducing the risk of thrombosis, and antioxidant properties of some drinks such as red wine have also been suggested. The proposed benefit of red wine over other drinks would only explain the potential increase in antioxidant levels as the effect of alcohol on HDL and haemostatic factors have been attributed to alcohol itself. A consumption of two units (one unit is equivalent to 8 g alcohol) a day of alcohol is believed to be beneficial in the risk of CHD, but the debate continues.[54]

5.4.7 Coffee and CHD risk

For over 20 years it has been suspected that caffeine or coffee consumption may contribute to the development of CHD, but the evidence remains inconsistent. There is little evidence that caffeine itself has any relation to CHD risk but there are other components of coffee, which might in part account for some observed associations. The Scandinavian practice of boiling coffee during its preparation appears to generate a hypercholesterolaemic fraction. Significant levels of these compounds have also been found in cafeteria coffee which have been found to increase plasma LDL cholesterol levels.[55] The relevance of this to the UK population, whose consumption of boiled coffee is very low, is unclear.

5.4.8 Diet and CHD risk

The diet is one of the modifiable risk factors associated with CHD risk. Recommendations for reducing total fat (especially saturated fat), increasing NSP intake and consumption of fruit and vegetables is advice that is likely to be associated with overall benefits on health. However, there is great inertia for dietary change, and many new products that claim to reduce the risk of CHD and other chronic diseases, without altering lifestyle factors such as diet, clearly attract a great deal of attention.

5.5 Effects of probiotics on blood lipids: the evidence

Current dietary strategies for the prevention of CHD advocate adherence to low fat/low saturated fat diets.[34] Although there is no doubt that under experimental conditions, low fat diets offer an effective means of reducing blood cholesterol concentrations, on a population basis they appear to be less effective, largely due to poor compliance attributed to low palatability and acceptability of these diets to the consumer. Due to the low consumer compliance, attempts have been made to identify other dietary components that can reduce blood cholesterol levels. These have included investigations into the possible hypocholesterolaemic properties of milk products, usually in a fermented form. The role of fermented milk products as hypocholesterolaemic agents in humans is still equivocal, as the studies performed have been of varying quality, design and statistical analysis with incomplete documentation being the major limitation of most studies. However, since 1974 when Mann and Spoerry[56] showed an 18% fall in plasma cholesterol after feeding 4–5 litres of fermented milk per day for three weeks to Masai warriors, there has been considerable interest in the effect of probiotics on human lipid metabolism.[56]

5.5.1 Evidence from the Masai

As epidemiological evidence suggested that an environmental agent that contributed to hypocholesterolaemia had been introduced into the Western world around 1900, Mann and Spoerry intended to investigate the effect of an exogenous surfactant material, known to be hypercholestrolaemic in animals.[56] The authors' original intention was to feed 4–5 litres of pasteurised European milk fermented with a wild culture of *Lactobacillus* to 24 male Masai warriors, for six days out of every week. However, demand rose to over 8.3 litres per day (23,000 KJ/day) and an exercise programme was started to prevent weight gain. However, eight of the subjects gained considerable weight (> 5 lb) after feigning injury to avoid this exercise. The eight subjects who gained weight surprisingly had a significant fall (18.2%) in serum cholesterol of 0.73 mmol/l. The total group's mean cholesterol level also significantly decreased (9.8%), as shown in Table 5.7. Although the marked reductions in serum cholesterol were striking, considering the weight increase (usually associated with a raised cholesterol concentration), this study is now considered simply as a curiosity. Due to the introduction of an exercise programme and the inability to control food intake, the work cannot lend much to the causality of the findings.

Table 5.7 Human studies to evaluate the hypocholesterolaemic properties of fermented milk products

Author	Subjects (n)	Product (vol/type)	Duration	Total cholesterol	LDL cholesterol
Mann et al.[56]	24M	8.3 l lacto/yog	3 weeks	−9.6% (P<0.001)	NA
Mann[57]	3 M 1F	4 l WMY	12 days	−16.8% (P<0.05)	NA
	3M 2F	2 l SMY	12 days	−23.2% (P<0.05)	NA
Howard and Marks[58]	10	3 l	3 weeks	5.5% (P<0.05)	NA
Hepner et al.[59]	6M 4F	720 ml (A)	4 weeks	−5.4% (P<0.01)	NA
	5M 3F	720 ml (B)	4 weeks	8.9% (P<0.01)	NA
Rossouw et al.[68]	11M	2l yoghurt	3 weeks	+16% (P<0.01)	+12% (P<0.001)
Thompson et al.[61]	13	1l UPY	3 weeks	NS	NS
Bazzare et al.[111]	5M 16F	550g yoghurt	1 week	−8.7% NA	NA
Massay[62]	30F	480 ml yoghurt	4 weeks	NS	NS
Jaspers et al.[64]	10M	681 g yoghurt	2 weeks	−11.6% transient (P<0.05)	NS
McNamara et al.[63]	18M	16 oz LFY	4 weeks	NS	NS
Agerbaek et al.[65]	58M	200 ml UPY	6 weeks	−6.1% (P<0.001)	−9.8% (P<0.001)
Richelsen et al.[66]	47M 43F	200 ml UPY	21 weeks	NA	−9% transient (P<0.05)
Sessions et al.[60]	78M 76F	200 ml UPY	12 weeks	NS	NS
Bertolami et al.[67]	11M 21F	200 ml UPY	8 weeks	−5.3% (P<0.004)	6.2% (P<0.001)

Notes:
F = female; M = male; WMY = whole milk yoghurt; UPY = unpasteurised yoghurt; SMY = skimmed milk yoghurt; PY = pasteurised yoghurt; LFY = low fat yoghurt; NA = data not available; NS = not significant.

Source:
Adapted from Taylor and Williams.[112]

5.5.2 Evidence for the 'milk factor'

As a follow-up to the Masai trial, Mann fed a small group of US volunteers (n = 4) 4 litres per day of yoghurt (microbiological activity unspecified) over a 12-day period and reported a significant fall of 37% in serum cholesterol values (however, the tabulated data indicated only a 16.8% fall).[57] When intake of the yoghurt was reduced to 2 litres the hypocholesterolaemic effect was maintained, although an intake of 1 litre per day resulted in a return to baseline cholesterol levels. The rate of cholesterol biosynthesis was monitored by measuring the specific activity of plasma digitonin-precipitated sterols, two hours after a pulse of [^{14}C] acetate. A 28% fall in acetate incorporation was reported by 16 days after a 12-day ingestion of the high dose of yoghurt (4 litres per day). Mann proposed the presence of a 'milk factor' to explain the fall in serum cholesterol, such as a 3HMG-CoA reductase inhibitor.[57] Investigating possible candidates for the 'milk factor', Howard and Marks fed lactose ± Ca/Mg, cheese whey or yoghurt to volunteers over a two-week period.[58] The yoghurt, but not the lactose ± Ca/Mg or cheese whey, significantly reduced plasma cholesterol by 5.5%. However, this trial was subject to the same problems of lack of dietary control with substantial changes from the volunteers' habitual diet resulting in a number of confounding factors.

Most of the early studies introduced confounding factors due to the lack of control of the subjects' diet. Hepner et al.[59] performed a study that attempted to control for these. This was a cross-over study in which 720 ml of yoghurt and 750 ml milk were given to the subjects for a four-week period. Significant reductions in plasma cholesterol were observed after the first week of both supplementation periods.[59] The observation that cholesterol levels can significantly fall after acceptance onto a study has been well documented. This is probably due to a conscious or even unconscious modification of the diet by the volunteer due to an awareness of dietary assessment. In an attempt to reduce this, baseline run-in periods are essential.[60] Of the early negative studies that have been published, those of Thompson et al.,[61] Massay[62] and McNamara et al.[63] incorporated a run-in period. The study performed by McNamara et al.[63] was one of the more carefully designed studies. They investigated the effects of the ingestion of 480 ml unspecified yoghurt and reported no significant cholesterol reduction. This was a well-controlled study which included a three-week run-in period and four-week intervention period, and investigated the effect of 16 oz of a low fat yoghurt (unspecified microbiological nature) and a non-fermented milk concentrate (as a control). Dietary intake and body weight remained constant and there was no change in serum cholesterol, LDL, HDL or TAG levels.[63] From the studies mentioned above it can be concluded that there is little evidence that fermented milk products affect serum lipid parameters per se.

5.5.3 Probiotic effect on lipid parameters

Hepner et al.[59] were the first to attempt to discern whether the presence of live bacteria was important for the reported affects of yoghurt on lipid parameters.

The aim of the study was to compare the effects of 750 ml pasteurised and unpasteurised yoghurt, using milk as a placebo. After a 12-week intervention period, all treatments significantly reduced plasma cholesterol levels, with milk resulting in a lesser reduction. Unfortunately, the nutritional and microbiological content of the products used was not reported which severely hampers comparison with other study data. Thompson et al.[61] assessed a wide range of milk-based products including milk laced with *Lactobacillus acidophilus* (titre 1.3×10^7 counts/ml), buttermilk (a milk product fermented with *Streptococcus cremoris* and *Streptococcus lactis* – titre 6.4×10^8 counts/ml) and a yoghurt (fermented with *Lactobacillus bulgaricus* and *Streptococcus thermophilus* – titre 1.2×10^9 counts/ml). One litre of supplement was fed for a three-week period, but no significant change was reported in serum total cholesterol, LDL or HDL. The possible importance of variation in yoghurt cultures stimulated Jasper et al.[64] to assess the effect of 681 g/day of three strains of a yoghurt fermented with a 1:1 ratio of *Lactobacillus bulgaricus* and *Streptococcus thermophilus*. Two strains (CH-I and CH-II) were taken separately over a 14-day period and two batches of a third strain (SH-IIIA and SH-IIIB) were taken separately over 14 days and 7 days which ran consecutively, with a 21-day 'washout period' between each of the intervention periods. Body weight remained constant in the subjects and there were only differences in the dietary intakes in minerals and vitamins. Significant falls in serum total and LDL cholesterol levels occurred after one week with one strain (CH-II) and two weeks with SH-IIIA strain. These transient changes could be explained by the effect of commencing a study as discussed previously, or this could be a true difference between the efficacious properties of different strains and indeed different types of probiotics.

Agerbaek et al.[65] tested the effect of 200 ml per day of a yoghurt that contained *Enterococcus faecium* which was shown to have hypocholesterolaemic properties when tested on animals. The study was a parallel design, and the active yoghurt was tested against identical yoghurt that had been chemically fermented with an organic acid (delta-gluco-lactone). The intervention period was for a six-week period in 58 middle-aged men with moderately raised cholesterol levels (5.0–6.5 mmol/l). They observed a 9.8% reduction in LDL cholesterol levels ($P < 0.001$) for the live yoghurt group, which was sustained over the intervention period (Table 5.7). This was a well-controlled study, which excluded many variables such as age, sex and body weight. However, an unforeseen skew in the randomisation resulted in a significantly different baseline total and LDL cholesterol levels in the two groups. The fall in these parameters observed in the live yoghurt group could be ascribed to a regression towards the mean. Another study performed using the same yoghurt and a similar design for a longer period (six months) was carried out in 87 men and women aged 50–70 years.[66] It was reported that at 12 weeks there was a significant drop in LDL cholesterol levels in the group taking the active yoghurt. These reductions were not sustained and this was partly explained by a reduction in the titre of the yoghurt at 12 weeks. At the end of the study, a non-significant reduction in LDL or total cholesterol levels was observed between the two groups. A recent publication investigating the same product used a 200 g/day ingestion of the yoghurt, for an eight-week period in a randomised double-blind placebo controlled trial, with 32 patients who had mild to moderate hypercholesterolaemia. The patients were asked to follow a lipid-lowering diet for eight weeks and were then given the test or control product for two eight-week periods. The results showed a significant reduction of 5.3% (P = 0.004) for total cholesterol and a 6.2% (P = 0.01) reduction in LDL cholesterol levels after the active product. However, the authors did question whether the average reduction of approximately 5% for total and LDL cholesterol was clinically important.[67]

A similar trial of the same product containing *E. faecium* was conducted in 160 middle-aged men and women with moderately raised cholesterol.[60] The study was a randomised, double-blind, multi-centre, placebo controlled parallel study. Volunteers consumed 200 ml per day of either the active or chemically fermented yoghurt for a 12-week period. Stratified randomisation was used to ensure that the groups were comparable for age, sex, body mass index (BMI) and baseline fasting cholesterol levels. The importance of not changing their dietary habits and lifestyle during the study was emphasised and adherence to the protocol confirmed by dietary assessment. Due to the importance of the titre of the bacterial content of the yoghurt, this was monitored throughout the study. The levels were found to be no lower than 1×10^6 counts/ml at any time tested. During the two-week run-in period, both groups showed significant reductions in blood cholesterol levels (P<0.05), but thereafter there was no further change in either of the groups or between the groups at any of the time points. These data are consistent with the conclusions drawn by Rossouw *et al.*[68] which indicated that apparent effects of some probiotics on blood cholesterol levels may be attributed to reductions in blood lipids observed in subjects who commence an intervention trial. While these reductions are well recognised but are difficult to prevent, they highlight the importance of the inclusion of a run-in period within such studies.

5.5.4 Possible mechanisms of action

Before the possible mechanisms are considered, it is important to highlight that since viable and biological active micro-organisms are usually required at the target site in the host, it is essential that the probiotics not only have the characteristics that are necessary to produce the desired biological effects, but also have the required viability and are able to withstand the host's natural barriers against ingested bacteria. The classic yoghurt bacteria, *Streptococcus thermophilus* and *Lactobacillus bulgaricus*, are technologically effective, but they do not reach the lower intestinal tract in a viable form. Therefore, intrinsic microbiological properties, such as tolerance to gastric acid, bile and pancreatic juice are important factors when probiotic organisms are considered.[69]

The mechanism of action of probiotics on cholesterol reduction is unclear, but there are a number of proposed possibilities. These include physiological actions of the end products of fermentation SCFAs, cholesterol assimilation, deconjugation of bile acids and cholesterol binding to bacterial cell walls. The SCFAs that are produced by the bacterial anaerobic breakdown of carbohydrate are acetic, propionic and butyric. The physiological effects of these are discussed in more detail in section 5.6.3.

It has been well documented that microbial bile acid metabolism is a peculiar probiotic effect involved in the therapeutic role of some bacteria. The deconjugation reaction is catalysed by conjugated bile acid hydrolase enzyme, which is produced exclusively by bacteria. Deconjugation ability is widely found in many intestinal bacteria including genera *Enterococcus, Peptostreptococcus, Bifidobacterium, Fusobacterium, Clostridium, Bacteroides and Lactobacillus.*[70] This reaction liberates the amino acid moiety and the deconjugated bile acid, thereby reducing cholesterol reabsorption, by increasing faecal excretion of the deconjugated bile acids. Many *in vitro* studies have investigated the ability of various bacteria to deconjugate a variety of different bile acids. Grill *et al.*[71] reported *Bifidobacterium longum* as the most efficient bacterium when tested against six different bile salts. Another study reported that *Lactobacillus* species had varying abilities to deconjugate glycocholate and taurocholate.[72] Studies performed on *in vitro* responses are useful but *in vivo* studies in animals and humans are required to determine the full contribution of bile acid deconjugation to cholesterol reduction. Intervention studies on animals and ileostomy patients have shown that oral administration of certain bacterial species led to an increased excretion of free and secondary bile salts.[73, 74]

There is also some *in vitro* evidence to support the hypothesis that certain bacteria can assimilate (take up) cholesterol. It was reported that *L. acidophilus*[75] and *Bif. bifidum*[76] had the ability to assimilate cholesterol in *in vitro* studies, but only in the presence of bile and under anaerobic conditions. However, despite these reports there is uncertainty whether the bacteria are assimilating cholesterol or whether the cholesterol is co-precipitating with the bile salts. Studies have been performed to address this question. Klaver and Meer[77] concluded that the removal of cholesterol from the growth medium in which *L. acidophilus* and a *Bifidobacterium sp.* were growing was not due to assimilation, but due to bacterial bile salt deconjugase activity. The same question was addressed by Tahri *et al.*,[78] with conflicting results, and they concluded that part of the removed cholesterol was found in the cell extracts and that cholesterol assimilation and bile acid deconjugase activity could occur simultaneously.

The mechanism of cholesterol binding to bacterial cell walls has also been suggested as a possible explanation for hypocholesterolaemic effects of probiotics. Hosona and Tono-oka[79] reported *Lactococcus lactis* subsp. *biovar* had the highest binding capacity for cholesterol of bacteria tested in the study. It was speculated that the binding differences were due to chemical and structural properties of the cell walls, and that even killed cells may have the ability to bind cholesterol in the intestine. The mechanism of action of probiotics on cholesterol reduction could be one or all of the above mechanisms with the ability of different bacterial species to have varying effects on cholesterol lowering. However, more research is required to elucidate fully the effect and mechanism of probiotics and their possible hypocholesterolaemic action.

5.6 The effects of prebiotics on coronary heart disease

5.6.1 Prebiotics

In recent years, there has been increasing interest in the important nutritional role of prebiotics as functional food ingredients. This interest has been derived from animal studies that showed markedly reduced TAG and total cholesterol levels when diets containing significant amounts of a prebiotic (oligofructose (OFS)) were fed. A prebiotic is defined as 'a non-digestible food ingredient that beneficially affects the host by selectively stimulating the growth and/or the activity of one or a number of bacteria in the colon, that has the potential to improve health'.[80] Prebiotics, most often referred to as non-digestible oligosaccharides, are extracted from natural sources (e.g. inulin and OFS) or synthesised from disaccharides (e.g. transgalacto-oligosaccharides). The most commonly studied of the prebiotics include inulin and OFS which are found in many vegetables, including onion, asparagus, Jerusalem artichoke and chicory root (Dysseler and Hoffem).[81] These consist of between 2 and 60 fructose molecules joined by β2-1 osidic linkages, which, due to the nature of this type of linkage, escape digestion in the upper gastrointestinal tract and remain intact but are selectively fermented by colonic microflora. Inulin is currently found as a food ingredient of bread, baked goods, yoghurt and ice-cream because it displays gelling and thickening properties and helps to improve the mouth feel and appearance of lower energy products.[81] In Europe, the estimated intake of inulin and OFS is between 2 g and 12 g per day.[82]

5.6.2 The effect of prebiotics on lipid metabolism in humans

Several studies that have investigated the effects of prebiotics on fasting plasma lipids have generated inconsistent findings (Table 5.8). In studies with individuals with raised blood lipids, three studies showed significant decreases in fasting total and LDL cholesterol, with no significant changes in TAG levels,[83–85] whereas one recent study in type II diabetics did not observe any change in cholesterol levels.[86] In normolipidaemic volunteers, only one study has demonstrated significant changes in both fasting TAG (-27%) and total cholesterol (-5%) levels with inulin[87] with another study showing a significant decrease only in TAG levels.[88] However, Luo et al.[89] and Pedersen et al.[90] have reported no effect of OFS or inulin treatment on plasma lipids levels in young healthy subjects. In a group of middle-aged men and women, lower plasma TAG levels were observed at eight weeks compared with a placebo.[91] It was suggested that the lack of lipid lowering noted in the studies of Pedersen et al.[90] and Luo et al.[89] may be due to insufficient duration of supplementation. In the study by Jackson et al.,[91] follow-up blood samples were taken four weeks after

Table 5.8 Summary of human studies to examine the effects of fructan supplementation on blood lipids

Author	Subjects	Fructan	Dose	Study design	Duration	Vehicle	Significant changes observed in blood lipids	glucose
Yashashati et al.[83]	8M and 10F NIDDM	OFS	8 g	DB, parallel	2 wks	Packed coffee drink Canned coffee jelly	↓TC ↓LDL-C	↓glucose
Hidaka et al.[84]	37 (M & F) hyperlipidaemic	OFS	8 g	DB, parallel	5 wks	Confectionery	↓TC	NS
Canzi et al.[87]	12 M normolipidaemic	Inulin	9 g	Sequential	4 wks	Breakfast cereal	↓TAG ↓TC	N/A
Luo et al.[89]	12 M normolipidaemic	OFS	20 g	DB cross-over	4 wks	100 g biscuits	NS	NS
Pedersen et al.[90]	66 F normolipidaemic	Inulin	14 g	DB cross-over	4 wks	40 g margarine	NS	N/A
Causey et al.[88]	9 M normolipidaemic	Inulin	20 g	DB cross-over	3 wks	Low fat ice-cream	↓TAG	NS
Davidson et al.[85]	21 M and F hyperlipidaemia	Inulin	18 g	DB cross-over	6 wks	Chocolate bar/paste or coffee sweetener	↓LDL-C ↓TC	N/A
Alles et al.[86]	9 M and 11 F Type II diabetes	OFS	15 g	SB cross-over	3 wks	Supplement not specified	NS	NS
Jackson et al.[91]	54 M and F normolipidaemic	Inulin	10 g	DB, parallel	8 wks	Powder added to food and drinks	TAG	↓insulin

Notes:
M, male; F, female; DB, double blind; N/A, not measured; NS, not significant; SB, single blind; TC, total cholesterol; LDL-C, LDL cholesterol; OFS, oligofructose; TAG, triacylglycerol.

completion of the inulin supplementation period by which time the concentrations of TAG had returned to baseline values, supporting the conclusion that inulin feeding may have been responsible. These findings are in line with observed effects of inulin on lipid levels in animals in which the predominant effect is on TAG rather than cholesterol concentrations.

Raised post-prandial TAG concentrations have also been recognised as a risk factor for CHD.[2] Data from studies in rats have shown a 40% reduction in post-prandial TAG concentrations when diets containing 10% OFS (w/v) were fed.[92] However, very little information regarding the effect of prebiotics on post-prandial lipaemia in human subjects are available, although one recent study in middle-aged subjects has shown no effect of inulin treatment on post-prandial TAG levels.[93]

The marked reduction in fasting lipid levels, notably TAGs, observed in animal studies have not been consistently reproduced in human subjects. Only two studies in normolipidaemic subjects have shown significant reductions in fasting TAG levels with inulin,[87, 88] with one study showing a significant effect of inulin treatment over time on fasting TAG levels compared with the placebo group.[91] The amount of fructans used in the human studies in Table 5.8 varies between 9 g and 20 g and this amount is small compared to that which is used in animal studies (50–200 g per kg of rat chow of OFS),[94] which is equivalent to a dose in humans of approximately 50–80 g of OFS/inulin per day. The prebiotic nature of OFS and inulin restricts its dosage in humans to 15–20 g per day since doses greater than this can cause gastrointestinal symptoms such as stomach cramps, flatulence and diarrhoea.[90] It is not known whether, at the levels used in human studies, significant effects would be observed in animals.[95]

The types of food vehicles used to increase the amount of OFS/inulin in the diet differ. In the case of Luo et al.,[89] 100 g of biscuits were eaten every day and for Pedersen et al.,[90] 40 g of margarine was consumed which may have contributed to the negative findings in blood lipids. In the case of Davidson et al.,[85] significant changes in total and LDL cholesterol levels were observed over six weeks with inulin in comparison with the placebo (sugar). The percentage change in each of the lipid parameters was calculated over each of the six-week treatment periods and, unexpectedly, there was an increase in total cholesterol, LDL cholesterol and TAG during the placebo phase. Non-significant falls in these variables were observed during inulin treatment and so when the net changes in the variables were calculated (change during inulin minus change during control treatment) there were significant differences in total and LDL cholesterol between the two treatments. The authors attributed the increase in total and LDL cholesterol levels in the placebo phase to be due to the increased intake of SFAs in the chocolate products that were used as two of the vehicles in the study.[85] In later studies, the use of inulin in its powder form enabled it to be added to many of the foods eaten in the subjects' normal diet without any need for dietary advice, thus avoiding changes in body weight. Since inulin has water binding properties, in its powder form it could be added to orange juice, tea, coffee, yoghurt and soup.[91]

The significant relationship between subjects' initial TAG concentration and percentage change in TAG levels over the eight-week study demonstrated by Jackson et al.[91] lends support to the hypothesis that initial TAG levels could be important in determining the degree of the TAG response to inulin. The lack of response in some individuals may be as a result of them being less responsive to inulin, variations in their background diet, or non-compliance with the study protocol. Speculation as to possible reasons for variability in response would be aided by a better understanding of the mechanism of action of inulin on plasma TAG levels.

The length of the supplementation period used in the studies in Table 5.8 may be another factor for inconsistent findings in changes in TAG levels in human subjects with inulin. The studies were conducted over two to eight weeks, with significant effects occurring in only two studies conducted over three to four weeks.[87, 88] The lack of lipid lowering noted in the studies of Alles et al.,[86] Pedersen et al.[90] and Luo et al.[89] may be due to insufficient duration of supplementation. In the study of Jackson et al.,[91] a trend for TAG lowering on inulin treatment was seen some time between four and eight weeks and this reflects the time needed for the composition of the gut microflora to be modified. A four-week wash-out seemed to be sufficient for the TAG concentrations to return to baseline values. This may provide an explanation for the significant findings in TAG levels in the studies of Canzi et al.[87] and Causey et al.[88] who used 3–4 week sequential and cross-over designs with very short wash-out periods.

While some of the studies, to date, support beneficial effects of inulin on plasma TAG, the findings are by no means consistent and more work is required to provide convincing evidence of the lipid-lowering consequences of prebiotic ingestion.

5.6.3 Mechanism of lipid lowering by prebiotics

Prebiotics have been shown to be an ideal substrate for the health-promoting bacteria in the colon, notably bifidobacteria and lactobacilli.[96] During the fermentation process a number of byproducts are produced including gases (H_2S, CO_2, H_2, CH_4), lactate and SCFAs (acetate, butyrate and propionate). The SCFAs, acetate and propionate enter the portal blood stream where they are utilised by the liver. Acetate is converted to acetyl CoA in the liver and acts as a lipogenic substrate for de novo lipogenesis, whereas propionate has been reported to inhibit lipid synthesis.[97, 98] Butyrate, on the other hand, is taken up by the large intestinal cells (colonocytes) and has been shown to protect against tumour formation in the gut.[99] The type of SCFAs that are produced during the fermentation process is dependent on the microflora which can be stimulated by the prebiotic. Inulin has been shown to increase both acetate and butyrate levels, whereas synthetically produced prebiotics, for example galacto-oligosaccharides, increase the production of acetate and propionate and xylo-oligosaccharides increase acetate only.[99]

Inulin and OFS have been extensively studied to determine the mechanism of action of prebiotics in animals. Early *in vitro* studies using isolated rat hepatocytes suggested that the hypolipaemic action of OFS was associated with the inhibition of *de novo* cholesterol synthesis by the SCFA propionate following impairment of acetate utilisation by the liver for *de novo* lipogenesis.[98] This is in agreement with human studies in which rectal infusions of acetate and propionate resulted in propionate inhibiting the incorporation of acetate into TAGs released from the liver.[100] Fiordaliso *et al.*[101] demonstrated significant reductions in plasma TAGs, phospholipids and cholesterol in normolipidaemic rats fed a rat chow diet containing 10% (w/v) OFS. The TAG-lowering effect was demonstrated after only one week of OFS and was associated with a reduction in VLDL secretion. TAG and phospholipids are synthesised in the liver by esterification of fatty acids and glycerol-3-phosphate before being made available for assembly into VLDL, suggesting that the hypolipidaemic effect of OFS may be occurring in the liver. The reduction observed in cholesterol levels in the rats was only demonstrated after long-term feeding (16 weeks) of OFS. Recent evidence has suggested that the TAG-lowering effect of OFS occurs via reduction in VLDL TAG secretion from the liver due to the reduction in activity of all lipogenic enzymes (acetyl-CoA carboxylase, fatty acid synthase, malic enzyme, ATP citrate lyase and glucose-6-phosphate dehydrogenase), and in the case of fatty acid synthase, via modification of lipogenic gene expression (see Fig. 5.5).[102]

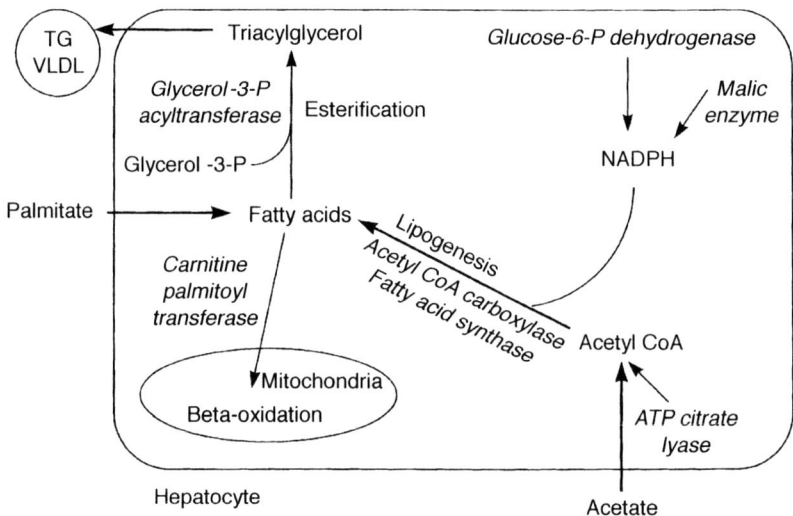

Fig. 5.5   Hepatic fatty acid metabolism

5.6.4 The effect of prebiotics on glucose and insulin levels

Very little is known about the effects of prebiotics on fasting insulin and glucose levels in humans. Of the supplementation studies conducted in humans, a significant reduction in glucose was observed in NIDDM subjects[83] and a trend for a reduction in glucose was observed in hyperlipidaemic subjects[84] with OFS. However, a recent study has reported no effect of OFS on blood glucose levels in type II diabetics.[86] A significant reduction in insulin levels was observed in healthy middle-aged subjects with inulin, although this was not accompanied by changes in plasma glucose levels.[91] The effect of the ingestion of acute test meals containing OFS on blood glucose, insulin and C-peptide levels in healthy adults showed a trend for a lower glycaemic response and peak insulin levels following the OFS enriched meals.[103]

The mechanism of action of prebiotics on lowering glucose and insulin levels has been proposed to be associated with the SCFAs, especially propionate. A significant reduction in post-prandial glucose concentrations was observed following both acute and chronic intakes of propionate-enriched bread.[104] The effect of propionate intake on post-prandial insulin levels was not investigated. A recent animal study has shown an attenuation of both post-prandial insulin and glucose levels following four weeks of feeding with OFS. These effects were attributed to the actions of OFS on the secretion of the gut hormones, glucose-dependent insulinotropic polypeptide (GIP) and glucagon-like peptide 1 (GLP-1).[92] These hormones are secreted from the small intestine (GIP) and the terminal ileum and colon (GLP-1) and contribute to the secretion of insulin following a meal in the presence of raised glucose levels.[105]

In summary, the mechanisms of action of prebiotics, especially inulin and OFS, have been determined largely from animal studies. Present data suggest inhibition of *de novo* lipogenesis as the primary mode of action of prebiotics in mediating their lipid-lowering effects via down regulation of the enzymes involved. If this is the case, more modest or inconsistent effects might be expected in humans, in whom *de novo* lipogenesis is extremely low, or variable depending on their background diet. In animal studies, rats are fed a diet that is low in fat and high in carbohydrate and so *de novo* lipogenesis is an up-regulated pathway in these animals for the synthesis of fatty acids. It is interesting to note that when rats are fed OFS along with a high fat diet typical of the Western-style diet, TAG levels are thought to be decreased by a different mechanism involving the enhanced clearance of TAG-rich lipoproteins. An increased GIP secretion in OFS-treated rats was observed by Kok *et al.*[92] and this gut hormone has been shown to enhance the activity of LPL, the principal enzyme involved in the clearance of TAG-rich lipoproteins following the ingestion of fat.[106] The release of GIP and GLP-1 in the intestine and colon may act as mediators of the systemic effect of prebiotics such as inulin and OFS, on blood lipid, insulin and glucose levels. However, further work is required to determine the metabolic pathways that are influenced by prebiotics. Their effect on gastrointestinal kinetics such as gastric emptying and its modification of the levels of TAG-rich lipoproteins (CMs) and glucose in the circulation has recently been proposed as a potential modulator of systemic effects.[107] Therefore the design of future studies to investigate the effect of prebiotics in humans should consider the choice of subjects, length of supplementation period and type of vehicle used to increase the intake of prebiotics in the diet, as these variables may influence the outcome of the study.

5.7 The effects of synbiotics on coronary heart disease

5.7.1 Synbiotics

A synbiotic is defined as 'a mixture of a prebiotic and a probiotic that beneficially affects the host by improving the survival and the implantation of live microbial dietary supplements in the gastrointestinal tract, by selectively stimulating the growth and/or by activating the metabolism of one or a limited number of health promoting bacteria'.[108] The use of synbiotics as functional food ingredients is a new and developing area and very few human studies have been performed looking at their effect on risk factors for CHD. Research conducted so far with synbiotics have looked at their effect on the composition of the gut microflora. In one study in healthy subjects, a fermented milk product containing a *Bifidobacterium spp.* with or without 18 g of inulin was given daily for 12 days.[109] The authors concluded that the administration of the fermented milk product (probiotic) substantially increased the proportion of bifidobacteria in the gut, but that this increase was not enhanced by the addition of 18 g of inulin. The composition of the gut microflora was then assessed two weeks after completing the supplementation period and it was found that subjects who received the fermented milk product and inulin maintained their bifidobacterial population in the gut compared with the subjects receiving the fermented milk product only. Although a synergistic effect on bifidobacteria in the gut was not observed with the synbiotic, these results suggest that either there was better implantation of the probiotic or a prebiotic effect on indigenous bifidobacteria.[109] Maintenance of high numbers of bifidobacteria in the gut may be beneficial in terms of healthy gut function; however, its effect on the lowering of blood lipid levels remains to be investigated. A more recent study has shown that a lower dose of prebiotic (2.75 g) added to a lactobacillus fermented milk was able to increase significantly the number of bifidobacteria when fed over a seven-week period in healthy human subjects.[108] If this effect was a result of the synbiotic product used in this study, the use of lower doses of prebiotics that can be used in synbiotic preparations should help to reduce gastrointestinal complaints observed when a prebiotic is used alone and improve the acceptability of these types of products by the general public.

5.8 Future trends

In recent years, a number of food manufacturers in the USA and Europe have been interested in the commercial opportunities for foodstuffs containing health-promoting probiotics and prebiotics. These food ingredients have received attention for their beneficial effects on the gut microflora and links to their systemic effects on the lowering of lipids known to be risk factors for CHD, notably cholesterol and TAG. Early attention was given to the incorporation of probiotics into dairy products such as fermented milk products (Yakult and Actimel Orange milk drink) and yoghurts, whose market is currently estimated at US$2 billion.[110] Prebiotics are currently gaining interest and this has opened up the market away from the dairy industry to other areas of the food industry since prebiotics can be baked into bread, cereals, cakes, biscuits and even added to soups. Synbiotics have also generated interest with some food manufacturers who are exploiting the effects of combining a prebiotic with a probiotic (Symbalance and PROBIOTIC plus oligofructose).

While consumers are interested in the concept of improving their health and well-being through diet, this is not quite so straightforward as originally thought. Recent bad press regarding food safety and the introduction of GM foods has made the public sceptical about new ingredients in foods. For progress to be made, the consumers need to be educated about the various health benefits and how they will be able to use these products in their own diet without adverse consequences. Although the introduction of probiotics onto the supermarket shelves are slowly being accepted in the UK population, carefully controlled nutrition studies need to be carried out to determine the beneficial effects of prebiotics, probiotics and synbiotics before substantial health claims can be made.

To make these foods attractive to the consumer, the products need to be priced in such a way that they are accessible to the general public. The low doses of prebiotics and probiotics needed to help maintain a healthy gut microflora should be made available to the general public, whereas products that contain higher amounts of prebiotics in order to help reduce blood lipids will need to be restricted in order for the appropriate population group to be targeted.

5.9 Sources of further information and advice

5.9.1 General biochemistry and metabolic regulation text books

DEVLIN, T.M. *Textbook of Biochemistry with Clinical Correlations*, 3rd edn, New York, John Wiley, 1992.

FRAYN, K.N. *Metabolic Regulation: A Human Perspective*, London, Portland Press, 1996.

5.9.2 Published reports on dietary intake and coronary heart disease

Department of Health, *Nutritional Aspects of Cardiovascular Disease, Report on Health and Social Subjects*, no. 46, London, HMSO.

5.9.3 Prebiotic, probiotic and synbiotic information

ADAMS, C.A. 'Nutricines', *Food Components in Health and Nutrition*, Nottingham, Nottingham University Press, 1999.

HASLER, C.M. and WILLIAMS, C.M. 'Prebiotics and probiotics: where are we today?', *BJN*, **80**, supp. 2.

LEEDS, A.R. and ROWLAND, I.R. *Gut Flora and Health: Past, Present and Future*, International Congress and Symposium Series 219, Royal Society of Medicine, 1996.

SADLER, M.J. and SALTMARSH, M. *Functional Foods: The Consumer, the Products and the Evidence*, Bath, Bookcraft, 1997.

5.10 References

1   KEYS, A. 'Coronary artery disease in seven countries', *Circulation*, 1970, **41**, I1–I211.

2   PATSCH, J.R., MEISENBÖCK, G., HOPFERWEISER, T., MULHBERGER, V., KNAPP, E., DUNN, J.K., GOTTO, A.M. and PATSCH, W. 'Relation of triglyceride metabolism and coronary artery disease: studies in the postprandial state', *Arterioscler Thromb*, 1992, **12**, 1336–45.

3   GRIFFIN, B.A. and ZAMPELAS, A. 'Influence of dietary fatty acids on the atherogenic lipoprotein phenotype', *Nut Res Rev*, 1995, **8**, 1–26.

4   GIBSON, G.R. and BEAUMONT, A. 'An overview of human colonic bacteriology in health and disease'. In A.R. Leeds and I.R. Rowland (eds), pp. 3–11, *Gut Flora and Health: Past, Present and Future*, International Congress and Symposium Series 219, London, Royal Society of Medicine, 1996.

5   KEYS, A. *Seven Countries: A Multivariate Analysis of Death and Coronary Heart Disease.*, Harvard University Press, Cambridge, MA, 1980.

6   World Health Organisation, 'World Health Statistics Annual 1989', Geneva, WHO, 1989.

7   MARTIN, M.J., BROWNER, W.S., WENTWORTH, J., HULLEY, S.B. and KULER, L.H. 'Serum cholesterol, blood pressure and mortality: implications from a cohort of 361,662 men', *Lancet*, 1986, **2**, 933–6.

8   SHEPHERD, J., COBBE, S.M., FORD, I., ISLES, C.G., LORIMER, A.R., MACFARLANE, P.W., MCKILLOP, J.H. and PACKARD, C.J. 'Prevention of coronary heart disease with pravastatin in men with hypercholesterolaemia', *New Engl J Med*, 1995, **333**(20), 1301–7.

9   SHAPER, A.G., POCOCK, S.J., PHILIPS, A.N. and WALKER, M. 'Identifying men at high risk of heart attacks – strategy for use in general practice', *BMJ*, 1986, **293** (6545), 474–9.

10 FIELDING, P.E. and FIELDING, C.J. 'Dynamics of lipoprotein transport in the circulatory system'. In D.E. Vance and J. Vance (eds), pp. 427–59, *Biochemistry of Lipids, Lipoproteins and Membranes*, Amsterdam, Elsevier, 1991.

11 SCHNEIDER, W.J. 'Removal of lipoproteins from plasma'. In D.E. Vance and J. Vance (eds), pp. 461–87 *Biochemistry of Lipids, Lipoproteins and Membranes*, Amsterdam, Elsevier, 1991.

12 DEVLIN, T.M. *Textbook of Biochemistry with Clinical Correlations*, 3rd edn, New York, John Wiley, 1992.

13 REDGRAVE, T.G. *Gastrointestinal Physiology IV*, Baltimore, University Park Press, 1983.

14 BRASAEMLE, D.L., CORNLEY-MOSS, K. and BENSADOUN, A. 'Hepatic lipase treatment of chylomicron remnants increases exposure of apolipoprotein E', *J Lipid Res*, 1993, **34**, 455–63.

15 KARPE, F. and HULTIN, M. 'Endogenous triglyceride-rich lipoproteins accumulate in rat plasma when competing with a triglyceride emulsion for a common lipolytic pathway', *J Lipid Res*, 1995, **36**, 1557–66.

16 GRIFFIN, B.A. and PACKARD, C.J. 'Metabolism of VLDL and LDL subclasses', *Curr Opin Lipidol*, 1994, **5**, 200–6.

17 TALL, A.R. 'Plasma cholesterol ester transfer protein', *J Lipid Res*, 1993, **27**, 361–7.

18 GENSINI, G.F., COMEGLIO, M. and COLELLA, A. 'Classical risk factors and emerging elements in the risk profile for coronary artery disease', *Eur Heart J*, 1998, **19** (supp. A), A52–A61.

19 ASSMANN, G., CULLEN, P. and SCHULTE, H. 'The Münster Heart Study (PROCAM): Results of follow-up at 8 years', *Eur Heart J*, 1998, **19** (supp. A), A2–A11.

20 AUSTIN, M.A. 'Plasma triglyceride and coronary artery disease', *Arterioscl Thromb*, 1991, **11**, 2–14.

21 WILSON, P.W.F. 'Established risk factors and coronary artery disease: the Framingham study', *Am J Hypertens*, 1994, **7**, 7S–12S.

22 O'MEARA, N.M., LEWIS, G.F., CABANA, V.G., IVERIUS, P.H., GETZ, G.S. and POLONSKY, K.S. 'Role of basal triglyceride and high density lipoprotein in determination of postprandial lipid and lipoprotein responses', *J Clin Endocrin Metab*, 1991, **75**, 465–71.

23 KARPE, F., STEINER, G., UFFELMAN, K., OLIVECRONA, T. and HAMSTEN, A. 'Postprandial lipoproteins and progression of coronary heart disease', *Atherosclerosis*, 1994, **106**, 83–97.

24 ZILVERSMIT, D. 'Atherogenesis: a postprandial phenomenon', *Circulation*, 1979, **60**, 473–85.

25 MEISENBÖCK, G. and PATSCH, J.R. 'Coronary artery disease: synergy of triglyceride-rich lipoproteins and HDL', *Cardiovascular Risk Factors*, 1991, **1**, 293–9.

26 AUSTIN, M.A., BRESLOW, J.L., HENNEKENS, C.H., BURLING, J.E., WILLETT, W.C. and KRAUSS, R.M. 'Low density lipoprotein subclass patterns and risk of myocardial infarction', *JAMA*, 1988, **260**, 1917–21.

27 AUSTIN, M.A., HOKANSON, J.E. and BRUNZELL, J.D. 'Characterisation of low-density lipoprotein subclasses: methodological approaches and clinical relevance', *Curr Opin Lipidol*, 1994, **5**, 395–403.

28   GRIFFIN, B.A. 'Low density lipoprotein heterogeneity', *Ballière's Clinical Endocrinology and Metabolism*, 1995, **9**, 687–703.

29   CHAPMAN, M.J., GUÉRIN, M. and BRUCKERT, E. 'Atherogenic, dense low-density lipoproteins: pathophysiology and new therapeutic approaches', *Eur Heart J*, 1998, **19** (supp. A), A24–A30.

30   REAVEN, G.M., CHEN, Y.-D.I., JEPPENSEN, J., MAHEUX, P. and KRAUSS, R.M. 'Insulin resistance and hyperinsulinaemia in individuals with small, dense, low density lipoprotein particles', *J Clin Invest*, 1993, **92**, 141–6.

31   MENSINK, R.P. 'Effects of individual saturated fatty acids on serum lipids and lipoprotein concentrations', *Am J Clin Nutr*, 1993, **57**(s), 711S–714S.

32   HEGSTED, D.M., ANSMAN, L.M., JOHNSON, J.A. and DALLAL, G.E. 'Dietary fat and serum lipids: an evaluation of the experimental data', *Am J Clin Nutr*, 1993, **57** 875–83.

33   HAYES, K.C. and KHOSLA, P. 'Dietary fatty acids thresholds and cholesterolaemia', *FASEB J*, 1992, **6**, 2600–7.

34   Department of Health, *Nutritional Aspects of Cardiovascular Disease: Report of the Cardiovascular Review Group Committee on Medical Aspects of Food Policy*, London, HMSO, 1994. Report on Health and Social Subjects 46.

35   GREGORY, J., FOSTER, K., TYLER, H. and WISEMAN, M. *The Dietary and Nutritional Survey of British Adults: A Survey of the Dietary Behaviour, Nutritional Status and Blood Pressure of Adults aged 16 to 64 living in Great Britain*', Office of Population Census and Surveys, Social Survey Division, London, HMSO, 1990.

36   GRUNDY, S.M., NIX, D., WHELAN, M.F. and FRANKLIN, L. 'Comparison of three cholesterol lowering diets in normolipidaemic men', *JAMA* 1986, **256**, 2351.

37   BERRY, E.M. 'The effects of nutrients on lipoprotein susceptibility to oxidation', *Current Opinions in Lipidology*, 1992, **3**, 5–11.

38   MENSINK, R.P. and KATAN, M.B. 'Effect of dietary *trans* fatty acids in high density and low density lipoprotein cholesterol levels in healthy subjects', *N Engl J Med*, 1990, **323**, 439–45.

39   DYBERG, J. and BANG, H.O. 'Haemostatic function and platelet polyunsaturated fatty acids in Eskimos', *Lancet*, 1979, **2**, 433–5.

40   BURR, M.L., FEHILY, A.M., GILBERT, J.F. *et al.* 'Effects of changes of fat, fish and fibre intakes on frequency of myocardial infarctions: DART Study', *Lancet*, 1989, **2**, 757–62.

41   HARRIS, W.S. '*n*-3 Fatty acids and serum lipoproteins: human studies', *Am J Clin Nutr*, 1997, **65** (S), 1645S–1654S.

42   SISCOVICK, D.S., RAGHUNATHAN, T.E., KING, I. and WEINMAN, S. 'Dietary intake and cell membrane levels of long chain *n*-3 polyunsaturated fatty acids and the risk of primary cardiac arrest', *JAMA*, 1996, **274**, 1363–7.

43   DE DECKERE, E.A.M., KORVER, O., VERSCHUREN, P.M. and KATAN, M.B. 'Health aspects of fish and n-3 polyunsaturated fatty acids from plant and marine origin', *Euro J Clin Nutr*, 1998, **52**, 749–53.

44 EEC Scientific Committee for Food, *Reference Nutrient Intakes for the European Community*, Brussels, EC, 1992.

45 MENSINK, R.P. and KATAN, M.B. 'Effects of monosaturated fatty acids versus complex carbohydrates on high density lipoproteins in healthy men and women', *Lancet*, 1987, **1**, 122–5.

46 GRUNDY, S.M. 'Comparison of monounsaturated fatty acids and carbohydrates for lowering plasma cholesterol', *N Engl J Med*, 1986, **314**, 745–8.

47 MORRIS, J.N., MARR, J.W. and CLAYTON, D.G. 'Diet and heart: a postscript'. *BMJ*, 1977, **2**, 1307–14.

48 KUSHI, L.H., LEW, R.A., STARE, F.J. *et al.*, 'Diet and 20-year mortality from coronary heart disease: the Ireland–Boston Diet–Heart Study', *N Engl J Med*, 1985, **312**, 811–18.

49 RIEMERSMA, R.A., WOOD, D.A., MACINTYRE, C.C., ELTON, R.A., GEY, K.F. and OLIVER, M.F. 'Risk of angina pectoris and plasma concentrations of vitamin A, C and E and carotene', *Lancet*, 1991, **337**, 1–5.

50 STEPHENS, N.G., PARSONS, A., SCHOFIELD, P.M., KELLY, F. and CHEESEMAN, K. 'Randomised controlled trial of vitamin E in patients with coronary disease: Cambridge Heart Antioxidant Study (CHAOS)', 1996, *Lancet*, **348**, 781–6.

51 ELLIOT, P., DYER, A. and STAMLER, J. 'Correcting for regression dilution in INTERSALT', *Lancet*, 1993, **342**, 1123.

52 LAW, M.R., FROST, C.D. and WALD, N.J. 'By how much does dietary salt reduction lower blood pressure? I-III- Analysis of observational data among populations', *BMJ*, 1991, **302**, 811–24.

53 GAZIANO, J.M., BURING, J.E., BRESLOW, J.L., GOLDHABER, S.Z., ROSNER, B., VANDENBURGH, M., WILLIET, W.C. and HENNEKENS, C.H. 'Moderate alcohol intake, increased levels of high density lipoprotein and its subfractions, and decreased risk of myocardial infarction', *New Eng J Med*, 1993, **329**, 1829–34.

54 LAW, M. and WALD, N. 'Why heart disease mortality is low in France: the time lag explanation', *BMJ*, 1999, **318**, 1471–80.

55 URGERT, R., MEYBOOM, S., KUILMAN, M., REXWINKEL, H., VISSERS, M.N., KLERK, M. and KATAN, M.B. 'Comparison of effect of cafetiere and filter coffee on serum concentrations of liver aminotransferases and lipids: six month randomised controlled trial', *BMJ*, 1996, **313**, 1362–6.

56 MANN, G.V. and SPOERRY, A. 'Studies of a surfactant and cholesteremia in the Maasai', *Am J Clin Nutr*, 1974, **27**, 464–9.

57 MANN, G.V. 'A factor in yoghurt which lowers cholesteremia in man', *Atherosclerosis*, 1977, **26**, 335–40.

58 HOWARD, A.N. and MARKS, J. 'Effect of milk products on serum-cholesterol', *Lancet*, 1979, **II**, 957.

59 HEPNER, G., FRIED, R., ST JEOR, S., FUSETTI, L. and MORIN, R. 'Hypocholesterolemic effect of yogurt and milk', *Am J Clin Nutr*, 1979, **32**, 19–24.

60 SESSIONS, V.A., LOVEGROVE, J.A., TAYLOR, G.R.J., DEAN, T.S., WILLIAMS, C.M., SANDERS, T.A.B., MACDONALD, I. and SALTER, A. 'The effects of a new

fermented milk product on total plasma cholesterol: LDL cholesterol and apolipoprotein B concentrations in middle aged men and women', *Proceedings of the Nutrition Society*, 1997, **56**, 120A.

61   THOMPSON, L.U., JENKINS, D.J.A., AMER, V., REICHERT, R., JENKINS, A. and KAMULSKY, J. 'The effect of fermented and unfermented milks on serum cholesterol', *Am J Clin Nutr*, 1982, **36**, 1106–11.

62   MASSEY, L.K. 'Effect of changing milk and yogurt consumption on human nutrient intake and serum lipoproteins', *J Dairy Sci*, 1984, **67**, 255–62.

63   MCNAMARA, D.J., LOWELL, A.E. and SABB, J.E. 'Effect of yogurt intake on plasma lipid and lipoprotein levels in normolipidemic males', *Atherosclerosis*, 1989, **79**, 167–71.

64   JASPERS, D.A., MASSEY, L.K. and LUEDECKE, L.O. 'Effect of consuming yogurts prepared with three culture strains on human serum lipoproteins', *J Food Sci*, 1984, **49**, 1178–81.

65   AGERBAEK, M., GERDES, L.U. and RICHELSEN, B. 'Hypocholesterolaemic effects of a new product in healthy middle-aged men', *Eur J Clin Nutr*, 1995, **49**, 346–52.

66   RICHELSEN, B., KRISTENSEN, K. and PEDERSEN, S.B. 'Long-term (6 months) effect of a new fermented milk product on the level of plasma lipoproteins: a placebo-controlled and double blind study', *Eur J Clin Nutr*, 1996, **50**, 811–15.

67   BERTOLAMI, M.C. 'Evaluation of the effects of a new fermented milk product (Gaio) on primary hypercholesterolemia', *Eur J Clin Nutr*, 1999, **53**, 97–101.

68   ROSSOUW, J.E., BURGER, E.-M., VAN DER VYVER, P. and FERREIRA, J.J. 'The effect of skim milk yoghurt, and full cream milk on human serum lipids', *Am J Clin Nutr*, 1981, **34**, 351–6.

69   HUIS IN'T VELD, J.H.J. and SHORTT, C. 'Selection criteria for probiotic microorganisms'. In A.R. Leeds and I.R. Rowland (eds), pp. 27–36, *Gut Flora and Health: Past, Present and Future*, International Congress and Symposium Series No. 219, London, New York, Royal Society of Medicine Press, 1996.

70   HYLEMOND, P.B. 'Metabolism of bile acids in intestinal microflora'. In H. Danielson and J. Sjovall (eds), pp. 331–43, *Sterols and Bile Acids*, New York, Elsevier Science, 1985.

71   GRILL, J.P., MANGINOT-DURR, C., SCHNEIDER, F. and BALLONGUE, J. 'Bifidobacteria and probiotic effects: action of *Bifidobacterium* species on conjugated bile salts', *Curr Microbiol*, 1995, **31**, 23–7.

72   GILLILAND, S.E., NELSON, C.R. and MAXWELL, C. 'Assimilation of cholesterol by *Lactobacillus acidophilus*', *Appl Environ Microbiol*, 1985, **49**(2), 377–81.

73   DE SMET, I., DE BOEVER, P. and VERSTRAETE, W. 'Cholesterol lowering in pigs through enhanced bacterial bile salt hydrolase activity', *BJN*, 1998, **79**, 185–94.

74   MARTEAU, P., GERHARDT, M.F., MYARA, A., BOUVIER, E., TRIVIN, F. and

RAMBAUD, J.C. 'Metabolism of bile salts by alimentary bacteria during transit in human small intestine', *Microbiol Ecol in Health & Disease*, 1995, **8**, 151–7.

75 GILLILAND, S.E., NELSON, C.R. and MAXWELL, C. 'Assimilation of cholesterol by *Lactobacillus acidophilus*', *Appl & Environ Microbiol*, 1985, **49** (2), 377–81.

76 RASIC, J.L., VUJICIC, I.F., SKRINJAR, M. and VULIC, M. 'Assimilation of cholesterol by some cultures of lactic acid bacteria and bifidobacteria', *Biotech Lett*, 1992, **14** (1), 39–44.

77 KLAVER, F.A.M. and VAN DER MEER, R. 'The assumed assimilation of cholesterol by lactobacilli and *Bifidobacterium bifidum* is due to their bile salt-deconjugating activity', *Appl Environ Microbiol*, 1993, **59**(4), 1120–4.

78 TAHRI, K., CROCIANI, J., BALLONGUE, J. and SCHNEIDER, F. 'Effects of three strains of bifidobacteria on cholesterol', *Lett Appl Microbiol*, 1995, **21**, 149–51.

79 HOSONO, A. and TONO-OKA, T. 'Binding of cholesterol with lactic acid bacterial cells', *Milchwissenschaft*, 1995, **50**(20), 556–60.

80 GIBSON, G.R. and ROBERFROID, M.B. 'Dietary modulation of the human colonic microbiota: introducing the concept of prebiotics', *J Nutr*, 1995, **125**, 1401–12.

81 DYSSELER, P. and HOFFEM, D. 'Inulin, an alternative dietary fibre: properties and quantitative analysis', *Eur J Clin Nutr,* 1995, **49**, S145–S152.

82 VAN LOO, J., COUSSEMENT, P., DE LEENHEER, L., HOEBREGS, H. and SMITS, G. 'On the presence of inulin and oligofructose as natural ingredients in the Western diet', *Crit Rev Food Sci and Nutr*, 1995, **35**, 525–52.

83 YAMASHITA, K., KAWAI, K. and ITAKURA, M. 'Effects of fructo-oligosaccharides on blood glucose and serum lipids in diabetic subjects', *Nutr Res,* 1984, **4**, 961–6.

84 HIDAKA, H., TASHIRO, Y. and EIDA, T. 'Proliferation of bifidobacteria by oligosaccharides and their useful effect on human health', *Bifidobacteria Microflora*, 1991, **10**, 65–79.

85 DAVIDSON, M.H., SYNECKI, C., MAKI, K.C. and DRENNEN, K.B. 'Effects of dietary inulin in serum lipids in men and women with hypercholesterolaemia', *Nutr Res,* 1998, **3**, 503–17.

86 ALLES, M.S., DE ROOS, N.M., BAKX, J.C., VAN DE LISDONK, E., ZOCK, P.L. and HAUTVAST, J.G.A.J. 'Consumption of fructooligosaccharides does not favourably affect blood glucose and serum lipid concentrations in patients with type 2 diabetes', *Am J Clin Nutr*, 1999, **69**, 64–9.

87 CANZI, E., BRIGHENTI, F., CASIRAGHI, M.C., DEL PUPPO, E. and FERRARI, A. 'Prolonged consumption of inulin in ready to eat breakfast cereals: effects on intestinal ecosystem, bowel habits and lipid metabolism', *Cost 92. Workshop on Dietary Fibre and Fermentation in the Colon*, Helsinki, 1995.

88 CAUSEY, J.L., GALLAHER, D.D. and SLAVIN, J.L. 'Effect of inulin consumption

on lipid and glucose metabolism in healthy men with moderately elevated cholesterol', *FASEB*, 1998, **12**, 4737.

89 LUO, J., RIZKALLA, S.W., ALAMOWITCH, C., BOUSSAIRI, A., BLAYO, A., BARRY, J.-L., LAFFITTE, A., GUYON, F., BORNET, F.R.J. and SLAMA, G. 'Chronic consumption of short-chain fructooligosaccharides by healthy subjects decreased basal hepatic glucose production but no effect on insulin-stimulated glucose metabolism', *Am J Clin Nutr*, 1996, **63**, 939–45.

90 PEDERSEN, A., SANDSTRÖM, B. and VAN AMELSVOORT, J.M.M. 'The effect of ingestion of inulin on blood lipids and gastrointestinal symptoms in healthy females', *BJN*, 1997, **78**, 215–22.

91 JACKSON, K.G., TAYLOR, G.R.J., CLOHESSY, A.M. and WILLIAMS, C.M. 'The effect of the daily intake of inulin on fasting lipid, insulin and glucose concentrations in middle-aged men and women', *BJN*, 1999, **82**, 23–30.

92 KOK, N.N., MORGAN, L.M., WILLIAMS, C.M., ROBERFROIOD, M.B., THISSEN, J.-P. and DELZENNE, N.M. 'Insulin, glucagon-like peptide 1, glucose dependent insulinotropic polypeptide and insulin-like growth factor 1 as putative mediators of the hypolipidemic effect of oligofructose in rats', *J Nutr*, 1998, **128**, 1099–103.

93 WILLIAMS, C.M. 'Effects of inulin on blood lipids in humans', *J Nutr*, 1998, 7, S1471–S1473.

94 ROBERFROID, M. 'Dietary fiber, inulin and oligofructose: a review comparing their physiological effects', *Crit Rev Food Sci and Nutr*, 1993, **33**, 102–48.

95 DELZENNE, N.M., KOK, N., FIORDALISO, M.-F., DEBOYSER, D.M., GOETHALS, F.M. and ROBERFROID, R.M. 'Dietary fructo-oligosaccharides modify lipid metabolism', *Am J Clin Nutr*, 1993, **57**, 820S.

96 GIBSON, G.R. and MCCARTNEY, A.L. 'Modification of gut flora by dietary means', *Biochem Soc Trans*, 1998, **26**, 222–8.

97 WOLEVER, T.M.S., BRIGHENTI, F., ROYALL, D., JENKINS, A.L. and JENKINS, D.J.A. 'Effect of rectal infusion of short chain fatty acids in human subjects', *Am J Gastroenterol*, 1989, **84**, 1027–33.

98 DEMIGNÉ, C., MORAND, C., LEVRAT, M.-A., BESSON, C., MOUNDRAS, C. and RÉMÉSEY, C. 'Effect of propionate on fatty acid and cholesterol synthesis and on acetate metabolism in isolated rat hepatocytes', *BJN*, 1995, **74**, 209–19.

99 VAN LOO, J., CUMMINGS, J., DELZENNE, N., ENGLYST, H., FRANCK, A., HOPKINS, M., KOK, N., MACFARLANE, G., NEWTON, D., QUIGLEY, M., ROBERFROID, M., VAN VLIET, T. and VAN DEN HEUVEL, E. 'Functional food properties of non-digestible oligosaccharides: a consensus report from the ENDO project (DGXII AIRII-CT94-1095)', *BJN*, 1999, **81**, 121–32.

100 WOLEVER, T.M.S., SPADAFORA, P.J., CUNNANE, S.C. and PENCHARZ, P.B. 'Propionate inhibits incorporation of colonic [1,2-^{13}C]acetate into plasma lipids in humans', *Am J Clin Nutr*, 1995, **61**, 1241–7.

101 FIORDALISO, M.-F., KOK, N., DESAGER, J.-P., GOETHALS, F., DEBOYSER, D., ROBERFROID, R.M. and DELZENNE, N. 'Dietary oligofructose lowers

triglycerides, phospholipids and cholesterol in serum and very low density lipoproteins in rats', *Lipids*, 1995, **30**, 163–7.

102 DELZENNE, N.M. and KOK, N. 'Effect of non-digestible fermentable carbohydrates on hepatic fatty acid metabolism', *Biochem Soc Trans*, 1998, **26**, 228–30.

103 RUMESSEN, J.J., BODE, S., HAMBERG, O. and GUDMAND-HOYER, E. 'Fructans of the Jerusalem artichokes : intestinal transport, absorption, fermentation, and influence on blood glucose, insulin, and C-peptide responses in healthy subjects', *Am J Clin Nutr*, 1990, **52**, 675–81.

104 TODESCO, T., RAO, A.V., BOSELLO, O. and JENKINS, D.J.A. 'Propionate lowers blood glucose and alters lipid metabolism in healthy subjects', *Am J Clin Nutr*, 1991, **54**, 860–5.

105 MORGAN, L.M. 'The role of gastrointestinal hormones in carbohydrate and lipid metabolism and homeostasis: effects of gastric inhibitory polypeptide and glucagon-like peptide-1', *Biochem Soc Trans*, 1998, **26**, 216–22.

106 KNAPPER, J.M., PUDDICOMBE, S.M., MORGAN, L.M. and FLETCHER, J.M. 'Investigations into the actions of glucose dependent insulinotrophic polypeptide and glucagon-like peptide-1 (7-36) amide on lipoprotein lipase activity in explants of rat adipose tissue', *J Nutr*, 1995, **125**, 183–8.

107 DELZENNE, N. 'The hypolipidaemic effect of inulin: when animal studies help to approach the human problem', *BJN*, 1999, **82**, 3–4.

108 ROBERFROID, M.B. 'Prebiotics and synbiotics: concepts and nutritional properties', *BJN*, 1998, **80** (supp. 2), S197–S202.

109 BOUHNIK, Y., FLOURIE, B., RIOTTOT, M., BISETTI, N., GAILING, M., GUIBERT, A., BORNET, F. and RAMBAUD, J. 'Effect of fructo-oligosaccharides ingestion on fecal bifidobacteria and selected metabolic indexes of colon carcinogenesis in healthy humans', *Nutrition and Cancer*, 1996, **26**, 21–9.

110 YOUNG, J. 'European market developments in prebiotic- and probiotic-containing foodstuffs', *BJN*, 1998, **80** (supp. 2), S231–S233.

111 BAZARRE, T.L., WU, S.L. and YUHAS, J.A. 'Total and HDL-cholesterol concentration following yoghurt and calcium supplementation', *Nutritional Reports International*, 1983, **28**, 1225–32.

112 TAYLOR, G.B.J. and WILLIAMS, C.M. 'Effect of probiotics and prebiotics on blood lipids', *BJN*, 1998, **80** (supp. 5), S225–S230.

6

Anti-tumour properties

I.T. Johnson, Institute of Food Research, Norwich

6.1 Introduction

Cancer is as old as the human race but what little evidence is available suggests that it was probably a relatively rare disease in the ancient world. In most populations, the principal causes of death are infant mortality, infectious disease and the chronic conditions of old age – principally cancer, heart disease and stroke. Deaths from the first two causes tend to decline dramatically with increasing prosperity, so cancer and cardiovascular disease inevitably cause a larger proportion of deaths in industrialised countries than they do in the developing world. Nevertheless, the precise reasons for the high levels of death from cancer experienced today in developed countries are controversial. Since cancer is largely a disease of old age, its prevalence will inevitably rise with the average longevity of the population but other factors seem to be at work in prosperous countries. Even in the nineteenth century it was possible for Tanchou to propose that increasing rates of cancer were a characteristic of urban societies,[1] and careful international studies of age-corrected rates for cancer continue to support this view.[2] A classic illustration of the historical association between increased industrialisation and cancer rates is provided by Japan, where until quite recently rates of breast and colorectal cancer were four to five times lower than in the USA and many countries of Northern Europe, whereas stomach cancer was several times more common. Since 1970 rates of breast and bowel cancer have risen steeply in Japan, but stomach cancer, as in many other industrialised countries, has declined. The explanation for these changes must lie in some aspect of environment or lifestyle, but despite decades of epidemiological and laboratory investigation we are still far from understanding the factors that determine the risk of cancer at sites other than the lung.

In their classic epidemiological analysis of this issue, Doll and Peto[3] estimated that diet was responsible for approximately 35% of cancers in the West; however, the uncertainty attached to this estimate was very high, and the precise causes virtually unknown. More recently, in an encyclopaedic report on nutrition and cancer, the World Cancer Research Fund[4] has confirmed the central importance of diet as a major determinant of many forms of cancer across the globe, and stated that the sharp increase in cancer rates in the developing world should be regarded as a global public health emergency.

The interactions between diet and the biological processes leading to the development of cancer are extremely complex but one can envisage three general factors that are potentially important in any human population. The first is the presence in food of carcinogenic compounds which play an active role in damaging cells and inducing tumours. This topic is largely beyond the scope of this chapter, but in any case its relevance to Western industrialised societies is questionable. Although there are many proven carcinogens in our diets, the human body is equipped with efficient defences, and the level of exposure is usually far too low to be of relevance to health. One obvious exception to this rule is the chronic exposure of many of us to ethanol from alcoholic drinks, but the decision to drink alcohol lies in the hands of the consumer, and there is evidence that there are protective effects of alcohol against heart disease,[5] and these may well outweigh the adverse effects on cancer.

The second issue is the adequacy of nutrient intake, and the possibility that certain deficiencies might influence an individual's susceptibility to cancer. The risks of cancer tend to be greater at the lower end of the socio-economic scale in many Western countries. The reasons for this are complex; part of the reason may be that though there is little evidence that this is due to malnutrition in the classical sense, it remains possible that optimal levels of certain nutrients may be higher than is currently accepted. Finally, susceptibility to cancer may be increased by an inadequate intake of biologically active food components that exert anti-carcinogenic effects, but which are not currently classified as nutrients in the conventional sense. Over the past two decades a large body of epidemiological evidence in favour of a protective effect of plant foods has appeared and become generally accepted by nutritionists and regulatory bodies.[4, 6, 7] The widespread promulgation of public health measures to encourage the consumption of five 80 g portions of fruits and vegetables per day has been one outcome of this consensus, and another has been a remarkable growth of interest in the possibility that the active principles in fruits, vegetables and cereals might be incorporated into functional foods. The purpose of this chapter is to review the nature of cancer, to explore the various ways in which diet can influence the initiation and development of this group of diseases, and to consider the potential role of functional food in their prevention.

6.2 The nature of tumour growth

The existence of cancer and the distinction between benign and malignant tumours were recognised by the early Greek physicians, who coined the term 'carcinoma', derived from the Greek *karkinos*, meaning 'crab', alluding to the creeping crab-like behaviour of a spreading tumour. The development of microscopy eventually led to the recognition that tumours contained cells that differed fundamentally in appearance and behaviour from those of the surrounding tissue. Oncology, the scientific investigation and clinical treatment of tumours, was founded in the early years of this century but it is only within the last two decades that the development of the cell and molecular sciences has enabled biologists to begin to acquire a deeper understanding of tumour biology. Much of this insight has been gained through the use of isolated tumour cells grown *in vitro*, and of animal models of carcinogenesis, which enable tumours to be studied within the complex environment of living tissue. Both of these approaches have their limitations and we are still far from a full understanding of cancer in human beings.

All cancers are diseases of abnormal cell proliferation, development and death. During the earliest stages of human life all of the embryonic cells divide constantly, and differentiate to form the specialised tissues and organs. Throughout infancy and childhood cell proliferation continues at whatever rates are necessary to fulfil the requirements of growth, but as maturity is reached organs such as the central nervous system, muscles and skeletal tissues cease to grow, and cell division becomes minimal. However, certain tissues continue to proliferate throughout life. These include the blood-forming tissues, the epithelia which line the surfaces of the body exposed to the environment, the glandular tissues which produce secretions, and the sexual organs which produce new reproductive cells. Cancer can affect virtually any organ of the body but tissues such as those of the lungs and gut, which have characteristically high rates of cell division and chronic exposure to the external environment, are particularly vulnerable.

6.2.1 Tumour cell biology

A tumour can be defined as any focal accumulation of cells beyond the numbers required for the development, repair or function of a tissue. Tumours may be benign or malignant. The former are usually relatively slow growing, but more importantly the cells tend to retain much of the specialisation and spatial localisation of the tissue from which they are derived. In contrast, malignant cells are characterised by a loss of differentiation, faster growth and a tendency to invade surrounding tissues and migrate to other organs to form secondary tumours or metastases. Thus cancer may be defined as the development, growth and metastatic spread of a malignant neoplasm. Malignant tumours derived from epithelial cells are called carcinomas, and those derived from connective or mesenchymal cells are called sarcomas. It is usually the secondary tumour that is lethal, so the early diagnosis of malignant primary tumours is essential for effective treatment.

6.2.2 Molecular biology

Regardless of their function in the body, all cells carry a complete set of genetic instructions for the development and function of the whole organism. The subset of genes which is expressed by any particular cell type determines its *phenotype,* the precise details of the structure, specialised functions and life cycle of the cell which enable it to exist in harmony with other cells as part of a tissue. The events that occur during the early stages of cancer development usually involve damage to the DNA coding for such crucial genes.

With the exception of certain cancers of childhood which often affect growing tissues such as the brain or bones, *carcinogenesis* – the development of cancer from normal cells – is usually a relatively slow process which occupies a substantial proportion of the lifetime of an individual. Tumour cells invariably contain a number of mutations affecting genes controlling the rate at which cells divide, differentiate or die, or the efficiency with which DNA damage is repaired.[8, 9] Such mutations may be inherited though the germ-line, and these form the basis for a number of recognised familial cancer syndromes, but most of the genetic abnormalities detectable in sporadic cancers, which are far more common, are somatic mutations acquired during carcinogenesis. Such damage may result from exposure to radiation or chemical mutagens, or through the effects of molecular species such as oxygen free radicals generated by the normal metabolism of the body. Whatever the source of the DNA damage, however, the defining characteristic of a pro-carcinogenic mutation is that it favours the proliferation and survival of an abnormal population of cells that have the potential for further evolution towards the malignant state.[10] Chemical carcinogens such as those present in tobacco smoke tend to be electrophiles – substances that can react easily with electron-rich regions of cellular proteins and DNA. The products formed by such interactions with DNA are called adducts. These are stable compounds which disrupt the synthesis of new DNA when the cell next divides, so that the sequence of genetic code in that region is damaged and the new cell carries a mutation. Many chemical carcinogens must be activated to an electrophilic form before they can act and, ironically, this often occurs as part of the sequence of events employed by the cell to detoxify the parent molecule or pro-carcinogen.

Many of the target genes that undergo mutation during carcinogenesis have been identified and their functions and interactions with other genes are at least partially understood.[11] The proto-oncogenes were first identified through their near-homology to the critical DNA sequences present in certain cancer-causing viruses which, when inserted into mammalian cells, would transform them into tumours. These so-called viral oncogenes have evolved through the 'capture' and exploitation of mammalian genes by viruses. In their original form such genes are essential components of normal mammalian cellular physiology and are expressed, usually to facilitate increased cellular proliferation, only at critical stages in the development or function of a tissue. When such 'proto-oncogenes' are activated inappropriately within the mammalian genome, without the intervention of a virus, they are termed 'oncogenes'. This can occur because of a mutation to the control sequence for the gene, causing over-expression of the normal product, or a mutation in the coding sequence itself, giving rise to a product that functions normally but which cannot be broken down. For example, the K-*ras* gene, which codes for a protein-regulating cell proliferation, is mutated and hence abnormally expressed early in the development of approximately 40% of human colorectal carcinomas.[12]

In contrast to the proto-oncogenes, over-expression of which creates conditions that favour tumour growth, it is the loss of expression of a tumour-suppressor gene that facilitates development of malignant characteristics in a cell. The *p53* gene is a good example.[13] The *p53* product is a protein of molecular weight 53 kD, which functions as a regulator of cell proliferation, and as a mediator of programmed cell death in response to unrepaired DNA damage. The absence of *p53*, or its presence in a mutated and therefore non-functional form, allows cells bearing other forms of DNA damage to continue dividing rather than undergoing apoptosis.[14, 15] There are familial forms of cancer caused by an inherited *p53* defect, and acquired mutations of this gene are among the most common genomic abnormalities found in a variety of human cancers.

According to the 'two hit hypothesis' for the functional role of tumour-suppressor genes, mutations at both alleles are required to fully inactivate the tumour suppressor activity of such genes.[16] However, another important mechanism for the induction of genetic abnormalities has attracted attention in recent years. Cytosine bases in the DNA backbone can acquire a methyl group which, if they lie within the promoter region of a gene, can cause it to be 'silenced' or, in effect, switched off.[17] This is a normal mechanism for the regulation of gene expression but it is becoming clear that abnormal DNA methylation can also occur and be transmitted across successive cell divisions. This provides a so-called 'epigenetic' mechanism for the inactivation of genes regulating tumour suppression or DNA repair, which can contribute to the complex series of events leading to the development of a tumour.[18]

6.3 Models of carcinogenesis

The simplest experimental model of carcinogenesis is the three-stage model consisting of initiation, promotion and progression.[19] At the initiation stage, a single cell is thought to acquire a mutation and then divide repeatedly so that the mutation is passed on to a clone of daughter cells, thus forming a focal lesion that can survive and grow at the expense of neighbouring cells. During promotion, the normal constraints on proliferation and spatial organisation within the affected tissue are disrupted further, and the appearance of further mutations to proto-oncogenes and tumour suppressor genes leads to a progressive loss of differentiation and orderly growth. The genes involved in this transition to cancer, and the functions they perform, are under intensive investigation and are particularly well characterised in the intestinal epithelium.[20]

At the progression stage the lesion has made the transition to malignancy and can give rise to secondary tumours at remote sites. Animal models have been used to identify specific carcinogenic substances which can act as mutagens at the initiation stage but do induce malignancy on their own, promoters which cannot initiate tumours but do accelerate tumour development after initiation, and complete carcinogens, which can do both. As we shall see later, this approach has also been used to identify inhibitors of carcinogenesis and to delineate their mode of action. The difficulty with animal models of carcinogenesis is that they usually require the application of large doses of carcinogens and promoters to groups of rodents, so that a high tumour yield is obtained during the course of the experiment. Such techniques are a poor model for induction of human cancers because these are usually caused by very prolonged exposure to a complex array of unknown carcinogenic stimuli over the course of a lifetime. However, there is no doubt that much of the fundamental understanding of tumour biology that has been gained from animal studies applies also to human disease.

6.4 Diet and gene interactions

As we have seen, carcinogenesis is a prolonged multi-stage process which usually occurs over many years. Because of its complexity there are, in principle, many critical steps at which food-related substances or metabolic processes may interact with the sequence of events so as to accelerate, delay or even reverse it. Diet-related anti-carcinogenesis can usefully be classified into *blocking mechanisms*, which operate during the initiation phase of carcinogenesis, and *suppressing mechanisms*, which delay or reverse tumour promotion at a later stage.[21, 22] A schematic illustration of these concepts and a summary of the mechanisms through which they may act is given in Fig. 6.1.

The principal blocking mechanism through which dietary constituents are thought to act is modulation of the Phase I and Phase II biotransformation enzymes which are expressed strongly in the gastrointestinal mucosa and in the liver and act as a first line of defence against toxic substances in the environment.[23] Phase I enzymes such as the cytochrome P450 complex catalyse oxidation, reduction and hydrolytic reactions, thereby increasing the solubility of potentially toxic compounds. However, this phase may also create electrophilic intermediates and hence activate pro-carcinogens. Phase II enzymes such as glutathione S-transferase act on the products of Phase I metabolism to form conjugates, which generally reduces their reactivity and increases their excretion. Thus, the biological activity of a carcinogen will often depend upon the relative activities of the Phase I and II enzymes involved in its

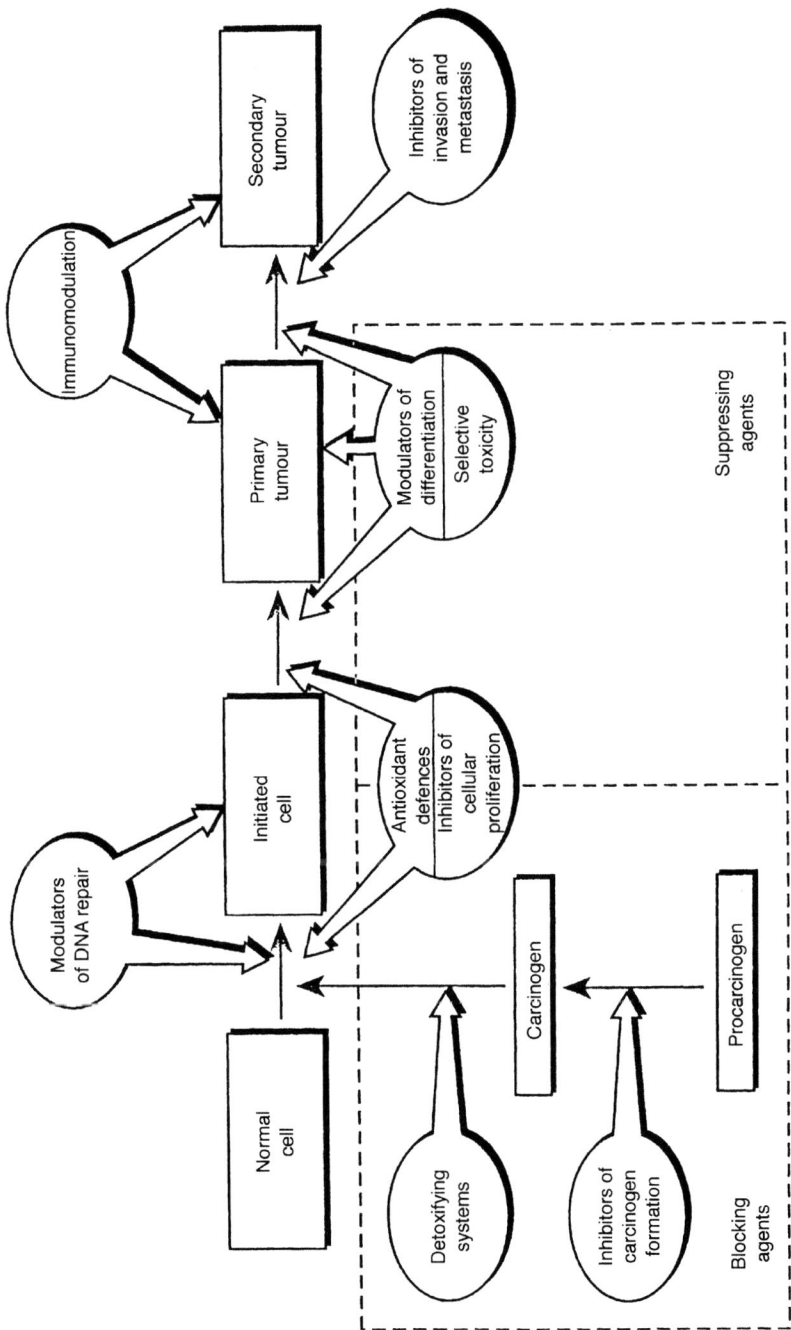

Fig. 6.1 Hypothetical sites of interaction between anti-carcinogenic substances in the diet and the progressive stages of carcinogenesis. Blocking agents are those acting to prevent initiation, whereas suppressing agents act to inhibit the development of tumours from initiated cells. (Reproduced from Johnson et al., 1994).[21]

metabolism. Pharmacological and dietary treatments can be used to block Phase I enzymes and enhance Phase II activity, so as to minimise the activation of carcinogens and increase their excretion. There is good evidence from experimental animal studies that this strategy can reduce DNA damage and tumour yield.[24]

Experimental animal studies have also shown that some substances can inhibit the appearance of tumours, even when given days or weeks after exposure to a chemical carcinogen.[25] Hence the mechanism of action cannot involve protection against DNA damage, but instead be due to some reduction in the rate at which initiated cells develop into tumours (Fig. 6.1). Suppression of carcinogenesis may involve inhibition of mitosis and increased expression of the differentiated phenotype, which serves to reduce the clonal expansion of initiated cells, or an increased susceptibility to undergo programmed cell death or apoptosis, which can eliminate pre-cancerous cells from the tissue.[26, 27]

6.5 Mechanisms of action: nutrients

6.5.1 General nutrition

Although prolonged energy, protein or micronutrient malnutrition may increase an individual's risk of developing cancer, perhaps by reducing the effectiveness of the immune system, life expectancy in societies with large malnourished populations is low, and infectious diseases are more likely to be the principal causes of illness and mortality. In prosperous Western societies, over-consumption of energy, coupled with inadequate exercise, appears to be a major risk factor for cancer. The World Cancer Research Fund report on diet and cancer[4] made some general recommendations on food supply, eating and related factors. For individuals, the general advice was to consume nutritionally adequate and varied diets based predominantly on fruits, vegetables, pulses and minimally processed starchy foods. Overweight, defined as body mass index (BMI: weight in kg/[height in metres]^2) in excess of 25 is associated with a rise in the relative risk of most cancers, and frank obesity is particularly associated with cancers of the breast and endometrium. For these reasons the report recommended that BMI should be maintained between 18.5 and 25. The committee did not consider that fat consumption was directly associated with cancer risk, but it did recommend that fat should contribute no more than 30% of total energy consumption, so as to reduce the risk of weight gain.

The general recommendations on energy and fat intake are similar to those for the avoidance of heart disease and are not in themselves very relevant to the concept of functional foods. However, the recommendation to consume a variety of fruits and vegetables is based partly on the putative presence of diverse protective factors in plant foods. This concept does provide, at least in principle, a rationale for the development of functional products with desirable biological effects beyond the simple provision of nutrients at a level that prevents symptoms of deficiency.

6.5.2 Antioxidant nutrients

As mentioned earlier, mutations can occur as a result of oxidative damage to DNA caused by free radicals generated as a damaging side-effect of aerobic metabolism.[28] Superoxide radicals are formed by the addition of an electron to molecular oxygen. These highly reactive species can then acquire a further electron and combine with protons to form hydrogen peroxide. In the presence of transition metal ions such as $Fe2^+$ and $Cu2^+$, hydrogen peroxide can break down to give even more highly reactive hydroxy radicals which may damage DNA directly, or participate in self-propagating chain reactions with membrane lipids. Plant and animal cells defend themselves against these effects by deploying so-called antioxidant compounds to trap or quench free radicals and hence arrest their damaging reactions. A variety of defence systems based on both water- and lipid-soluble antioxidant species and on antioxidant enzymes are deployed throughout the intra- and extracellular environment, at the sites most vulnerable to pro-oxidant damage. Many of those in the human body are dependent upon antioxidants derived from the diet. The theory that free radicals are a major cause of human cancer and that the risk of disease can be reduced by increased consumption of food-borne antioxidants has prompted an enormous growth of interest in antioxidant nutrients and other antioxidant substances in food.[29] It is worth noting, however, that the role of mutagenesis due to oxygen free radicals in the pathogenesis of human cancers remains largely hypothetical,[28] and attempts to prevent cancer by intervention with high doses of antioxidant vitamins have been largely unsuccessful.[30, 31]

Vitamin E

The major lipid-soluble antioxidant is vitamin E, first isolated from wheatgerm oil and obtained principally from nuts, seed oils and cereals. Vitamin E is actually a collective term for eight compounds: a-, b-, g- and d- tocopherol, and a-, b-, g- and d- tocotrienol, but RRR-a-tocopherol, accounts for 90% of endogenous vitamin E activity in humans. All the tocopherols and tocotrienols contain a hydroxyl-bearing aromatic ring structure, which enables them to donate hydrogen to free radicals, and thus act as biological antioxidants. The unpaired electron which results from hydrogen donation is delocalised into the ring structure of the tocopherol, rendering it relatively stable and unreactive. Chain reactions initiated by hydroxy radicals can be broken by the formation of a stable radical as a result of interaction with vitamin E.[32] Vitamin E is readily incorporated into cell membranes, which, being rich in polyunsaturated fatty acids, are highly susceptible to damage by free radicals derived from metabolic activity. In humans, frank symptoms of vitamin E deficiency are only seen in premature infants or malabsorption states, but intakes higher than are required to protect against deficiency may provide additional protection against free-radical mediated DNA damage. Epidemiological studies show a strong inverse correlation between risk of cancer and vitamin E intake at the population level, but the association is not corroborated by studies of individuals taking supplements.[33] Moreover a well-controlled investigation designed to test the hypothesis that dietary supplementation with vitamins C and E would reduce the recurrence of adenomas in patients who had undergone polypectomy showed no evidence of a protective effect.[31] Similarly a prolonged placebo-controlled intervention with vitamin E or vitamin E and beta-carotene failed to prevent the development of lung cancer in smokers.[30]

Carotenoids

Approximately 500 carotenoids have been identified in vegetables and fruits used as human foods, but the vast majority of these compounds occur at low concentrations and are probably of little nutritional importance. By far the most well-known and intensively studied of the carotenoids is beta-carotene,[34] which is a precursor for vitamin A, but the increased interest in dietary antioxidants in recent years has focused attention on other carotenoids such as lycopene and lutein which are abundant in tomatoes and coloured vegetables.[35, 36] The molecular structure of the carotenoids includes an extended chain of double bonds which enables them to function as antioxidants. Carotenoids are released from plant foods in the small intestine and absorbed in conjunction with dietary fat. Beta-carotene is converted into vitamin A by enzymes in the intestinal mucosa but it is detectable in human plasma, at levels that are related positively to the dietary intake of fruits and vegetables, and at least ten other carotenoids have also been recorded in human blood.

There is good epidemiological evidence for an inverse association between intake of carotenoids and lung cancer, and weaker evidence for protective effects against cancers of the alimentary tract.[37] The possibility that carotenoids might express antioxidant activity in human tissues, thereby protecting cell membranes, proteins and DNA against damage by free radicals, provides a plausible rationale for these associations, but once again the causal link has not been proven and the possibility remains that carotenoids are acting as markers for fruit and vegetable intake which may be beneficial for other reasons.[36] Intervention trials with beta-carotene have proved disappointing. The Alpha-Tocopherol Beta-Carotene (ATBC) study, which involved over 29,000 male smokers, and included a cohort given 20 mg beta-carotene daily for up to eight years, produced no evidence for a protective effect against cancer at any site. On the contrary, there was a higher incidence of lung, prostate and stomach cancer in the beta-carotene group.[30] Similarly the CARET study, in which subjects received 30 mg beta-carotene and 25,000 international units of retinol per day, was terminated because of an increase in deaths from lung cancer in the treatment group.[38] There is no suggestion that beta-carotene is toxic in any other circumstances, even when given at pharmacological doses for long periods to treat photosensitivity disorders,[39] but the evidence suggests that it may act as a tumour promoter when taken by subjects already harbouring pre-cancerous lesions induced by chronic exposure to tobacco smoke. Under these circumstances it is obviously inappropriate to encourage the development and consumption of functional foods designed to provide consumers with high doses of carotenoids, but the general advice to increase fruit and vegetable consumption remains valid.

Vitamin C

Vitamin C occurs as L-ascorbic acid and dihydroascorbic acid in fruits, vegetables and potatoes, as well as processed foods to which it has been added as an antioxidant. The only wholly undisputed function of vitamin C is the prevention of scurvy. Although this is the physiological rationale for the currently recommended intake levels, there is growing evidence that vitamin C may provide additional protective effects against other diseases including cancer, and the RDA may be increased in the near future. Scurvy develops in adults whose habitual intake of vitamin C falls below 1 mg/d, and under experimental conditions 10 mg/d is sufficient to prevent or alleviate symptoms.[40] The recommended dietary allowance (RDA) is 60 mg per day in the USA, but plasma levels of ascorbate do not achieve saturation until daily intakes reach around 100 mg.[41] Ascorbate is probably the most effective water-soluble antioxidant in the plasma. It scavenges and reduces nitrite, thus inhibiting the formation of carcinogenic *N*-nitroso compounds in the stomach, and *in vitro* studies suggest that it plays a protective role against oxidative damage to cell constituents and circulating lipoproteins.[42] The epidemiological evidence is consistent with a protective effect of vitamin C against cancers of the stomach, pharynx and oesophagus in particular,[43] but the evidence for causality remains inconclusive because of the sheer complexity of the composition of fruits and vegetables, which are the main source of the vitamin in the unsupplemented diet. Byers and Guerrero[33] considered the collective evidence from a large series of case-control and cohort studies in which intakes of fruits and vegetables, and of vitamins C and E from food or from supplements, were determined. There was a strong and consistent protective effect of fruits and vegetables against cancers of the alimentary tract and lung and a correlation with estimated vitamin C intake based on fruit and vegetable composition. However, there were considerable confounding effects of other dietary constituents and the evidence for a protective effect of vitamin C from supplements was less convincing. Most of the ascorbate in human diets is derived from natural sources, and consumers who eat five portions, or about 400–500 g, of fruits and vegetables per day could obtain as much as 200 mg of ascorbate. Nevertheless, given the low cost and low toxicity of ascorbate, it seems likely that there will be a continuing trend towards supplementation of foods.

6.5.3 Folate

In historical terms, folates are among the most recently identified of the vitamins. Wills was the first to describe a form of anaemia associated with pregnancy and malnutrition which could be cured by yeast or liver extract.[44, 45] The active constituent of these dietary supplements was eventually isolated as folic acid (pteroylglutamic acid), a water-soluble substance containing a pteridine ring linked to *para*-aminobenzoic acid and glutamic acid. Naturally occurring folates originate from green plants and yeast cells, and are plentiful in liver and kidney. They are usually reduced and substituted in the pteridene moiety, and contain up to seven glutamate residues. Dietary folates are deconjugated to the monoglutamic form at the surface of the intestinal mucosa, actively transported and mostly metabolised by the epithelial cells to the main circulating form which is 5-methyltetrahydrofolic acid. The principal metabolic role of folates and their derivatives is to act as coenzymes in reactions involving transfer of single carbon groups during the synthesis of amino acids and DNA. This accounts for their vital role in the support of growth, pregnancy and the production of blood cells. It has been conclusively established that an inadequate supply of folates during the early stages of embryonic development increases the risk of neural tube defects,[46] and a number of foods, including breakfast cereals and bread, are now routinely enriched with folic acid. Growing interest in the relationship between human folate status and the long-term risk of disease will probably ensure that this trend continues.

It is well established that folate-deficient diets are associated with increased risk of hepatic cancer in animal models.[47] Rats fed diets deficient in methyl donating groups have higher rates of cell proliferation, increased DNA damage and a higher susceptibility to experimentally induced cancers, which appears to result from changes in gene expression associated with abnormalities of DNA synthesis.[48] The precise relationship between folate metabolism and carcinogenesis is unclear, but the link may lie in the role that folate coenzymes play in the control of DNA methylation. In mammals and many other organisms the cytosine nucleotides in the DNA backbone frequently become methylated by the enzyme DNA-methyltransferase (DNA-MTase) after replication. As mentioned earlier, the methylation pattern of the cytosine residues is now believed to be an important determinant of gene expression. Much remains to be learned about this topic, but in general, loss of methylation could cause abnormal expression of oncogenes controlling cell proliferation, whereas inappropriate methylation of cytosine-rich regions of DNA in the promoter regions of tumour suppressor genes could cause loss of function.[49]

Issa et al.[50] demonstrated that methylation of CpG islands in the estrogen receptor gene (ER) occurs in a very high proportion of colorectal tumours, and that the same site-specific abnormality occurs progressively with age in the otherwise normal colorectal mucosa of human subjects with no colorectal neoplasia. The same authors have also shown that expression of ER in tumour cells slows mitosis and should perhaps be regarded as a tumour suppressor gene, the silencing of which may be an early 'field' event inducing hyperproliferation and predisposing the colorectal mucosa to induction of neoplasia. There is no direct evidence that human folate metabolism is involved with these phenomena, but there is circumstantial evidence that inadequate folate nutrition is a risk factor for cancer, particularly of the bowel and cervix.[51] Recently Ma et al.[52] explored the relationship between risk of colorectal carcinoma and a common mutation affecting the activity of the enzyme 5,10-methylenetetrahydrofolate reductase (MTHFR) in a large cohort study. The presence of a homozygous mutation was shown to reduce the risk of colerectal cancer in men with adequate folate levels, but the protection was absent in men with low overall folate status. One possible explanation for this effect is that low levels of MTHFR expression shunt folates into DNA synthesis, thereby helping to maintain normal patterns of DNA methylation. Low levels of folate might favour hypomethylation of cytosines, and possibly cause a compensatory upregulation of DNA-MTase, leading to hypermethylation of CpG islands, but this remains highly speculative. Nevertheless the growing epidemiological evidence that inadequate folate nutrition increases the risk of cancer, whereas long-term use of folate supplements reduces risk,[53] will ensure that interest in the preventive role of folate-supplemented foods will continue.

6.6 Mechanisms of action: phytochemicals

The discovery that in industrialised societies diets that are deficient in fruits and vegetables can effectively double the risk of developing many different types of cancer has focused renewed attention on the beneficial properties of these foods.[6, 54] As we have seen, plant foods are rich in micronutrients, but they also contain an immense variety of biologically active secondary metabolites providing colour, flavour and natural toxicity to pests and sometimes humans.[21] The chemistry and classification of such substances is still a matter for much research and debate, but this has not prevented attempts to isolate and exploit substances that have variously been termed 'protective factors', 'phytoprotectants' and 'nutraceuticals'. Commercial applications tend to be confined to the health food market at the present time. The non-nutrient carotenoids mentioned earlier fall into the present category, as do a host of compounds containing phenol rings, phytosterols, sulphur-containing compounds found in onions and their relatives, and another group of sulphur compounds, the glucosinolates from brassica vegetables. Only a few of the more important examples will be discussed here.

6.6.1 Phenolic compounds

A huge variety of biologically active phenolic compounds containing one or more aromatic rings are found naturally in plant foods, where they provide much of the flavour, colour and texture. The simpler phenolic substances include monophenols with a single benzene ring, such as 3-ethylphenol and 3,4-dimethylphenol found in fruits and seeds, the hydroxycinnamic acid group which contains caffeic and ferulic acid, and the flavonoids and their glycosides which include catechins, proanthocyanins, anthocyanidins and flavonols. The tannins are a complex and poorly defined group of water-soluble phenolics with high molecular weights. The daily intake of phenolic substances may be as high as 1 g per day, but the quantity of defined flavonoids in the diet probably amounts to no more than a few tens of milligrams per day.

Flavonoids

As long ago as 1936, Rusznyàk and Szent-Györgi[55] proposed that the flavonols were an essential dietary factor contributing to the maintenance of capillary permeability. This is no longer thought to be true, but recent interest in dietary antioxidants and metabolically active phytochemicals has focused renewed attention on the possible beneficial effects of flavonoids.[56, 57] Flavonoids are very effective antioxidants and it has been proposed that they protect against cardiovascular disease by reducing the oxidation of low density lipoproteins. There is some epidemiological evidence for this, but flavonoids are generally poorly absorbed from food, and their effects on the overall antioxidant capacity of the plasma remains to be established. Nevertheless flavonoids and other phenolic substances may exert local anti-carcinogenic effects in the intestine where, in addition to acting as intraluminal antioxidants, they may induce Phase II xenobiotic metabolising enzymes, suppress the production of biologically active prostaglandins by inhibiting the arachidonic acid cascade,[58] and inhibit mitosis by inhibiting intracellular protein kinases.[59]

Although briefly under suspicion as a natural carcinogen,[60] the ubiquitous flavonol quercetin is now regarded as a possible protective factor against cancers of the alimentary tract.[61]

Phytoestrogens

The phytoestrogens are diphenolic compounds derived from plant foods and which bear a structural similarity to mammalian estrogens.[62] The glycosides genistin and daidzin, and their methylated derivatives biochanin A and formononetin, which are found principally in soya products, are broken down by the intestinal microflora to yield genistein, daidzein, and in some individuals, equol, all of which are absorbed into the circulation, and they or their breakdown products can be detected in human urine.[63] The lignan precursors matairesinol and secoisolariciresinol occur more commonly in cereal seeds such as flax. They are also degraded in the gut to yield the active lignans enterolactone and enterodiol. These compounds exert weak hormone-like activity and may bind to oestrogen receptors *in vivo*, thereby effectively blocking the more potent activity of endogenous oestrogens. In human feeding trials with soy products, isoflavones have been shown to modify the menstrual cycle, and there is much interest in the possibility that these compounds could suppress the growth of hormone-dependent tumours of the breast and reproductive organs.[62] There are also epidemiological associations suggesting a protective effect of soy-based diets against prostate cancer in males,[64] but once again the causal mechanisms have not been proven and there is a strong possibility of confounding by other dietary factors.

Genistein may also suppress tumour growth by other non-oestrogenic mechanisms including suppression of cell turnover by inhibition of protein kinases involved in the regulation of mitosis. On the other hand, it is less widely recognised that genistein is an inhibitor of topoisomerase II, an enzyme that helps to maintain the structure of DNA during mitosis. Both synthetic topoisomerase poisons and genistein are known to be mutagenic *in vitro*, but the biological significance of this is unclear.[65] There is no epidemiological evidence to suggest any adverse effect of soy products in humans, but caution is obviously necessary when considering the incorporation of such biologically active compounds into functional foods.

6.6.2 Glucosinolates

Interest in glucosinolates stems from epidemiological and experimental evidence showing that brassica vegetables such as cabbage, sprouts, kale and broccoli seem to offer particularly strong protection against cancer of the lung and gastrointestinal tract.[7, 66] The brassicas, and a few other edible plants drawn from the order *Capparales*, are the source of all the glucosinolates in the human diet. Around 100 different compounds have been identified, all of which possess the same fundamental structure comprising a β-D-thioglucose group, a sulphonated oxime moiety and a variable side-chain.[67] Glucosinolates occur throughout the plant, although the concentration varies between tissues, and they are stable under normal conditions. However, when the plant tissue is physically damaged, for example by food preparation or chewing, they come into contact with an enzyme – myrosinase – which is released from intracellular vacuoles. Myrosinase hydrolyses the glucosinolates to release glucose and an unstable product which then undergoes further degradation to release a complex variety of breakdown products. The most important from the nutritional point of view are the isothiocyanates, a group of hot and bitter compounds, commonly termed 'mustard oils'. These compounds, which are often volatile with an acrid smell, are the principal source of flavour in mustard, radishes and the milder vegetables.[67] High levels of glucosinolates reduce the palatability of plant tissues for generalist herbivores such as birds and molluscs, but specialist invertebrate herbivores have adapted to their presence and may be attracted specifically to feed on plants containing particular compounds.[68] Glucosinolates with an aliphatic side-chain containing a beta-hydroxy group yield isothiocyanates which spontaneously cyclise to form stable oxazolidine-2-thiones. These compounds are goitrogenic to domestic livestock, and this is an important limiting factor in the commercial exploitation of brassica feedstuffs.[69]

There is ample evidence from both animal experiments and tissue cultures studies to show that brassica vegetables and their constituents selectively induce Phase II enzymes. Evidence for the induction of Phase II enzymes by two classes of glucosinolate breakdown products, the isothiocyanates and indole-3-carbinole, has been systematically reviewed recently by Verhoeven *et al.*[70] Particular attention has been paid to induction of Phase II enzymes by sulphorophane, an isothiocyanate derived from broccoli,[71] but other isothiocyanates derived from other common brassica vegetables probably exert comparable levels of biological activity.[72]

Wattenberg[25] showed that both cruciferous vegetables and benzyl isothiocyanate could inhibit the appearance of tumours in experimental animals long after the initial exposure to a carcinogen. Suppressing mechanisms are still poorly understood but one possibility is that glucosinolate breakdown products modulate the level of apoptosis in target tissues. Isothiocyanates have been shown recently to induce apoptosis in tissue culture, and in the colorectal crypts of the rat after treatment with the carcinogen dimethylhydrazine, an effect which is associated with a reduction in pre-cancerous lesions.[27]

6.7 Mechanisms of action: other factors

Apart from recognised nutrients and the emerging plethora of potentially biologically active secondary plant metabolites or phytoprotectants, a variety of other food-borne factors that are difficult to classify may play some role in the prevention of cancer. For example, epidemiological evidence suggests that consumption of a relatively high ratio of fish and poultry to red meat significantly decreases the risk of bowel cancer.[73] The reasons for this are unclear. Such diets may provide a favourable balance of amino acids or minerals, a relatively low intake of potentially pro-oxidant iron, or a relatively high intake of certain polyunsaturated fatty acids. However, far more research will be necessary before any underlying principles can be exploited for use in the context of functional foods.

Dietary fibre, which comprises all the non-digestible structural carbohydrates of plant cell walls and any associated lignin, provides a further example of a complex food-borne factor which cannot be classified as a nutrient, and which continues to generate debate over such issues as definition and analytical techniques. However, whatever the unresolved complexities, dietary fibre has a lengthy history and had proved itself eminently suitable as a component of functional food products long before the term was even coined.

6.7.1 Dietary fibre

The concept of dietary fibre as an anti-carcinogenic food constituent was first proposed by Burkitt[74] who based his initial hypothesis on observations of disease incidence among rural Africans, claiming that the various non-digestible polysaccharides of plant cell walls in their traditional, largely plant-based diets were protective against a range of diseases including cancer of the large bowel. On the whole this hypothesis has been supported by case-control studies. The limited evidence from large prospective studies has been somewhat less convincing, but the recent reports from the World Cancer Research Fund,[4] the European Cancer Prevention Organization[75] and the UK Department of Health[76] have all agreed that the evidence that dietary fibre protects against colorectal cancer is at least moderately convincing.

Burkitt's original hypothesis was based largely on the concept of faecal bulk. His field observations in Africa, where cancer and other chronic bowel diseases were rare, suggested that populations consuming traditional rural diets rich in vegetables and cereal foods produced stools that were bulkier and more frequent than those of persons living in the industrialised West. Some cell wall polysaccharides are readily metabolised by the faecal microflora and converted into bacterial mass, whereas others remain intact and help to retain faecal water. Burkitt argued that consumption of highly processed cereals subjected Westerners to a form of chronic constipation which led to a variety of conditions associated with straining to pass stool. Moreover a low volume of faecal material and infrequent bowel movements would lead to prolonged exposure of the colonic epithelial cells to faecal mutagens. In the years since it was proposed, this hypothesis has become widely accepted by the medical profession and the general public, and it certainly has never been disproved. The mildly laxative effects of dietary fibre are now well recognised, and numerous human intervention trials have confirmed that dietary supplements containing wheat bran or isphagula can increase the volume of faecal material and reduce the colonic transit time.[77] Human faecal water is genotoxic *in vitro*, and a number of known carcinogens including heterocyclic amines and N-nitroso compounds are present at low concentrations in the faecal stream.[78, 79] It has not been conclusively established that these substances initiate colorectal carcinogenesis in humans, but a high consumption of fibre will certainly tend to reduce their concentration still further. Moreover the plausibility of the faecal bulking hypothesis has been strengthened by epidemiological study of Cummings *et al.*[80] which showed a statistically significant inverse relationship between average stool weight and risk of bowel cancer across a range of populations. The faecal bulking hypothesis provides the principal rationale for the current Department of Health recommendations for dietary reference values in the UK which suggest that adults should consume an average of 18 g fibre per day.

The realisation that colorectal carcinogenesis is a prolonged multi-stage process involving a complex set of genetic changes has raised a host of new questions about the interactions that can occur between the colonic epithelium, dietary fibre or its breakdown products, and other constituents of the faecal stream. For example, it has long been suspected that bile salts may cause chronic irritation in the colon and hence act as endogenous tumour promoters.[81] Certainly bile salts stimulate colonic mucosal cell proliferation, both in tissue culture and in animals. Moreover, high fat diets tend to increase the level of bile acids in the faecal stream, and this effect could explain the adverse effect of total fat consumption on the risk of bowel cancer.[73] Conversely, fibre may dilute faecal bile acids by increasing bulk, and the non-fermentable particulate components of plant cell walls may also provide a finely dispersed solid phase upon which bile salts can be adsorbed, thereby reducing their concentration in faecal water.[82]

Those components of dietary fibre that are vulnerable to fermentation by faecal micro-organisms may exert another, more active anti-carcinogenic effect. The main products of carbohydrate fermentation in the colon are the short chain fatty acids acetate, propionate and butyrate. These substances can be absorbed and utilised as metabolic substrates.[83] Butyrate is known to be utilised preferentially by the colonic mucosa, and a steady supply of butyrate appears to be essential for mucosal integrity.[84] Recently it has emerged that besides supplying metabolic energy, butyrate may increase the extent to which colonic epithelial cells are differentiated and induce apoptosis of tumour cells.[85] If this hypothesis is correct, then prolonged consumption of fermentable carbohydrates may be an important dietary strategy for reducing the risk of colorectal cancer. However, rapidly fermentable oligosaccharides may disappear too rapidly after entering the right colon to provide a supply of butyrate to the more distal regions of the large bowel. Lignified plant cell walls, and also starches which are resistant to digestion in the small bowel, are fermented much more slowly and so probably deliver butyrate to a greater surface area of mucosa.

Although the colon seems the most likely site for fibre to exert its anti-carcinogenic effects, there is also some evidence that it may protect against cancer of other organs, especially the breast. For example, Howe et al.[86] reviewed ten case-control studies of breast cancer and diet and concluded that a 20 g increase in fibre was associated with a statistically significant reduction in risk of breast cancer of about 15%. This is a relatively small effect associated with an increase in fibre consumption somewhat in excess of the average consumption of fibre in Northern Europe and the USA, but the association raises the interesting issue of how fibre might exert anti-carcinogenic effects in tissues remote from the gut lumen. One possibility is that diets very rich in fibre lead to reductions in post-prandial glucose and insulin, and lower plasma oestrogen levels. These effects may inhibit the growth of hormone-dependent tumours.[87]

In spite of the generally positive epidemiological evidence for a protective effect of fibre against cancer, it is not entirely clear that real benefits can be achieved at the levels of fibre consumption typical of the industrialised West. A long-term prospective study conducted with a large cohort of American nurses has recently failed to demonstrate any protective effect of fibre intake against bowel cancer or adenomatous polyps,[88] perhaps because even the highest level of fibre intake (24.9 ± 5.5 g/d in the top quintile of the population) was too low to provide a measurable biological effect. This interpretation is supported by a study of dietary trends and the changing rates of colorectal cancer in Japan and the USA, showing that the steeply rising incidence in Japan in recent years coincided with a decline in fibre intake below 20 g per day.[89] For consumers there seems little reason to deviate from current nutritional advice to increase the intake of dietary fibre by consuming a variety of sources including cereals, vegetables and fruit, but it is not certain that the protective effects of dietary fibre can be readily achieved by consumption of conventional fibre-rich foods. High-fibre breakfast cereals are among the oldest and most well-established functional foods on the market, but further development of such products will require careful selection of polysaccharides to provide an optimal combination of palatability and biological effect.

6.8 Conclusion: the role of functional food

Great progress has been made towards a better understanding of the relationship between diet and cancer since Doll and Peto published their study on the causes of human cancer in 1981,[3] but the practical application of this knowledge in the fight against human disease remains frustratingly limited. As should now be clear, cancer is not a single disease arising from one causal event. In most cases the victim acquires the disease only after years of exposure to a host of environmental factors which will have interacted with his or her unique genome, throughout a large fraction of their lifespan. Even in the case of carcinoma of the lung, which is the most frequent cause of death from cancer in most Western countries, and which has a known and avoidable cause, it has required many years of patient epidemiological investigation to establish this relationship beyond doubt, and it is still not possible to predict any individual smoker's particular level of risk with certainty. The problem of diet and cancer is immensely more difficult because of the variety of diseases involved and the complexity of human diets, and because the task requires the recognition and understanding of an array of protective factors rather than any single source of carcinogens.

As we have seen, some of the most compelling evidence for a protective effect of diets against cancer to emerge in recent years is that for fruit and vegetables.[6, 90] Despite the difficulties of disentangling the effects of diet from other aspects of lifestyle such as smoking, exercise and alcohol consumption, most authorities agree that, compared to those at the other end of the scale, the highest consumers of fruits and vegetables in most populations have about half the risk of developing most types of cancer.

In an age of convenience foods and pre-cooked meals, many consumers find a high consumption of fresh vegetables difficult to achieve. At first sight this seems to provide an excellent opportunity for the development of functional food products which could provide the protective effects of fresh vegetables without the need for greatly increased bulk or frequency of consumption. The difficulty lies in the sheer complexity of plants and the bewildering variety of diseases to which the protective effects seem to apply. There have been brave attempts to confront this problem with the development of a unifying hypothesis such as the dietary fibre model, or more recently the antioxidant theory, but attempts to prove these hypotheses have failed. Diet is inescapably complex, and food often seems to exert biological effects greater than the sum of its parts. No doubt the anti-carcinogenic mechanisms that underlie the protective effects of plant foods are susceptible to experimental investigation but we seem far from the isolation of a single substance or group of substances that can be incorporated into functional food products with any confidence.

6.9 Future trends

What of the future? First, there is ample room for optimism that the expansion of basic knowledge in the field of human cancers and their causes will continue, and probably accelerate. It follows that our understanding of the relationship between conventional nutrition, other protective substances in food, and cancer will continue to develop and provide greater insight into the role of diet across the lifetime of the individual. With this knowledge we will be better able to assess the role of individual foods within the diet, and hence to optimise the composition of such foods to increase their impact.

The second major factor is the rapid progress that is being achieved in the related fields of human genomics and the genetic manipulation of organisms used for human food. In time, our increasing knowledge of the human genome will shed more light on the interplay of genes and environment which determines an individual's risk of disease, and this should lead to an increasing degree of 'personalisation' of dietary advice. At the same time our ability to manipulate the genome of other organisms will give food producers and manufacturers the power to enhance the composition of plant foods to maximise their protective effects. This is, of course, an optimistic assessment of future trends; the inherent difficulties of this approach to human diets in terms of consumer confidence must by now be obvious to all. Already it is possible to predict much of a person's genetically determined risk of disease, but such knowledge can be an emotional burden to the individual concerned, and an excuse for damaging discrimination by institutions and potential employers. At the time of writing, the issue of genetic modification of plant foods has gripped the public imagination, and products containing such ingredients are rapidly disappearing from the marketplace. It remains to be seen whether a second or third generation of products carrying proven benefits to health will, given time, become acceptable to public opinion. In any event we must try to ensure that the premature release of commercial products that prove to be ineffectual or, far worse, actually harmful, does not lead to a general debasement of the whole concept of dietary strategies for the avoidance of cancer.

6.10 Sources of further information and advice

British Nutrition Foundation, *Report of the Task Force on Protective Substances in Food*, in press.

JOHNSON, I.T. and FENWICK, G.R. (eds) 'Dietary Anticarcinogens and Antimutagens: Chemical and Biological Aspects', *Proceedings of Food and Cancer Prevention III*, Cambridge, Royal Society of Chemistry, in press.

Department of Health, *Nutritional Aspects of the Development of Cancer*, London, HMSO, 1998.

American Institute for Cancer Research, *Food, Nutrition and the Prevention of Cancer: A Global Perspective*, Washington DC, 1997.

WALDRON, K.W., JOHNSON, I.T. and FENWICK, G.R. (eds) *Food and Cancer Prevention: Chemical and Biological Aspects*, Cambridge, Royal Society of Chemistry, 1993.

6.11 References

1 TANCHOU, S. 'Recherches sur la fréquence du cancer', *Gazette des hôpitaux*, July 1843, 6.

2 World Health Organization, *The World Health Report*, Geneva, WHO, 1997.

3 DOLL, R. and PETO, R. 'The causes of cancer: quantitative estimates of avoidable risks of cancer in the United States today', *J Nat Cancer Inst*, 1981, **66**, 1191–308.

4 World Cancer Research Fund, 'Colon, rectum', *Food, Nutrition and the Prevention of Cancer: A Global Perspective*, pp. 216–51, Washington DC, American Institute for Cancer Research, 1997.

5 GAZIANO, J.M., HENNEKENS, C.H., GODFRIED, S.L., SESSO, H.D., GLYNN, R.J., BRESLOW, J.L. and BURING, J.E. 'Type of alcoholic beverage and risk of myocardial infarction', *Am J Cardiol*, 1999, **83**, 52–7.

6 BLOCK, G., PATTERSON, B. and SUBAR, A. 'Fruit, vegetables, and cancer prevention: a review of the epidemiological evidence', *Nutr Cancer*, 1992, **18**, 1–29.

7 STEINMETZ, K.A. and POTTER, J.D. 'Vegetables, fruit, and cancer prevention: a review', *J Am Diet Assoc*, 1996, **96**, 1027–39.

8 ANDERSON, M.W., YOU, M. and REYNOLDS, S.H. 'Proto-oncogene activation in rodent and human tumors', *Adv Exp Med Biol*, 1991, **283**, 235–43.

9 FEARON, E.R. and VOGELSTEIN, B. 'A genetic model for colorectal tumorigenesis', *Cell*, 1990, **16**, 759–67.

10 NOWELL, P.C. 'The clonal evolution of tumour cell populations', *Science*, 1976, **194**, 23–8.

11 ANDERSON, M.W., REYNOLDS, S.H., YOU, M. and MARONPOT, R.M. 'Role of proto-oncogene activation in carcinogenesis', *Environ Health Perspect*, 1992, **98**, 13–24.

12 BOS, J.L., FEARON, E.R., HAMILTON, S.R., VERLAAN DE VRIES, M., VAN BOOM, J.H., VAN DER EB, A.J. and VOGELSTEIN, B. 'Prevalence of ras gene mutations in human colorectal cancers', *Nature*, 1987, **327**, 293–7.

13 DONEHOWER, L.A. and BRADLEY, A. 'The tumor suppressor p53', *Biochim Biophys Acta*, 1993, **1155**, 181–205.

14 BAKER, S.J., FEARON, E.R., NIGRO, J.M., HAMILTON, S.R., PREISINGER, A.C., JESSUP, J.M., VAN TUINEN, P., LEDBETTER, D.H., BARKER, D.F., NAKAMURA, Y. *et al.* 'Chromosome 17 deletions and p53 gene mutations in colorectal carcinomas', *Science*, 1989, **244**, 217–21.

15 GERWIN, B.J., SPILLARE, E., FORRESTER, K., LEHMAN, T.A., KISPERT, J., WELSH, J.A., PFEIFER, A.M., LECHNER, J.F., BAKER, S.J., VOGELSTEIN, B. *et al.* 'Mutant

p53 can induce tumorigenic conversion of human bronchial epithelial cells and reduce their responsiveness to a negative growth factor, transforming growth factor beta 1', *Proc Natl Acad Sci USA*, 1992, **89**, 2759–63.

16 KNUDSON, A.G. Jr. 'The ninth Gordon Hamilton-Fairley memorial lecture. Hereditary cancers: clues to mechanisms of carcinogenesis', *Br J Cancer*, 1989, **59**, 661–6.

17 KASS, S.U., PRUSS, D. and WOLFFE, A.P. 'How does DNA methylation repress transcription?', *Trends Genet*, 1997, **13**, 444–9.

18 JONES, P.A. and LAIRD, P.W. 'Cancer epigenetics comes of age', *Nat Genet*, 1999, **21**, 163–7.

19 PITOT, H.C. and DRAGAN, Y.P. 'The multistage nature of chemically induced hepatocarcinogenesis in the rat', *Drug Metab Rev*, 1994, **26**, 209–20.

20 STAPPENBECK, T.S., WONG, M.S., SAAM, J.R., MYSOREKAR, I.U. and GORDON, J.I. 'Notes from some crypt watchers: regulation of renewal in the mouse intestinal epithelium', *Current Opinion Cell Biol*, 1998, **10**, 702–9.

21 JOHNSON, I.T., WILLIAMSON, G.M. and MUSK, S.R.R. 'Anticarcinogenic factors in plant foods: a new class of nutrients?', *Nutr Res Rev*, 1994, **7**, 175–204.

22 WATTENBERG, L. 'Inhibition of carcinogenesis by minor anutrient constituents of the diet', *Proc Nutr Soc*, 1990, **49**, 173–83.

23 GREENWALD, P., NIXON, D.W., MALONE, W.F., KELLOFF, G.J., STERN, H.R. and WITKIN, K.M. 'Concepts in cancer chemoprevention research', *Cancer*, 1990, **65**, 1483–90.

24 PRIMIANO, T., EGNER, P.A., SUTTER, T.R., KELLOFF, G.J., ROEBUCK, B.D. and KENSLER, T.W. 'Intermittent dosing with oltipraz: relationship between chemoprevention of aflatoxin-induced tumorigenesis and induction of glutathione S-transferases', *Cancer Res*, 1995, **55**, 4319–24.

25 WATTENBERG, L.W. 'Inhibition of carcinogen-induced neoplasia by sodium cyanate, tert-butylisocyanate and benzyl isothiocyanate administered subsequent to carcinogen exposure', *Cancer Res*, 1981, **41**, 2991–4.

26 CHAN, T.A., MORIN, P.J., VOGELSTEIN, B. and KINZLER, K.W. 'Mechanisms underlying nonsteroidal antiinflammatory drug-mediated apoptosis', *Proc Natl Acad Sci USA*, 1998, **95**, 681–6.

27 SMITH, T.K., LUND, E.K. and JOHNSON, I.T. 'Inhibition of dimethylhydrazine-induced aberrant crypt foci and induction of apoptosis in rat colon following oral administration of the glucosinolate sinigrin', *Carcinogenesis*, 1998, **19**, 267–73.

28 FEIG, D.I., REID, T.M. and LOEB, L.A. 'Reactive oxygen species in tumorigenesis', *Cancer Res*, 1994, **54**, 1890s–4s.

29 MCLARTY, J.W. 'Antioxidants and cancer: the epidemiological evidence'. In *Antioxidants and Disease Prevention*, H.S. Garewal (ed.), pp. 45–65, Boca Raton, CRC Press, 1997.

30 ALBANES, D., HEINONEN, O.P., HUTTUNEN, J.K., TAYLOR, P.R., VIRTAMA, J., EDWARDS, B.K., HAAPAKOSKI, J., RAUTALATHI, M., HARTMAN, A.M. and PALMGREN, J. 'Effects of alpha-tocopherol and beta carotene supplements on cancer incidence in the alpha-tocopherol beta-carotene cancer prevention

study', *Am J Clin Nutr,* 1995, **62**, 1427S–30S.

31 GREENBERG, E.R., BARON, J.A., TOSTESON, T.D., FREEMAN, D.H., Jr., BECK, G.J., BOND, J.H., COLACCHIO, T.A., COLLER, J.A., FRANKL, H.D., HAILE, R.W. *et al.* 'A clinical trial of antioxidant vitamins to prevent colorectal adenoma', *N Engl J Med,* 1994, **331**, 141–7.

32 BURTON, G.W., JOYCE, A. and INGOLD, K.U. 'First proof that vitamin E is the major lipid-soluble chain-breaking antioxidant in human blood plasma', *Lancet,* 1983, **2**, 327–8.

33 BYERS, T. and GUERRERO, N. 'Epidemiologic evidence for vitamin C and vitamin E in cancer prevention', *Am J Clin Nutr,* 1995, **62**, 1385S–92S.

34 WANG, X.D. 'Review: absorption and metabolism of beta-carotene', *J Am Coll Nutr,* 1994, **13**, 314–25.

35 KHACHIK, F., BEECHER, G.R. and SMITH, J.C. Jr. 'Lutein, lycopene, and their oxidative metabolites in chemoprevention of cancer', *J Cell Biochem Supp,* 1995, **22**, 236–46.

36 GIOVANNUCCI, E. 'Tomatoes, tomato-based products, lycopene, and cancer: review of the epidemiologic literature', *J Natl Cancer Inst,* 1999, **91**, 317–31.

37 VAN POPPEL, G. and GOLDBOHM, R.A. 'Epidemiological evidence for beta-carotene and cancer prevention', *Am J Clin Nutr,* 1995, **62**, 1393S–402S.

38 ROWE, P.M. 'Beta-carotene takes a collective beating', *Lancet,* 1996, **347**, 249.

39 DIPLOCK, A. 'The safety of beta-carotene and the antioxidant vitamins C and E'. In *Antioxidants and Disease Prevention,* H.S. Garewal (ed.), pp. 3–17, Boca Raton, CRC Press, 1997.

40 BARTLEY, W., KREBS, H.A. and O'BRIEN, J.P. *Vitamin C Requirements of Human Adults,* London, HMSO, 1953.

41 BATES, C.J., RUTISHAUSER, I.H.E., BLACK, A.E., PAUL, A.A., MANDAL, A.R. and PATNAIK, B.K. 'Long-term vitamin status and dietary intake of healthy elderly subjects', *Brit J Nutr,* 1979, **42**, 43–56.

42 FREI, B., ENGLAND, L. and AMES, B.N. 'Ascorbate is an outstanding antioxidant in human plasma', *Proc Natl Acad Sci, USA,* 1989, **86**, 6377–81.

43 BLOCK, G. 'Vitamin C and cancer prevention: the epidemiologic', *Am J Clin Nutr,* 1991, **53**, 270S–82S.

44 WILLS, L. 'The nature of the haemopoeitic factor in Marmite', *Lancet,* 1933, **1**, 1283–5.

45 WILLS, L., CLUTTERBUCK, P.W. and EVANS, P.D.F. 'A new factor in the production and cure of certain macrocytic anaemias', *Lancet,* 1937, **1**, 311–14.

46 SCOTT, J.M., KIRKE, P.N. and WEIR, D.G. 'The role of nutrition in neural tube defects', *Ann Rev Nutr,* 1990, **10**, 277–95.

47 DIZIK, M., CHRISTMAN, J.K. and WAINFAN, E. 'Alterations in expression and methylation of specific genes in livers of rats fed a cancer promoting methyl-deficient diet', *Carcinogenesis,* 1991, **12**, 1307–12.

48 POGRIBNY, J.P., BASNAKIAN, A.G., MILLER, B.J., LOPATINA, N.G., POIRIER, L.A.

and JAMES, S.J. 'Breaks in genomic DNA and within the p53 gene are associated with hypomethylation in livers of folate/methyl-deficient rats', *Cancer Res,* 1995, **55**, 1894–901.

49 BAYLIN, S.B., HERMAN, J.G., GRAFF, J.R., VERTINO, P.M. and ISSA, J.P. '-Alterations in DNA methylation: a fundamental aspect of neoplasia', *Adv Cancer Res,* 1998, **72**, 141–96.

50 ISSA, J.P., OTTAVIANO, Y.L., CELANO, P., HAMILTON, S.R., DAVIDSON, N.E. and BAYLIN, S.B. 'Methylation of the oestrogen receptor CpG island links ageing and neoplasia in human colon', *Nat Genet,* 1994, **7**, 536–40.

51 FREUDENHEIM, J.L., GRAHAM, S., MARSHALL, J.R., HAUGHEY, B.P., CHOLEWINSKI, S. and WILKINSON, G. 'Folate intake and carcinogenesis of the colon and rectum', *Int J Epidemiol,* 1991, **20**, 368–74.

52 MA, J., STAMPFER, M.J., GIOVANNUCCI, E., ARTIGAS, C., HUNTER, D.J., FUCHS, C., WILLETT, W.C., SELHUB, J., HENNEKENS, C.H. and ROZEN, R. 'Methylene-tetrahydrofolate reductase polymorphism, dietary interactions, and risk of colorectal cancer', *Cancer Res,* 1997, **57**, 1098–102.

53 GIOVANNUCCI, E., STAMPFER, M.J., COLDITZ, G.A., HUNTER, D.J., FUCHS, C., ROSNER, B.A., SPEIZER, F.E. and WILLETT, W.C. 'Multivitamin use, folate, and colon cancer in women in the Nurses' Health Study', *Ann Intern Med,* 1998, **129**, 517–24.

54 PATTERSON, B.H., BLOCK, G., ROSENBERGER, W.F., PEE, D. and KAHLE, L.L. 'Fruit and vegetables in the American diet: data from the NHANES II survey', *Am J Public Health,* 1990, **80**, 1443–9.

55 RUSZNYÀK, S. and SZENT-GYÖRGI, A. 'Vitamin nature of flavones', *Nature,* 1936, **139**, 798.

56 HOLLMAN, P.C. and KATAN, M.B. 'Absorption, metabolism and health effects of dietary flavonoids in man', *Biomed Pharmacother,* 1997, **51**, 305–10.

57 MANACH, C., REGERAT, F., TEXIER, O., AGULLO, G., DEMIGNE, C. and REMESY, C. 'Bioavailability, metabolism and physiological of 4-oxo-flavonoids', *Nutr Res,* 1996, **16**, 517–44.

58 FORMICA, J.V. and REGELSON, W. 'Review of the biology of quercetin and related bioflavonoids', *Food & Chem Toxicol,* 1995, **33**, 1061–80.

59 YOSHIDA, M., SAKAI, T., HOSOKAWA, N., MARUI, N., MATSUMOTO, K., FUJIOKA, A., NISHINO, H. and AOIKE, A. 'The effect of quercetin on cell cycle progression and growth of human gastric cancer cells', *Febs Lett,* 1990, **260**, 10–13.

60 MACGREGOR, J.T. 'Genetic and carcinogenic effects of plant flavonoids: an overview', *Adv Exp Med Biol,* 1984, **177**, 497–526.

61 DESCHNER, E.E., RUPERTO, J.F., WONG, G.Y. and NEWMARK, H.L. 'The effect of dietary quercetin and rutin on AOM-induced acute colonic epithelial abnormalities in mice fed a high-fat diet', *Nutr Cancer,* 1993, **20**, 199–204.

62 SETCHELL, K.D.R. and CASSIDY, A. 'Dietary isoflavones: Biological effects and relevance to health', *J Nutr,* 1999, **129**, 758S–67S.

63 AXELSON, M., KIRK, D.N., FARRANT, R.D., COOLEY, G., LAWSON, A.M. and SETCHELL, K.D.R. 'The identification of the weak oestrogen equol (17-

hydroxy-3-{4'-hydroxyphenyl}chroman) in human urine', *Biochem J,* 1982, **201**, 353–7.

64 DENIS, L., MORTON, M.S. and GRIFFITHS, K. 'Diet and its preventive role in prostatic disease', *Eur Urol,* 1999, **35**, 377–87.

65 KAUFMANN, W.K. 'Human topoisomerase II function, tyrosine phosphorylation and cell cycle checkpoints', *Proc Soc Exp Biol Med,* 1998, **217**, 327–34.

66 VERHOEVEN, D.T., GOLDBOHM, R.A., VAN POPPEL, G., VERGAGEN, H. and VAN DEN BRANDT, P.A. 'Epidemiological studies on brassica vegetables and cancer risk', *Cancer Epidemiol Biomarkers Prev,* 1996, **5**, 733–48.

67 FENWICK, G.R., HEANEY, R.K. and MULLIN, W.J. 'Glucosinolates and their breakdown products in food and food plants', *Crit Rev Food Sci Nutr,* 1983, **18**, 123–201.

68 GIAMOUSTARIS, A. and MITHEN, R. 'The effect of modifying the glucosinolate content of leaves of oilseed rape (*Brassica-napus* ssp oleifera) on its interaction with specialist and generalist pests', *Annals Appl Bio,* 1995, **126**, 347–63.

69 HEANEY, R.K. and FENWICK, G.R. 'Natural toxins and protective factors in brassica species, including rapeseed', *Nat Toxins,* 1995, **3**, 233–7.

70 VERHOEVEN, D.T., VEREHAGEN, H., GOLDBOHM, R.A., VAN DEN BRANDT, P.A. and VAN POPPEL, G.A. 'Review of mechanisms underlying anticarcinogenicity by brassica vegetables', *Chem Biol Interact,* 1997, **103**, 79–129.

71 TALALAY, P., FAHEY, J.W., HOLTZCLAW, W.D., PRESTERA, T. and ZHANG, Y. 'Chemoprotection against cancer by phase 2 enzyme induction', *Toxicol Lett,* 1995, **82–3**, 173–9.

72 HECHT, S.S. 'Chemoprevention of cancer by isothiocyanates, modifiers of carcinogen metabolism', *J Nutr,* 1999, **129**, 768S–74S.

73 WILLET, W.C., STAMPFER, M.J., COLDITZ, G.A., ROSNER, B.A. and SPEIZER, F.E. 'Relation of meat, fat and fiber intake to the risk of colon cancer in a prospective study among women', *N Engl J Med,* 1990, **323**, 1664–72.

74 BURKITT, D.P. 'Epidemiology of cancer of the colon and rectum', *Lancet,* 1971, **28**, 3–13..

75 European Cancer Prevention Organization, 'Consensus meeting on cereals, fibre and colorectal and breast cancers', *Euro J Cancer Prev,* 1998, **6**, 512–14.

76 Department of Health, *Nutritional Aspects of the Development of Cancer,* London, HMSO, 1998.

77 SMITH, A.N., DRUMMOND, E. and EASTWOOD, M.A. 'The effect of coarse and fine Canadian red spring wheat and French soft wheat bran on colonic motility in patients with diverticular disease', *Am J Clin Nutr,* 1981, **34**, 2460–3.

78 BINGHAM, S.A. 'Epidemiology and mechanisms relating diet to risk of colorectal cancer', *Nutr Res Rev,* 1996, **9**, 197–239.

79 BINGHAM, S.A., PIGNATELLI, B., POLLOCK, J.R.A., ELLUL, A., MALAVEILLE, C., GROSS, G., RUNSWICK, S., CUMMINGS, J.H. and O'NEILL, I.K. 'Does increased

endogenous formation of N-nitroso compounds in the human colon explain the association between red meat and colon cancer?', *Carcinogenesis,* 1996, **17**, 515–23.

80 CUMMINGS, J.H., BINGHAM, S.A., HEATON, K.W. and EASTWOOD, M.A. 'Fecal weight, colon cancer risk, and dietary intake of nonstarch polysaccharides (dietary fibre)', *Gastroenterol,* 1992, **103**, 1783–9.

81 NARISAWA, L.F., MAGADIA, N.E., WEISBURGER, J.H. and WYNDER, E.L. '-Promoting effect of bile acids on colon carcinogenesis after intrarectal instillation of MNNG in rats', *J Natl Cancer Inst,* 1975, **55**, 1093–7.

82 STORY, J.A. and KRITCHEVSKY, D. 'Comparison of the binding of various bile salts in vitro by several types of fiber', *J Nutr,* 1976, **106**, 1292–4.

83 CUMMINGS, J.H., POMARE, E.W., BRANCH, W.J., NAYLOR, C.P.E. and MACFARLANE, G.T. 'Short chain fatty acids in human large intestine, portal, hepatic and venous blood', *Gut,* 1987, **28**, 1221–7.

84 ROEDIGER, W.E.W. 'Role of anaerobic bacteria in the metabolic welfare of the colonic mucosa in man', *Gut,* 1980, **21**, 793–8.

85 HAGUE, A., BUTT, A.J. and PARASKEVA, C. 'The role of butyrate in human colonic epithelial cells: an energy source or inducer of differentiation and apoptosis', *Proc Nutr Soc,* 1996, **55**, 937–43.

86 HOWE, G.R., HIROHATA, T. and HISLOP, T.G. 'Dietary factors and the risk of breast cancer', *JNCI,* 1990, **82**, 561–9.

87 GERBER, M. 'Fibre and breast cancer', *Euro J Cancer Prev,* 1998, **7** (supp. 2), S63–S7.

88 FUCHS, C.S., GIOVANUCCI, E.L., COLDITZ, G.A., HUNTER, D.J., STAMPFER, M.J., ROSNER, B., SPEIZER, F.E. and WILLET, W.C. 'Dietary fibre and the risk of colorectal cancer and adenoma in women', *New Engl J Med,* 1999, **340**, 169–76.

89 HONDA, T., KAI, I. and OHI, G. 'Fat and dietary fiber intake and colon cancer mortality: a chronological comparison between Japan and the United States', *Nutr Cancer,* 1999, **33**, 95–9.

90 STEINMETZ, K.A. and POTTER, J.D. 'Vegetables, fruit, and cancer. I. Epidemiology', *Cancer Causes Control,* 1991, **2**, 325–57.

7

Functional foods and acute infections
Probiotics and gastrointestinal disorders

E. Isolauri and S. Salminen, University of Turku

7.1 Introduction

The primary role of the gastrointestinal tract is digestion and absorption of nutrients. In addition, its epithelial layer forms an important interface between the body and the external environment. The gastrointestinal tract is constantly exposed to harmful antigens such as allergens and potentially pathogenic micro-organisms. A unique defence system has developed to resist uncontrolled and excessive penetration by these substances.[1, 2] Mucosal immunity has developed two important lines of host defence: immune exclusion as performed by secretory antibodies, and specific immunosuppression to avoid local and peripheral inflammatory responses.

Immunophysiological regulation in the gut (Fig. 7.1), and the normal interaction between the internal environment and foreign antigens, depends on the establishment of indigenous microflora. As a result, in the healthy host, the gut-associated lymphoid tissue enables the generation of an efficient immune response to pathogens while concomitantly maintaining hyporesponsiveness to dietary antigens. In gastrointestinal disease, the two opposite functions of the gastrointestinal tract, antigen absorption and the barrier function, are in conflict. This is particularly clear in food allergy (dietary antigens disturb the barrier) and chronic inflammatory bowel disease (inflammation in the mucosa interferes with the absorption of nutrients).

Probiotics, defined as live microbial food ingredients beneficial to health,[3] are normal commensal bacteria of the healthy human gut microflora. Probiotic functional foods are an attractive means of maintaining the nutritional state of the host with impaired gut barrier functions. Promotion of the gut barrier function is ensured by normalisation of increased intestinal permeability and

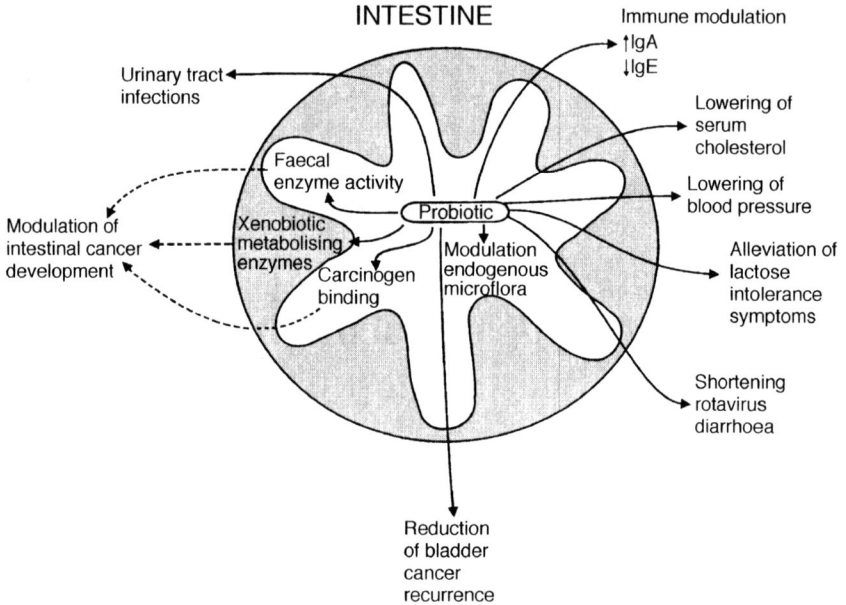

Fig. 7.1   Proposed effects of probiotics mediated through the intestinal tract.

altered gut microecology. Improvement of the intestinal immunological barrier is manifest in enhanced intestinal immunoglobulin (Ig)A responses, providing a first line of immune defence against foreign micro-organisms, and alleviation of intestinal inflammatory response, as well as in re-establishment of the balance of pro-inflammatory and anti-inflammatory cytokines, which direct immune responses by promoting the activation of antigen-specific and non-specific effector mechanisms.

7.2   The background

7.2.1   Antigen handling in the gastrointestinal tract

The small intestine is challenged by a myriad of potentially harmful intraluminal antigens as well as rapid and constant changes in the composition of the antigen load. The mucosal barrier in the gut excludes most antigens.[1] Together with non-immunological factors such as saliva, gastric acid, peristalsis, mucus, intestinal proteolysis, intestinal flora and epithelial cell membranes with intercellular junctional complexes, the secretory immuno-globulin system contributes to the exclusion of antigens. Nevertheless, there are specialised antigen transport mechanisms in the villous epithelium. This creates a second line of defence, immune elimination, which directs towards the removal of antigens that have penetrated the mucosa and controls antigen transfer.

Antigens are absorbed across the epithelial layer by transcytosis. The main degradative pathway entails lysosomal processing of the antigen. A minor pathway allows the transport of unprocessed antigens.[4] Peyer's patches are covered by M cells, and antigen transport across this epithelium is characterised by rapid uptake and reduced degradation. Antigens are then presented to subjacent lymphocytes or transported to interfollicular T cell areas of Peyer's patches or mesenteric lymph nodes. These differentiate into effector cells, which mediate active immune suppression and promote the differentation of IgA-secreting B-cells. As a result of a specific absorption process across the intestinal mucosa, most dietary antigens are excluded or actively eliminated (see Fig. 7.1).

7.2.2 Microbes and gut defence

The vast majority of intraluminal and mucosal micro-organisms are normal components of the gut microflora and facilitate barrier function of the gastrointestinal tract. This barrier function, commonly referred to as colonisation resistance, prevents colonisation of the gut with potential pathogens. Thus, a main function of the microflora is as part of the host–microbe interactions taking place in the gastrointestinal tract. This interaction may be disturbed in gastrointestinal inflammatory states in such a way that specific members of the normal microflora become either pathogenic or opportunistic pathogens, the pattern of infection that may be caused by commensal or other normally non-pathogenic agents, when host defence mechanisms are compromised. The difference between a normal microbe and an opportunistic pathogen depends on microbial virulence factors and host health status.

To become a pathogen, a microbe has to fulfil one or more of the following criteria:

- be able to survive in the gastrointestinal tract and to invade the surface epithelium
- to multiply in numbers to break the colonisation resistance
- to invade or translocate the epithelium to cause diseases
- to have the ability to be detrimental to the host
- to elaborate cellular or other toxins.

Attachment of pathogens may happen in different ways (including by specific receptors), resulting in the penetration of the microbe through the mucus and adherence on the epithelium by surface proteins or different pili-like structures. To have an effect on the host, the microbe has to compete with the resident microflora for nutrients and invade host cells. For this purpose probiotics, beneficial members of the gut microflora, may compete for adhesion sites and protect the host by producing antimicrobial components and/or bacteriocins.

7.2.3 Competition between pathogens and probiotics

Both probiotics and pathogens may adhere to intestinal mucus and intestinal mucosa. Both need to survive gastric conditions and to multiply in the gut for any effects on health. This may also result in the competitive exclusion of the pathogen by an effective probiotic, either by means of colonising the surface, production of anti-microbial substances or by direct interaction with the pathogen. In this respect, intestinal bacteria are very different and even closely related strains may behave differently.

Some strains of probiotic lactic acid bacteria have been described in cases of clinical infection.[5] In most, if not all cases, bacteremia has been described in immunocompromised patients and patients with rapid, fatal, underlying disease. In such cases, lactobacilli may be identified, perhaps since they are among the most common bacteria in the gastrointestinal tract and mucosal surfaces of the human. They do not appear to have pathogenic potential, but rather fight pathogens as has been described in several articles on successful probiotics.[6] Consequently, it is important to select probiotic bacteria that are safe and effective.

For organisms that are pathogenic, some virulence factors may be needed. Such virulence factors have not been found when studying lactic acid bacteria in clinical bacteremia cases.[5, 6] Enterococci such as *Enterococcus faecium* are known to be causes of infection in humans and they are identified in clinical cases over one hundred times more often that lactic acid bacteria or bifidobacteria. Even so, they are classified as opportunistic unlike accepted pathogens such as *Shigella* or Salmonella. In case of such pathogenic microbes, probiotics have been shown to protect the host and selectively inhibit the transfer and translocation of such pathogens. In other cases, lactic acid bacteria may be able to protect the host by binding microbial toxins in the gastrointestinal tract.[7] Thus, probiotic lactic acid bacteria and bifidobacteria can act as promoters of a strong gut mucosal barrier and improved protection against disease.

All intraluminal and mucosal bacterial antigens, both harmful and beneficial,[3] elicit specific responses in the gut-associated lymphoid tissue. This has been explained by their capacity to bind to epithelial cells and thus allow antigen entry via enterocytes, escaping tolerance induction in Peyer's patches. Strong adhesion has been associated with enhanced gut immune responses. Inflammatory responses associated with pathogenic bacteria are also explained by triggering phagocytic activity and the generation of pro-inflammatory cytokines such as interleukin (IL)-6, IL-12 and interferon-γ. Elimination of pathogenic agents from the mucosae also involves the interaction of IgA antibodies with the inflammatory response.

Recent data suggest that immune responses directed towards indigenous gut microflora and probiotics differ from that directed to pathogens. Evidence exists of distinctive B-cell populations secreting different types of IgA to these microorganisms.[8] Distinct microbial factors and the evolving immune responses may explain the persistence of the gut microflora in the intestine and the beneficial effects of probiotics, while pathogens are effectively eradicated from the gut lumen and mucosa.

7.2.4 Immune regulation in the gastrointestinal tract

The surface of mucosal membranes is protected by a local adaptive immune system. The mucosal immune system consists of a protective network of tissues, lymphoid cells and effector molecules.[9] The gut-associated lymphoid tissue comprises an important element of the total immunological capacity of the host in recognising and selectively handling foreign antigens for the initiation of immune responses. The regulatory function of the intestinal immune response takes place in different compartments: aggregated in follicles and Peyer's patches, distributed within the mucosa and in the intestinal epithelium, as well as in secretory sites. The best-characterised component of the mucosal immune defence is the secretory IgA system. IgA antibody production is abundant at mucosal surfaces and is thought to provide the host with a first line of immune defence. Secretory IgA is resistant to intraluminal proteolysis and does not directly activate complement or inflammatory responses, which makes secretory IgA ideal for protecting mucosal surfaces. In humans, there are two isotypes: IgA1, which predominates in the small intestine, and IgA2, resistant to most bacterial proteases and thus frequent in the colonic mucosa.

Immune regulation is directed towards hyporesponsiveness to antigens such as food proteins, a phenomenon called oral tolerance, which is a hallmark of the intestinal immune system. The second unique feature is the common mucosal immune system. Immune response, initiated in the gut-associated lymphoid tissue, affects immune responses at other mucosal surfaces including respiratory tract and lacrimal, salivary and mammary glands. The migration of lymphocytes into tissues is targeted by homing receptors on lymphocytes that interact with their ligands on the endothelial cells.

Oral tolerance is the immunological hyporesponsiveness to antigens formerly encountered by the enteric route.[10] Studies in experimental animals demonstrate that the dose and frequency of antigen fed influence the course of acquisition of tolerance. Feeding high doses results in clonal deletion and/or energy in the periphery whereas feeding low doses of antigen results in active suppression subsequent to induction of regulatory T cells in Peyer's patches. Oral tolerance has been taken to be a concomitant effect of immune exclusion and suppression of systemic immune response, possibly attributed to the suppressor cytokine transforming growth factor-β.[11] The tolerogenicity of orally administered antigen depends on the age and immunological state of the host.

On activation, immune cells respond with release of a host of cytokines that then direct the subsequent immune responses. CD4+T helper (Th) cells have been divided into phenotypic subsets based on the cytokines they produce. Th1 cells secrete interferon-γ, IL-2 and lymphotoxin and promote immunity to intracellular pathogens. Th2 cells secrete IL-4, IL-5, IL-6, IL-10 and IL-13 and promote immune response to helminth infections as well as IgE production.

Once an immune response begins to deviate toward either the Th1 or Th2 phenotype, there is potential for further polarisation of the immune response by the cytokines themselves: IL-4 is obligatory for the establishment of the Th2-type immunity, which leads to enhanced IgE production, eosinophilia and atopic disease. Thus the Th1 or Th2 subset, respectively, has the capability to promote its own expansion while preventing that of the other.

Many of the immunoregulatory aberrations favouring sensitisation instead of the maturation of oral tolerance prevail in early infancy. The immature immunological protection manifests itself in reduced capacity to generate IgA-producing cells. In the newborn, the cytokine production profile is directed away from cell-mediated immunity toward humoral immunity, and the abundance of IL-4-generating cells may divert the immunological T-cell memory to Th2 phenotype, which leads to enhanced IgE production and possibly to atopic sensitisation. The constitutively polarised immune regulation partly explains the increased risk of atopic disease in infancy.[12] The immature gut barrier may lead to aberrant antigen transfer and immune responses and thus explain the vulnerability to breakdown of oral tolerance at an early age.[1] At an early age, such antigens are frequently derived from food, and allergic reactions to foods are common.[13] The predisposition to acute gastrointestinal infectious disease is again associated with immaturity and dysfunction of the gut defence barrier.

Intestinal permeability can be secondarily increased as a result of inflammation in the intestinal mucosa induced by viruses, bacteria or dietary antigens. A greater amount of antigens may traverse the mucosal barrier and the routes of transport may be altered. During the ensuing mucosal dysfunction, the normal pattern of antigen handling is impaired, which may evoke aberrant immune responses and lead to inflammatory response beyond the gastrointestinal tract, as well as sensitisation to intraluminal antigens – abrogation of tolerance to indigenous microflora and dietary antigens.[14]

7.3 Probiotics and the immune system

The indigenous gut microflora are an important component of the gut defence barrier. The capacity to generate IgA-producing cells increases in response to the establishment of the gut microflora.[15] First, the micro-organisms have been shown to translocate to mesenteric lymph node, but the number of translocating bacteria begins to drop with the onset of specific IgA response, reflecting maturation of the intestine's immunological defence mechanisms.

Gut microflora have been shown to induce and maintain oral tolerance in experimental animal models.[16] In contrast to control mice, germ-free animals maintain a production of IgE antibodies to orally administered dietary antigens. The IgE response could be corrected by the reconstitution of the microflora at the neonatal stage, but not at a later age. These results suggest that, in affecting the development of gut-associated lymphoid tissue at the neonatal stage, the gut microflora direct the maturation of the oral tolerance mechanisms.

Recent studies following the microflora development in vaginally born infants and in infants born by caesarean section indicate major differences in culturable microflora (Grönlund, unpublished data). Colonisation was associated with the maturation of humoral immune mechanisms, particularly of circulating IgA- and IgM-secreting cells.

The recognition and the regulation of the immune response to antigens is an important mechanism for the prevention of life-threatening infections and inflammatory responses. Faced with the fact that foreign antigens constantly challenge the intestine's mucosal surfaces, it is obvious, as recently demonstrated,[17] that even in health, intestinal T cells express activation markers and spontaneously secrete pro-inflammatory cytokines. Thus any interference with the mucosal barrier function brings about a risk of disease.

Probiotic functional foods can improve specific physiological functions in the human gastrointestinal tract, for example the host immune defence, and thereby reduce the risk of contracting certain avoidable illnesses.

7.3.1 Probiotics and the modulation of the immune system

Probiotic bacteria have been shown to promote the endogeneous host defence mechanisms. In addition to effects on the non-immunological gut defence, characterised by stabilisation of the gut microflora,[18] probiotic bacteria have been shown to enhance non-specific host resistance to microbial pathogens.[19] Several strains of lactic acid bacteria have been shown to induce *in vitro* the release of pro-inflammatory cytokines, tumour necrosis factor-α and IL-6, reflecting stimulation of non-specific immunity.[20] Enhanced phagocytosis has also been reported in humans by *Lactobacillus acidophilus* strain Lal[21] and *Lactobacillus rhamnosus* GG.[22] Phagocytosis is responsible for early activation of the inflammatory response before antibody production. Recently, probiotic bacteria were shown to modulate phagocytosis differently in healthy and allergic subjects, in the former an immunostimulatory effect while in the latter down regulation of the inflammatory response was detected,[22] substantiating the immunoregulatory role of the gut microflora in the gut-associated lymphoid tissue.

Probiotic strains have been shown to modulate the host's specific humoral immune responses to potentially harmful antigens, and thereby further promote the intestine's immunological barrier.[19] Oral introduction of *Bifidobacterium bifidum* has been shown to enhance the antibody response to ovalbumin,[23] and *Bifidobacterium breve* to stimulate IgA response to cholera toxin in mice,[24] and an increased humoral immune response including an increase in rotavirus-specific antibody-secreting cells in the IgA class has been detected in children with acute rotavirus diarrhoea who received *Lactobacillus rhamnosus* GG during the acute phase of diarrhoea compared with controls.[25] The mean serum rotavirus IgA antibody concentrations at the convalescent stage were also higher in those receiving *Lactobacillus rhamnosus* GG.[26] In accordance, oral introduction of lactobacilli to suckling rats sensitised with cow milk increased the number of cells secreting antibodies to β-lactoglobulin.[4]

Recently, probiotics have been shown to modulate the hosts' immune responses to foreign antigens with a potential to dampen hypersensitivity reactions.[19] Unheated and heat-treated homogenates were prepared from probiotic strains, including *Lactobacillus rhamnosus* GG, *Bifidobacterium lactis, Lactobacillus acidophilus, Lactobacillus delbrückii* subsp. *bulgaricus* and *Streptococcus thermophilus*.[27] The phytohemagglutinin-induced proliferation of mononuclear cells was suppressed in these homogenates compared to controls with no homogenate indicating that probiotic bacteria possess heat-stable anti-proliferative component(s), which could be therapeutically exploited in inflammatory conditions.

7.3.2 Prevention of gastrointestinal infection

Oral introduction of probiotics can enhance non-specific host resistance to microbial pathogens and thereby facilitate the exclusion of pathogens in the gut. This was clinically manifested in a reduction in the number of diarrhoeal episodes in infants given *Lactobacillus helveticus* and *Streptococcus thermophilus*-fermented formula[28] or *Lactobacillus acidophilus* and *Lactobacillus casei*-fermented milk[29] compared to a group given non-fermented formula or milk. In a like manner, Saavedra *et al*.[30] also demonstrated this effect in a double-blind, placebo-controlled trial in hospitalised infants given a standard infant formula or a formula supplemented with *Bifidobacterium bifidum* and *Streptococcus thermophilus*. Over a 17-month follow-up, 31% of the patients given the standard infant formula, but only 7% of those receiving the probiotic-supplemented formula, developed diarrhoea, and the prevalence of rotavirus shedding was significantly lower in those receiving probiotic-supplemented formula.

Anti-microbial treatment disturbs colonisation resistance of the gut micro-flora, which may induce clinical symptoms, most frequently diarrhoea. Evidence from the available studies indicates that probiotic fermented milks may be of value in the prevention of antibiotic-associated diarrhoea. The preventive potential of probiotics on antibiotic-associated diarrhoea in children was recently studied.[31] To avoid confusion caused by recent anti-microbial treatments, the incidence of diarrhoea after single anti-microbial treatment and the effect of probiotics was evaluated in children with no history of anti-microbial use during the previous three months. The incidence of diarrhoea was 5% in the group given *Lactobacillus rhamnosus* GG and 16% in the placebo group, substantiating the efficacy of the probiotic approach.

The value of probiotic preparations for the prophylaxis for traveller's diarrhoea has been studied using *Lactobacillus acidophilus, Bifidobacterium bifidum, Lactobacillus bulgaricus* and *Streptococcus termophilus*,[32] but the results have been conflicting, due to differences in probiotic species and vehicles used, in dosage schedule, as well as in travel destinations in which the studies have been conducted. Recent double-blind, placebo-controlled studies indicate, however, that there is evidence that some strains of lactic acid bacteria may provide protection against traveller's diarrhoea.[33]

7.4 Probiotic functional foods and the treatment of gastrointestinal disorders

7.4.1 Treatment of gastrointestinal infection

Rotavirus is the most common cause of acute childhood diarrhoea. Rotavirus infection results in partial destruction of the intestinal mucosa, with loss of microvilli, and alterations in the composition of the intestinal microflora. *Lactobacillus rhamnosus* GG as a fermented milk or as a freeze-dried powder has been shown to reduce significantly the duration of diarrhoea compared to fermented-then-pasteurised milk product as a placebo.[34] The beneficial clinical effect was accompanied by stabilisation of the indigenous microflora,[18] reduction in the duration of rotavirus shedding[35] and reduction of increased gut permeability caused by rotavirus infection.[4] In addition to these effects on the non-immunological gut barrier, the gut immune defence was also promoted by probiotic therapy as documented by a significant increase in IgA-secreting cells to rotavirus.[25, 26] The specific IgA response could contribute to the preventive potential of probiotics, and also against reinfections.

7.4.2 Treatment of inflammation

There is an increasing appreciation of the role of cytokines in regulation of the inflammatory responses at local and systemic levels. Ingestion of probiotic bacteria has the potential to stabilise the immunological barrier of gut mucosa by reducing the generation of local pro-inflammatory cytokine such as tumour necrosis factor-α.

Intestinal inflammation is constantly accompanied with imbalance of the intestinal microflora. There is also evidence to suggest that the trigger for the inflammatory response or maintenance of the inflammation could be the bacterial flora residing in the gut. Durchmann *et al.*[36] have confirmed that healthy individuals are tolerant to their own microflora, and that such tolerance is abrogated in patients with inflammatory bowel disease. In support of this, alteration of the properties of the indigenous microflora by probiotic therapy reversed some disturbances of the gut immune responses characteristic of these conditions.[37] Thus probiotic therapy may help balance the gut microbial environment,[18] and thereby prevent the generation of inflammatory mediators, a secondary response of the gut-associated lymphoid tissue to altered intraluminal milieu, which may sustain the loss of intestinal integrity.[38]

The intestinal microflora contribute to the processing of food antigens in the gut. Probiotic bacteria-derived proteases have the ability to degrade cow milk casein and thereby to generate peptides with suppressive effects on lymphocyte proliferation in healthy individuals.[39] To characterise the immunomodulatory effect of probiotics in allergic inflammation, a study was made to investigate whether caseins degraded by probiotic bacteria-derived enzymes could modulate the cytokine production by anti-CD3 antibody-induced peripheral blood mononuclear cells in atopic infants with cow milk allergy.[40] Unhydrolysed casein increased the production of IL-4 in cultures from patients with atopic dermatitis while *Lactobacillus rhamnosus* GG-hydrolysed casein reduced the production of IL-4. These results indicate that probiotics modify the structure of potentially harmful antigens and reduce their immunogenicity.

To evaluate the clinical effect of probiotic therapy in food allergy,[41] infants with atopic dermatitis and challenge-proven cow milk allergy were given extensively hydrolysed whey formula or an extensively hydrolysed whey formula containing probiotics. There was a significant improvement in the clinical course of atopic dermatitis in the group given probiotic-supplemented elimination diet, and in parallel, markers of intestinal[41] and systemic[42] allergic inflammation decreased significantly. Parallel results have been obtained in milk-hypersensitive adults.[22] In these, a milk challenge in conjunction with a probiotic strain prevented the immunoinflammatory response characteristic to the challenge without probiotics.

7.5 Future trends

Probiotic functional foods may offer a new direction in the search for future treatment and prevention strategies as well as nutrition for patients with intestinal barrier dysfunction such as food allergy and inflammatory bowel diseases. For this purpose, identification of the effects of candidate probiotics on the immunophysiological regulation in the gastrointestinal tract is of utmost importance. Recent studies comparing the effects of different probiotic strains indicate that strain-specific mechanisms exist.[27] Therefore, disease-specific probiotic functional foods may be developed.

Thus far studies on probiotic functional foods have focused on yoghurts and fermented drinks and juices; however, possibilities for alternatives are numerous. Improved understanding on the microbe–host interactions again may uncover novel probiotic strains for such products.

Safety studies have indicated no significant risk or virulence factors attached to probiotic lactic acid bacteria or bifidobacteria. Recommendations for the relevant procedures have been made outlining the targets and the steps necessary in the safety assessment of both natural and novel probiotics. These recommendations cover mainly probiotics from traditional sources and include also a discussion on how the novelty of a probiotic should be defined and taken into account in safety assessment procedures.[43] Table 7.1 summarises important studies and methodologies that can be applied to probiotic safety assessment. It is also important to consider the possibilities of using non-viable probiotic microbes and microbe preparations for disease-specific applications as also non-

Table 7.1   Examples of studies and safety effects with probiotic bacteria

Type of study	Effects
In vitro studies	Invasion potential, prevention of pathogen invasion Mucus degradation Influence on pathogen growth
Animal studies	Safety assessment in animal models
Clinical studies	Side-effects or harmful effects, safety of probiotic use in disease-specific conditions
Epidemiological studies	Probiotic-related infections, surveillance of safety of product in use

viable probiotics have been reported as effective ingredients for many applications.[44] Such preparations may require less safety studies as non-viable bacteria are not likely to cause infections.

7.6 Sources of further information and advice

Further sources of information can be obtained, for example, from the functional foods working group documents[3] and the consensus document.[45] These reviews and statements were developed by an ILSI Europe-coordinated, EU-sponsored programme on functional food science in Europe and cover extensive state-of-the-art reviews on probiotics. Recent compendiums on probiotic properties and different uses can be found in references 19, 38, 46 and 47.

7.7 References

1 SANDERSON, I.R. and WALKER, W.A. 'Uptake and transport of macromole-cules by the intestine: possible role in clinical disorders (an update)', *Gastroenterol*, 1993, **104**, 622–39.
2 BRANDTZAEG, P. 'Molecular and cellular aspects of the secretory immunoglobulin system', *APMIS*, 1995, **103**, 1–19.
3 SALMINEN, S., BOULEY, C., BOUTRON-RUAULT, M.C., CONTOR, L., CUMMINGS, J.H., FRANCK, A., GIBSON, G.R., ISOLAURI, E., MOREAU, M.C., ROBERFROID, M. and ROWLAND, I. 'Functional food science and gastrointestinal physiology and function', *Br J Nutr*, 1998, **80**, S147–71.
4 ISOLAURI, E., MAJAMAA, H., ARVOLA, T., RANTALA, I., VIRTANEN, E. and ARVILOMMI, H. '*Lactobacillus casei* strain GG reverses increased intestinal permeability induced by cow milk in suckling rats', *Gastroenterol*, 1993, **105**, 1643–50.

5 SAXELIN, M., CHUANG, N.H., CHASSY, B., RAUTELIN, H., MÄKELÄ, P.H., SALMINEN, S. and GORBACH, S.L. '*Lactobacilli* and bacteremia in Southern Finland 1989–1992', *Clin Infect Dis*, 1996, **22**, 564–6.

6 KIRJAVAINEN, P.V., CRITTENDEN, R.G., DONOHUE, D.C., HARTY, D.W.S., MORRIS, L.F., OUWEHAND, A.C., PLAYNE, M.J., RAUTELIN, H., SALMINEN, S.J. and TUOMOLA, E.M. 'Adhesion and platelet aggregation properties of bacteremia-associated *lactobacilli*', *Infec and Immun*, 1999, **67**, 2653–5.

7 EL-NEZAMI, H., KANKAANPÄÄ, P., SALMINEN, S. and AHOKAS, J. 'Ability of dairy strains of lactic acid bacteria to bind food carcinogens', *Food Chem Toxicol*, 1998, **36**, 321–6.

8 MESTECKY, J., RUSSELL, M.W. and ELSON, C.O. 'Intestinal IgA: novel views on its function in the defence of the largest mucosal surface', *Gut*, 1999, **44**, 2–5.

9 MCGHEE, J.R. 'Mucosa-associated lymphoid tissue'. In P.J. Delves and I.M. Roitt (eds) *Encyclopedia of Immunology*, London, Academic Press, 1998, **3**, 1774–80.

10 STROBEL, S. and MOWAT, A.M. 'Immune responses to dietary antigens: oral tolerance', *Immunol Today*, 1998, **19**, 173–81.

11 WEINER, H.L., FRIEDMAN, A., MILLER, A., KHOURY, S.J., AL-SABBAGH, A., SANTOS, L., SAYEGH, M., NUSSENBLATT, R.B., TRENTHAM, D.E. and HAFLER, D.A. 'Oral tolerance: immunologic mechanisms and treatment of animal and human organ-specific autoimmune diseases by oral administration of autoantigens', *Annu Rev Immunol*, 1994, **12**, 809–37.

12 COOKSON, W.O.C.M. and MOFFATT, M.F. 'Asthma: an epidemic in the absence of infection?', *Science*, 1997, **275**, 41–2.

13 ISOLAURI, E., TAHVANAINEN, A., PELTOLA, T. and ARVOLA, T. 'Breast-feeding of allergic infants', *J Pediatr*, 1999, **134**, 27–32.

14 ISOLAURI, E. 'Cow milk allergy', *Environ Toxicol Pharmacol*, 1997, **4**, 137–41.

15 SHROFF, K.E., MESLIN, K. and CEBRA, J.J. 'Commensal enteric bacteria engender a self-limiting humoral mucosal immune response while permanently colonizing the gut', *Infect Immun*, 1995, **63**, 3904–13.

16 SUDO, N., SAWAMURA, S., TANAKA, K., AIBA, Y., KUBO, C. and KOGA, Y. 'The requirement of intestinal bacterial flora for the development of an IgE production system fully suscepticle to oral tolerance induction', *J Immunol*, 1997, **159**, 1739–45.

17 CAROL, M., LAMBRECHTS, A., VAN GOSSUM, A., LIBIN, M., GOLDMAN, M. and MASCART-LEMONE, F. 'Spontaneous secretion of interferon and interleukin 4 by human intraepithelial and lamina propria gut lymphocytes', *Gut*, 1998, **42**, 643–9.

18 ISOLAURI, E., KAILA, M., MYKKÄNEN, H., LING, W.H. and SALMINEN, S. 'Oral bacteriotherapy for viral gastroenteritis', *Dig Dis Sci*, 1994, **39**, 2595–600.

19 Reviewed in OUWEHAND, A., SÜTAS, Y., SALMINEN, S. and ISOLAURI, E. 'Probiotic therapies: present and future', *Int Semin Paediatr Gastroenterol Nutr*, 1998, **7**, 7–15.

20 MIETTINEN, M., VUOPIO-VARKILA, J. and VARKILA, J. 'Production of human tumor necrosis factor alpha, interleukin-6, and interleukin-10 is induced by lactic acid bacteria', *Infect Immun*, 1996, **64**, 5403–5.

21 SCHIFFRIN, E.J., ROCHAT, F., LINK-AMSTER, H., AESCHLIMANN, J.M. and DONNET-HUGHES, A. 'Immunomodulation of human blood cells following the ingestion of lactic acid bacteria', *J Dairy Sci*, 1994, **78**, 491–7.

22 PELTO, L., SALMINEN, S., LILIUS, E.M. and ISOLAURI, E. 'Milk hypersensitivity – key to poorly defined gastrointestinal symptoms in adults', *Allergy*, 1998, **53**, 307–10.

23 MOREAU, M.C., HUDAULT, S. and BRIDONNEAU, C. 'Systemic antibody response to ovalbumin in gnotobiotic C3H/HeJ mice with *Bifidobacterium bifidum* or *Escherichia coli.*', *Microecol Ther*, 1990, **20**, 309–12.

24 YASUI, H., NAGAOKA, N., MIKE, A., HAYAKAWA, K. and OHWAKI, M. 'Detection of *Bifidobacterium* strains that induce large quantities of IgA', *Microb Ecol Health Dis*, 1992, **5**, 155–62.

25 KAILA, M., ISOLAURI, E., SOPPI, E., VIRTANEN, E., LAINE, S. and ARVILOMMI, H. 'Enhancement of the circulating antibody secreting cell response in human diarrhea by a human lactobacillus strain', *Pediatr Res*, 1992, **32**, 141–4.

26 MAJAMAA, H., ISOLAURI, E., SAXELIN, M. and VESIKARI, T. 'Lactic acid bacteria in the treatment of acute rotavirus gastroenteritis', *J Pediatr Gastroenterol Nutr*, 1995, **20**, 333–9.

27 PESSI, T., SÜTAS, Y., SAXELIN, M., KALLIOINEN, H. and ISOLAURI, E. 'Antiproliferative effects of homogenates derived from five strains of candidate probiotic bacteria', *Appl Environ Microb*, in press.

28 BRUNSER, O., ARAYA, M., ESPINOZA, J. GUESRY, P.R., SECRETIN, M.C. and PACHECO, I. 'Effect of an acidified milk on diarrhoea and the carrier state in infants of low socio-economic stratum', *Acta Paediatr Scand*, 1989, **78**, 259–64.

29 GONZALEZ, S., ALBARRACIN, G., LOCASCIO DE RUIZ PESCE, M., MALE, M., APELLA, M.C., PESCE DE RUIZ HOLGADO, A. and OLIVER, G. 'Prevention of infantile diarrhoea by fermented milk', *Microbiologie-Aliments-Nutrition*, 1990, **8**, 349–54.

30 SAAVEDRA, J.M., BAUMAN, N.A., OUNG, I., PERMAN, J.A. and YOLKEN, R.H. 'Feeding of *Bifidobacterium bifidum* and *Streptococcus thermophilus* to infants in hospital for prevention of diarrhoea and shedding of rotavirus', *Lancet*, 1994, **344**, 1046–9.

31 ARVOLA, T., LAIHO, K., TORKKELI, S., MYKKÄNEN, H., SALMINEN, S., MAUNULA, L. and ISOLAURI, E. 'Prophylactic *Lactobacillus* GG reduces antibiotic-associated diarrhea in children with respiratory infections: a randomised study', *Pediatrics*, in press.

32 SALMINEN, S., DEIGHTON, M., GORBACH, S. and BENNO, Y. 'Lactic acid bacteria in health and disease'. In S. Salminen and A. von Wright (eds), pp. 211–54, *Lactic Acid Bacteria: Microbiology and Functional Aspects*, New York, Marcel Dekker, 1998.

33 HILTON, E., KOLAKOVSKI, P., SINGER, C. and SMITH, M. 'Efficacy of

Lactobacillus GG as a diarrheal preventive in travelers', *J Travel Med*, 1997, **4**, 41–3.

34   ISOLAURI, E., JUNTUNEN, M., RAUTANEN, T., SILLANAUKEE, P. and KOIVULA, T. 'A human Lactobacillus strain (*Lactobacillus* GG) promotes recovery from acute diarrhea in children', *Pediatrics*, 1991, **88**, 90–7.

35   CANANI, R.B., ALBANO, F., SPAGNUOLO, M.I., DI BENEDETTO, L., STABILE, A. and GUARINO, A. 'Effect of oral administration of *Lactobacillus* GG on the duration of diarrhea and on rotavirus excretion in ambulatory children', *J Pediatr Gastroenterol Nutr*, 1997, **24**, 469.

36   DUCHMANN, R., KAISER, I., HERMANN, E., MAYET, W., EWE, K. and MEYER ZUM BÜSCHENFELDE, K.H. 'Tolerance exists towards resident intestinal flora but is broken in active inflammatory bowel disease (IBD)', *Clin Exp Immunol*, 1995, **102**, 448–55.

37   MALIN, M., SUOMALAINEN, H., SAXELIN, M. and ISOLAURI, E. 'Promotion of IgA immune response in patients with Crohn's disease by oral bacteriotherapy with *Lactobacillus* GG', *Ann Nutr Metab*, 1996, **40**, 137–45.

38   ISOLAURI, E. 'Probiotics and gut inflammation', *Curr Opin Gastroenterol*, in press.

39   SÜTAS, Y., SOPPI, E., KORHONEN, H., SYVÄOJA, E.L., SAXELIN, M., ROKKA, T. and ISOLAURI, E. 'Suppression of lymphocyte proliferation *in vitro* by bovine caseins hydrolysed with *Lactobacillus* GG-derived enzymes', *J Allergy Clin Immunol*, 1996, **98**, 216–24.

40   SÜTAS, Y., HURME, M. and ISOLAURI, E. 'Downregulation of antiCD3 antibody-induced IL-4 production by bovine caseins hydrolysed with *Lactobacillus* GG-derived enzymes', *Scand J Immunol*, 1996, **43**, 687–9.

41   MAJAMAA, H. and ISOLAURI, E. 'Probiotics: a novel approach in the management of food allergy', *J Allergy Clin Immunol*, 1997, **99**, 179–86.

42   ISOLAURI, E., ARVOLA, T., SÜTAS, Y. and SALMINEN, S. 'Probiotics in the management of atopic eczema', *Clin Exp Allergy*, in press.

43   SALMINEN, S., VON WRIGHT, A., MORELLI, L., MARTEAU, P., BRASSARD, D., DE VOS, W., FONDÉN, R., SAXELIN, M., COLLINS, K., MOGENSEN, G., BIRKELAND, S.E. and MATTILA-SANDHOLM, T. 'Demonstration of safety of probiotics – a review', *Int J Food Microbiol*, 1998, **44**, 93–106.

44   OUWEHAND, A.C. and SALMINEN, S.J. 'The health effects of viable and non-viable cultured milks', *Int Dairy J*, 1998, **8**, 749–58.

45   DIPLOCK, A.T., AGGETT, P.J., ASHWELL, M., BORNET, F., FERN, E.F. and ROBERFROID, M.B. 'Scientific concepts of functional foods in Europe: consensus document', *Br J Nutr*, 1999, **81**, S1–27.

46   SALMINEN, S.J. and VON WRIGHT, A. *Lactic Acid Bacteria: Microbiology and Functional Properties*, New York, Marcel Dekker, 1998.

47   LEE, Y.K., GORBACH, S.L., NUMITA, N. and SALMINEN, S. *Handbook of Probiotics*, New York, John Wiley, 1999.

Part III

Developing functional food products

8

Maximising the functional benefits of plant foods

D.G. Lindsay, Institute of Food Research, Norwich

8.1 Introduction

Overwhelming proportions of the world's population are dependent on plants as their principal, if not exclusive, source of food. In such populations the incidence of disease due to vitamin deficiencies is widespread. It has been estimated that over 100 million children world-wide are vitamin A deficient, and improving the vitamin A content of their food could prevent as many as two million deaths annually in young children.[1] This is apart from the deficiencies in iodine intake, resulting in goitre and in iron-deficient anaemia which are estimated to affect millions in the developing world. There is also an important need to improve the amino acid content of legume proteins that are deficient in essential sulphur amino acids.

In contrast to the developing world, the incidence of known nutritional deficiency disorders in the developed world is low and can be discounted as a major cause of diet-related disease. Even in the case of vegetarians there appears to be no appreciable problem. Nutritional deficiency diseases have been avoided through the widespread fortification of food. Fortification is also utilised to replace nutrients lost in the heat processing of foods and through oxidation. In addition the use of nutritional supplements is becoming more and more common.

Diet has been implicated as an important risk factor in the initiation or progression of those diseases that are the greatest contributors to ill health in the developed countries, namely cardiovascular disease and cancer. It has also been implicated as a factor in other diseases where environment influences the outcome of the disease such as maturity onset diabetes.

One of the most striking and consistent observations, in terms of the relationship to health, has been the decrease in cancer risk associated with an increasing intake of fruit and vegetables in the diet.[2] There appears to be no single explanation for this effect but understanding the basis for the protective effects of plant constituents on carcinogenesis is the subject of intensive research internationally.

8.2 The concept of functionality

It might be argued that since fruit and vegetables are known to reduce the risk of the development of cancer, the only action that is required is to encourage greater consumption of these foods. Under such circumstances the need to consider any specific enhancement of their functional benefits is pointless. This argument ignores the fact that:

- Ninety per cent of the world's population suffers from nutritional deficiency diseases. While for them the definition of functionality may differ from that applied to the remaining 10% of the population, the augmentation of certain nutrients will have health benefits.
- Consumer choice in the developed world will depend on socio-economic and cultural constraints. The greater freedom of choice ensures that foods are selected that are enjoyable and available and these may not always be healthy.
- The consumption of fruit and vegetables may not provide optimal protection against the risk of disease.
- Plant food composition is constantly changing as new varieties are marketed. Since it is not known what the exact protective mechanisms are that can be induced by eating fruit and vegetables, it is not possible to link composition to specific functional mechanisms. No criteria could be applied to the development of plant varieties, in terms of their composition, other than that they remain the same. This is an unsatisfactory basis on which to base the future of the plant breeding industry. Phytochemicals or vitamins vary by an order of magnitude or more in the gene pool. It could help in the prevention of disease to know in which direction this pool should be altered, and with what likely consequences.

There needs to be a systematic examination of those bioactive, protective phytochemicals (including nutrients) that will:

- improve knowledge about their uptake, metabolism and their localisation in tissues and cells, as well as understanding the basis of their activity
- define the steps that determine their biosynthesis in the plant and their turnover
- enable the intakes to be determined that will maximise their protective effects without causing toxicity.

8.3 Functional effects deliverable by plants

It is really only in the last 10–15 years that there has been an interest in understanding the basis for the health benefits associated with the consumption of non-nutritive components of plant foods. Prior to this period bioactive, secondary metabolites of food plants were considered to be undesirable. For example, the use of the term 'mycotoxin' was applied to any metabolite occurring in plants as a result of fungal growth. Many of these metabolites had been identified because of their toxicity to farm animals, but under such circumstances the exposure was high. It was never considered that at low exposures to these bioactive substances there might be beneficial effects. But there is clear evidence that one such compound, zearalenone, a product of the growth of *Fusarium moniliforme* on maize, is a weak oestrogen. It is likely to have effects following ingestion that are similar, if not identical, to those produced through the consumption of isoflavones. Isoflavones are found in some soya health food products and have been shown to be weak oestrogens that can prolong the oestrus cycle in women who consume soya products. This is not necessarily a toxic effect. Low dose exposures may result in benefits since there is a lower incidence of hormonally related cancers in women living in societies with a high consumption of soya.[3]

There is a consistent body of data which suggests that those consumers in the developed world who have a consistently high intake of plant-derived foods, have a much reduced incidence of cancer and probably of other environmentally related disease. It is hypothesised that a fundamental contributor to the causes of these diseases is the generation of reactive oxidative species (ROS), which are generated through normal metabolism, and in response to stress and infection as well as exposure to some toxic chemicals.[4] ROS are highly reactive free radicals that are generated by specific scavenging cells as a natural response to eliminate pathogens. Under normal conditions it is essential that their production is tightly regulated because of their toxicity to cells. Even so, it is clear that the processes are not 100% efficient and oxidatively damaged cellular macromolecules and their degradation products can be detected in human fluids and tissues, and their proportion increases with age.[5, 6]

Any component of the diet that is capable of acting as an antioxidant or of inducing antioxidant protective mechanisms might be expected to offer protection against the damaging effects of ROS generation in susceptible cells or tissues. Similarly components of the diet that inhibit specific cell division processes, or stimulate the immunological surveillance mechanisms could offer protection against the adverse effects of oxidative damage.

The health benefits of consuming plant foods are likely to be attributable to a number of effects that act in concert, rather than to be attributable to a single group of compounds. The occurrence of high levels of antioxidant vitamins in plants could act directly to reduce oxidative damage to human cells. Plants synthesise several classes of antioxidants, including vitamin C, as well as phenolic compounds, e.g. flavonoid pigments, carotenoids and tocopherols (principally vitamin E). In the plant they serve as protectants against environmental stress and in the delay and control of senescent processes. Increasing levels could have the triple advantage of improving nutrition, on the plant performance during growth and in post-harvest quality preservation. The potential benefits both to farmers and consumers make them very interesting targets for enhancement.

Apart from the direct ability of phytochemicals to inhibit free radicals, it is known that they are capable of inhibiting certain phase I enzymes that can activate pro-carcinogens to carcinogens (see Fig. 8.1). Phytochemicals also upregulate the synthesis of the enzymes that deactivate carcinogens, or other toxic metabolites, such as quinone reductase, those that inactivate free radicals such as catalase or superoxide dismutase, or those involved with regulating the synthesis of glutathione (glutathione reductase and glutathione peroxidase) and its conjugation (glutathione transferase). It has also been demonstrated that phytochemicals can inhibit cell division and stimulate immune responsiveness.[7]

The application of targeted genetic manipulations in plants will need to satisfy food regulatory bodies that the enhancement of levels will provide health benefits to all sections of the population, or conversely that there will be no risks to certain population subgroups. This will be a difficult challenge. Conventional plant breeding may have resulted in major compositional changes in food plants, which have not been well documented, but there is no evidence of any adverse

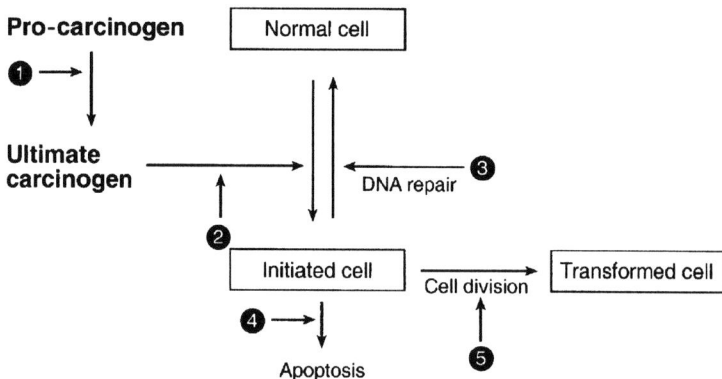

Key:
❶ Act as substrates/inhibitors of activating enzymes blocking the activation of the pro-carcinogen.
❷ Inactivate the ultimate carcinogenic species directly or by inducing deactivating enzymes, e.g. quinone reductase, catalase, superoxide dismutase, glutathione peroxidase, UDP gluconosyltransferases (UDPGT), glutathione-S-transferase, etc.
❸ Induce specific DNA repair enzymes.
❹ Stimulate the process of apoptosis in initiated cells.
❺ Inhibit cell division or regulate the induction and activity of specific hormones or membrane receptors for growth factors and nuclear gene expression systems.

Fig. 8.1   Potential mechanisms and sites for the inhibition of carcinogenesis by protective phytochemicals.

health effects. Indeed the evidence is overwhelmingly for health benefits. However, to put improvements in food quality through genetic manipulation into a rational framework, the effect on composition will need to be evaluated. This can only be done if it is known what the effects will be on the uptake, distribution and metabolism in target cells and tissues. Currently there is very little information available for most phytochemicals. At the present time it is possible to market novel foods if they are 'substantially equivalent' to traditionally consumed foods. This is a pragmatic basis for control but in order to put the issue of nutritional enhancement into a scientific framework, much more information about the impact of compositional changes on bioavailability will need to be known.

8.4 Plant sources of functional compounds

While many health authorities are encouraging the consumption of five portions of fruit and vegetables a day for the promotion of healthy eating, it is not the case that all fruit and vegetables act as important sources of the compounds that show beneficial effects. Some compounds are very specific to certain types of fruit or vegetable whereas others can be widely present in plants.

Plants provide the major sources of vitamins C, E and folates in the diet. In the Western diet practically all of the vitamin C is derived from fruit and vegetables. It has been estimated that 85% of intake in the UK is derived from fruit, fruit juices and vegetables. Until recently the seasonal availability of fruit and vegetables, together with the significant losses of vitamin C that occur on storage, meant that intakes of the vitamin were seriously deficient at certain times of the year. Interestingly the most important contributor of vitamin C to the diet is the potato – not because it is rich in vitamin C but because of its high consumption.

Tocopherols are found in a variety of plant foods such as nuts, seeds, plant oils, fruits, vegetables and cereals. The most important sources are the plant oils, especially given their wide utilisation in the manufacture of foods. Fruit and vegetables are much poorer sources of vitamin E, ranging in levels from 0.2 to 18 mg vit. E activity as α-TE compared with 100–500 mg vitamin E activity as α-TE. Highly processed oils can result in a loss of up to 50% of the tocopherol content of virgin oils.

The phenolics present in plants cover a wide range of chemical classes, each with interesting beneficial effects. Common antioxidant phenolics found in fruit and vegetables include flavonols, anthocyanins, flavan-3-ols (catechins) and hydroxycinnamates. Flavonols range from 4–100 mg kg^{-1} fresh weight (f.w.) in pome and stone fruits to 10–350 mg kg^{-1} f.w. in berry fruits. Anthocyanins are particularly high in cherries and berry fruits. Levels can reach up to 5,000 mg kg^{-1} f.w. Flavon-3-ols range from 1 to 250 mg kg^{-1} f.w. in fruits. Hydroxycinnamates range from 10 to 1,500 mg kg^{-1} f.w. in most fruits. The flavonol content of vegetables is highest in leafy vegetables but high levels are also found in alliceae and brassicae. Hydroxycinnamates are somewhat lower in vegetables compared with fruits, with ranges varying from 1 to 1,600 mg kg^{-1} f.w. The isoflavones are principally found in soybeans and products derived from them. Lentils and flaxseed are important sources for some communities. Most Western diets are likely to provide plant oestrogens from the lignols present in fruit and vegetables.

Some other potentially beneficial compounds, such as organosulphides (predominantly found in allium foods such as garlic, onions and leeks) and glucosinolates (present in cruciferous vegetables), are of limited interest in terms of enhancement of levels due to their strong flavours.

8.5 The delivery of functional effects

Food plants provide a regulated source of delivery of functional compounds. Most of the bioactive substances that might provide health benefits also have specific functions within the plant. Plant secondary metabolites function (a) as pollinator attractants (anthocyanins, flavonoids), (b) in infestation control (phytoalexins), and (c) as UV-protectants (carotenoids and flavonoids).

In general their production is under strict regulatory control and is tissue specific. Any attempt to upregulate their biosynthesis substantially might result in adverse effects elsewhere in the plant and toxicity. For example, the over-expression of glutathione synthesis in plants can result in the symptoms of oxidative stress in the plant.[8] Thus there is an inbuilt form of control that automatically limits concentrations and therefore intake when consumed as a food. This is not so with supplements.

Localisation of secondary metabolites in the cell wall or tightly bound to other structures normally acts to limit bioavailability, or to ensure that the phytochemical passes through the small intestine and reaches the lower bowel. This can affect the time course of release. The problem with rapid absorption, which could occur with supplements, is that there is the risk that the phytochemical might be delivered to the target or non-target sites in concentrations in excess of those required to optimise the effect. The greatest benefits are probably achieved through slow release, so that the effects extend for a longer period.

8.6 Enhancing functional effects

The overwhelming majority of the phytochemicals of interest, in terms of their potential health protective effects, are synthesised in the plant by two principal biosynthetic pathways – the phenylpropanoid and isoprenoid pathways – with some common links. The phenylpropanoid pathway leads to the production of lignins and their phenolic ester precursors, the flavones and related compounds, and isoflavones (see Fig. 8.2).

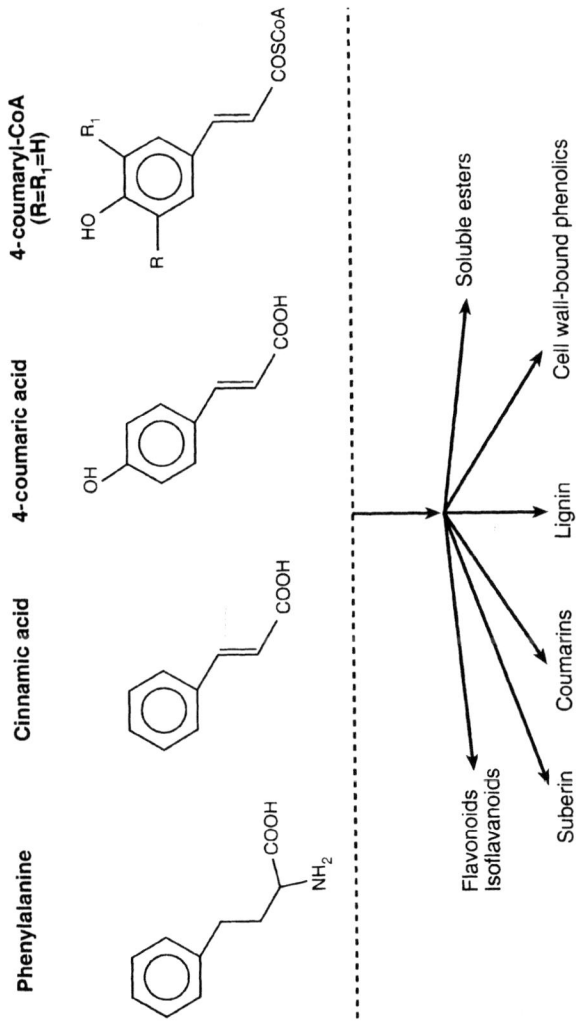

Fig. 8.2 Phytochemical synthesis via the phenylpropanoid pathway.

Acetyl-CoA

| 3-hydroxy-3-methylglutaryl CoA | HMG-CoA

Mevalonate

| Isopentenyl diphosphate | IPP

| Geranyl diphosphate | GPP   → | Monoterpenes |

| Farnesyl diphosphate | FPP   → | Sterols |

| Geranylgeranyl diphosphate | GGPP   → | Carotenoids |

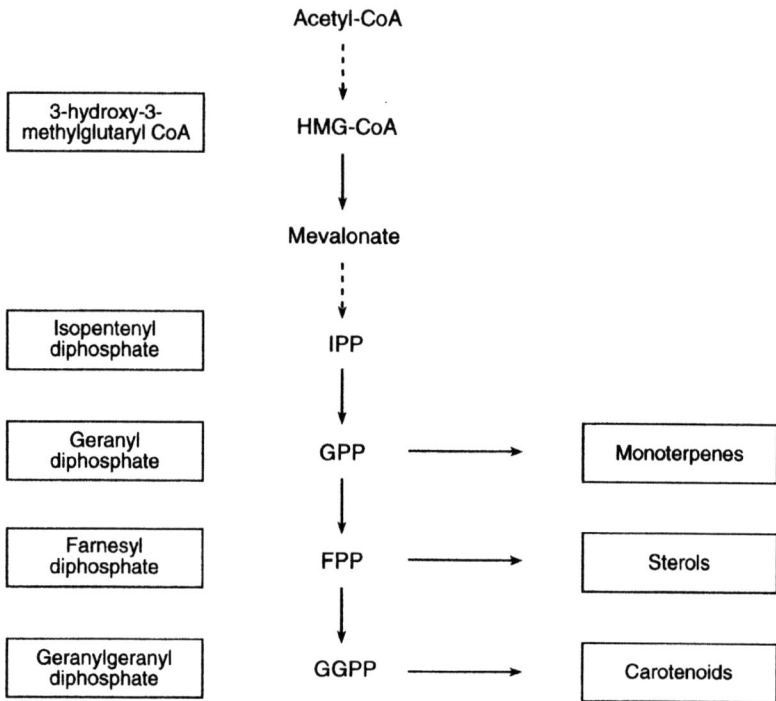

Fig. 8.3 Phytochemical synthesis via the isoprenoid pathway.

The isoprenoid pathway leads to the formation of terpenes, sterols, carotenoids, and the tocopherols (see Fig. 8.3).

The synthesis of specific metabolites, which can be very plant specific, is controlled through highly branched pathways and is carefully regulated. Given the wide diversity in structure and function of these metabolites in the plant, major differences in temporal and spatial distribution of the metabolite can occur, depending on the stage of development of the plant and between different plant organs and cell types.

There are a number of ways in which the concentrations of functionally active compounds can be increased by genetic manipulation. The most traditional approach, and one that has much to recommend it, is the use of 'classical' plant breeding techniques. Plant varieties have not been selected to date on the basis of nutritional qualities but there are wide natural variations that can be found in the gene pool of crop plants. In the case of the pro-vitamin A carotenoids, plants provide highly variable amounts depending on their colour. Varieties of sweet potato may contain levels varying from 0.13 mg to 11.3 mg g^{-1} dry weight of betacarotene.[9] Similar variations in levels can be found in carrots and cassava. In the case of the tomato, genes have been identified that are associated with high and low lycopene content. Incorporation of genes that increase lycopene content, or elimination of genes that decrease the lycopene content, can be done by pedigree selection and back-cross programmes. Such techniques have produced hybrids with a three- or four-fold content of lycopene in tomato fruits.[10]

Genetic engineering is now being applied to enhance levels of functional compounds in food crops. Indeed for some purposes it will be the only approach feasible, especially where there are widespread deficiency diseases and the population is dependent on staple crops that are not sources of the nutrient required. The introduction of a pro-vitamin A carotenoid into rice[11] is a major step forward in providing health benefits to those communities where rice is a staple food. However, there is strong opposition to the application of the technology for food production in Europe.

Potential strategies for the enhancement of specific metabolites could target upon the following:

- over-expression of enzymes that control the final steps in the biosynthesis of a metabolite
- over-expression of rate-limiting enzymes
- silencing of genes whose expression causes the metabolite to be degraded
- increased expression of genes that are not subject to metabolic feedback control
- increasing the number of plastids in a plant
- increasing metabolic flux into the pathway of interest
- expression in storage organs using site-specific promoters.

The strategy that has had the greatest success at present is the first one but this presupposes that the metabolite of interest is the final one in a particular pathway. In practice, if a substantial increase in the concentration of a metabolite is required, the use of specific promoters directing the synthesis to a particular organelle normally used for storage purposes, or where the plant normally synthesises the metabolite, is essential. Failure to do so could cause toxicity in the plant by interfering with the production or function of other essential metabolites.

No strategies have yet been applied where multiple gene insertions are necessary to produce the metabolite, or where plastid numbers have been increased. However, rapid accumulation of sequence data of both chromosomal DNA and expressed sequence tags of plants and other species is providing rapid advances in knowledge of the genetic make-up and functions of several plants and it is expected that these other possibilities will soon be feasible.

Food processing technologies, which are safe but do not involve excessive heat treatment or the risk of oxidative destruction of vitamins, need to be applied to assess the effects on specific functional compounds. The fact that some compounds, such as lycopene, are actually more bioavailable following high temperature processing than in raw or lightly processed food means that careful attention has to be given to the factors that influence bioavailability and the method of its production.

8.7 Factors affecting the intake of functional compounds

While food processing normally leads to a reduction in the levels of vitamins – the more rigorous the process, the greater the reduction in levels – in some instances processing has a dramatic effect on availability.

The diet plays an important role in the uptake of specific nutrients and phytochemicals. Those that are lipophilic are absorbed much more readily from a lipid-rich diet. Frying tomatoes in oil dramatically improves the uptake of lycopene compared with the consumption of fresh tomatoes.[12] Raw carrots, which have high levels of pro-vitamin A carotenoids, are poorer sources of betacarotene than gently cooked carrot.[13] The bioavailability of certain trace elements is increased on cooking or processing, such as the increased bioavailability of iron in canned spinach.[14] The chemical form of the phytochemical present in food is very important in determining the uptake through the gastrointestinal tract. Quercitin-β-glucoside is more easily absorbed than the aglycone quercitin. Isorhamnetin-β-glucoside, which is chemically similar to quercitin, differing only by a single methoxyl group, is much more readily absorbed. Flavonoid rutinosides (rhamnosyl 1-6 glucosides) are not easily absorbed.[15]

The chemical form of the phytochemical is of profound importance when considering the biological relevance of specific chemicals and their levels in the diet. Whilst some phenols might be better antioxidants than others when tested in *in vitro* systems, this is of little significance in terms of health relevance. What matters is whether the compounds are easily absorbed, are not quickly degraded in tissues, and are able to reach the target sites. Flavonoids (see Fig. 8.4) that are not absorbed undergo extensive degradation by gut micro-organisms, and may play a limited role in preventing oxidative damage in the colon.

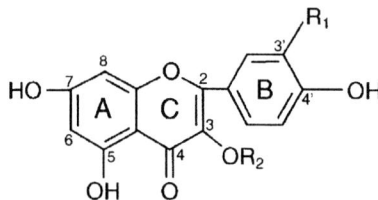

Fig. 8.4   Structure of flavonoids.

8.8 Enhancing macronutrient quality

The focus of much of the genetic engineering work to date has been on improving the overall protein and lipid profiles in pulses and oilseeds. While the impetus for this work has been principally to realise new market opportunities in the animal feedstuffs and industrial chemical sectors, there are potential applications with nutritional benefits.

8.8.1 Alterations in the fatty acid composition of oilseeds

The manipulation of oilseed fatty acid composition was one of the early successes of the application of genetic engineering. Commercial cultivation of a genetically engineered lauric oil rapeseed was achieved in 1995 in the USA.[16] This success reflected the relative ease of the manipulation of genes into *Brassicae napus*, sufficient knowledge about the metabolic pathways involved in storage oil biosynthesis, and the potential to alter composition through single gene insertions.

The commercial driving force for this product was not, however, a nutritional one but as a potential replacement for palm and coconut oils in soap and detergent manufacture. There are major commercial constraints on the modification of plant oil seeds for nutritional purposes. This is not only because of the lack of sufficient categorical evidence for health benefits and the diversity of needs within the population, but also because of the expense of applying the technologies available. There is still insufficient knowledge about the full implications of genetic modification on the biochemical regulation of lipid biosynthesis. Special promoters must be used in any construct to ensure that the target for modification is the oil storage bodies and not the membrane lipids that are essential for plant growth and survival. Multiple gene insertions are also required for some applications, increasing the overall costs of production and seriously affecting the economic feasibility of the process.

In general commercial oilseeds accumulate long chain fatty acids containing 16 or 18 carbons with one to several double bonds, although higher chain lengths can occur in some plants. Synthesis occurs in the plastids through a two-carbon addition to a growing acyl-carrier protein (ACP) linked via a covalent thioester bond eventually to C18-ACP (palmitoyl-ACP) (see Fig. 8.5). Acyl-ACP thioesterases cleave the acyl group from the ACP. Free acyl CoAs are formed that are transferred to the cytoplasm where further desaturation and elongation can occur to form other fatty acids that can be utilised in triacylglycerol biosynthesis. In general the acyl-ACP thioesterases which are present in commercial oilseeds only cleave ACP bond at the C16:0, C18:0 and C18:1 stages.

A novel oil has been synthesised through the transfer of the California bay tree gene for a lauryl acyl carrier protein thioesterase into rapeseed. The thioesterase from the Californian bay tree shows maximal activity for 12C-ACP thioesters and can intercept the biosynthesis and divert the pathway to the formation of the free lauric acid for triacylglycerol (TAG) synthesis.

The free fatty acid pool serves as a source of fatty acids used in the synthesis of the TAGs. Formation of TAG begins with the acylation of glyceryl-3-phosphate catalysed by an enzyme (glycerol-3-phosphate acyltransferase), which is most active in acylating saturated FAs. A second enzyme, lysophosphatidic acid transferase, is usually highly selective and shows preferential activity towards unsaturated FAs, if these are present in the free FA pool, resulting in the preferential insertion of the unsaturated fatty acid in the middle of the triacylglycerol position (the sn2 position). Such lipids, known as structured lipids, are claimed to have nutritional benefits over unstructured

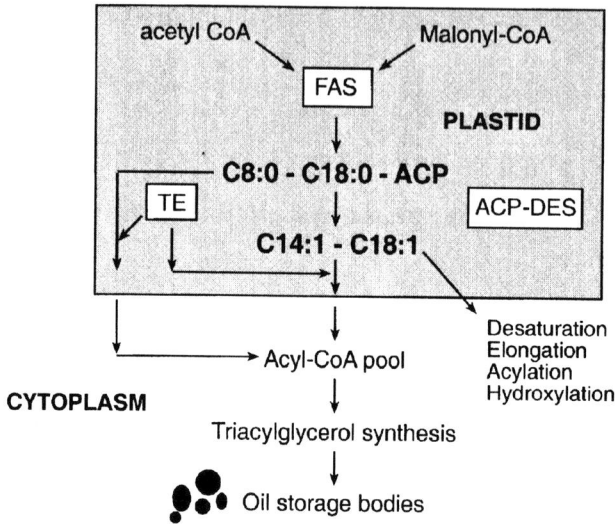

Fig. 8.5   Biosynthesis of plant lipids. (FAS: fatty acid synthase complex. ACP-DES: acyl-carrier protein desaturases. TE: acyl carrier protein thioesterases.)

lipids, although it is presently doubtful that these effects are superior to the benefits that can be obtained from the mixture of various types of oil for parenteral nutrition purposes.[17]

Eicosopentanoic acid (EPA; 20:5) and docosahexaenoic acid (DHA; 22:6), are polyunsaturated fatty acids (PUFAs) of particular interest since they are normally only available from fish oil sources, and their isolation is expensive. Although humans can synthesise them from the essential PUFA α-linolenic acid (18:3n-3), the conversion efficiency is low and consumption of EPA and DHA directly is more efficient at increasing their levels in plasma. The nutritional interest lies in the fact that they are beneficial as precursors for the synthesis of certain eicosanoids that have pro- and anti-inflammatory properties.

Consumption of fish oil causes a replacement of arachidonic acid (AA) in membranes with EPA and DHA. In most conditions AA is the principal precursor of eicosanoids (class II) that are more potent than those derived from dihomo-γ-linoleic acid (class I) or EPA (class III) (see Fig. 8.6). EPA-derived eicosanoids reduce the tendency for platelets to aggregate due to the production of weaker thromboxanes. These inhibit the stronger aggregator thomboxanes derived from AA decreasing the risk of atherosclerosis. Also EPA inhibits Δ-6 desaturase that decrease the amount of dietary linoleic acid converted to AA. EPA and DHA competitively inhibit the oxygenation of AA by cyclooxygenase which is the first step in the synthesis of the Type II eicosanoids. There is evidence linking an increased intake of these PUFAs to protection against cardiovascular disease,[18] to improvements in the immune response,[19] and even longevity.[20]

The introduction of the genes for the biosynthesis of specific ω-3 PUFAs will be a major challenge to molecular biologists since the PUFA synthetic pathways

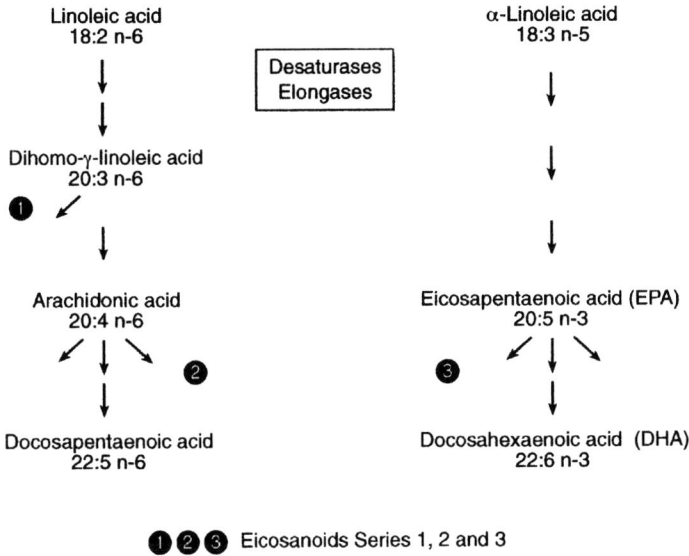

Fig. 8.6   Biosynthesis of eicosanoid precursors.

in algal and fungal sources of these PUFAs are poorly defined, and the enzymes and substrates involved are uncharacterised at the genomic level. In addition the multiple gene transfers not only add to the costs of production but can lead to instability in gene expression (co-suppression effects).

It is difficult to predict how to engineer a plant to produce DHA given the complexity of controlling biosynthesis in a multi-gene pathway. A significant breakthrough has been the synthesis of γ-linoleic acid (GLA; 18:3) in tobacco as a result of the upregulation of the Δ6-desaturase gene.[21] Very recently there has been a report of the isolation of a Δ5-desaturase gene from yeast which converts di-homo-γ-linolenic acid to arachidonic acid, and which is the principal precursor for the production of the eicosonoids.[22]

8.8.2 Alteration in amino acid content of proteins

Legumes are one of the most important sources of proteins in human diets. The major protein in bean seeds is phaseolin, which comprises 40% of the total protein content. It contains only three methionine residues and is seriously deficient in this essential amino acid when compared with the major egg protein, ovalbumin.

To improve the nutritional value of phaseolin, a 45bp oligonucleotide containing six methionine codons was introduced into the third exon of the phaseolin gene,[23] but the resulting seeds contained little phaseolin. Subsequent three-dimensional analysis of the protein indicated that the introduction of extra methionine residues would destabilise the phaseolin and stop it from folding correctly during its synthesis in the vacuole.[24]

Examination of the amino acid sequences of various related storage proteins to phytohemagglutinin showed that there were variable and conserved regions in the molecule. Introduction of methionine codons into the variable region by site-directed mutagenesis did not affect the stable accumulation of phytohemagglutinin into the vacuoles of the transgenic tobacco seed.[25]

Care has to be taken, however, in any such manipulations from the risk of creating sites of allergenicity. A methionine-rich albumin gene from the brazil nut was ligated into the promoter region of the phaseolin gene and the chimeric gene introduced into tobacco where it resulted in a 30% increase in methionine content in the seed.[26] Similar success was found with its introduction into soybean.[27] However, ligation of the gene into the promoter region of the concavalin gene in French beans only produced a limited amount of the brazil nut protein in seeds, showing the difficulty in developing generic approaches.[28] In addition the brazil nut protein has been shown to be an allergen,[29] casting doubt over the value of pursuing such an approach. A more promising approach is to use the protein isolated from sunflower seeds with a high methionine content and which is not allergenic.[30]

The metabolic demands that occur in expressing high levels of sulphur-rich proteins appear to cause competition for the formation of other sulphur-containing compounds in the plant. The total sulphur content of the legumes are little changed as a result of these manipulations.[30] For example, in the case of soya there is a suppression of the synthesis of other methionine-containing proteins including a protease inhibitor protein. There is a lack of knowledge of sulphur flux, the control of pathways of sulphur metabolism, the mechanisms by which amino acids can be channelled from one synthetic pathway to another, and the control of gene expression by the amino acid supply. The unexpected reduction in protease inhibitor in soybean has a nutritional benefit, however, since the reduction of these inhibitors in legumes increases digestibility and improves trace element uptake.

Further information on the regulation of seed protein gene expression is necessary to construct a strong promoter, as well as improvements in the stable accumulation of engineered proteins into seeds of transgenic legume plants, before nutritionally improved legumes are feasible. Above all, care will have to be exercised in assessing the safety of the resulting food.

Other approaches that could lead to an improvement in the nutritional content of such crops would be to upregulate glutathione biosynthesis (see Fig. 8.7). Apart from providing an extra source of sulphur it is considered to be a key component in the defence of the plant against oxidative stress. Its manipulation could lead to both agronomic and nutritional benefits. The biosynthesis of glutathione has been well studied. A number of the DNA sequences coding important enzymes in its biosynthesis are available from bacterial, animal and plant sources.

The upregulation of glutathione synthatase did not increase the glutathione content of transgenic plants. But if γ-glutamylcysteine synthatase was enhanced, there was a sevenfold increase in foliar glutathione levels. However, signs of

Glutamate   Cysteine

γ-EC

Glycine   γ-Glutamylcysteine

GSH-synthatase

Ascorbate ←——————→ GSH ———————→ NADP+

DHAR   GPx   GR

Dehydroascorbate ———————— GSSG ←———————— NADPH

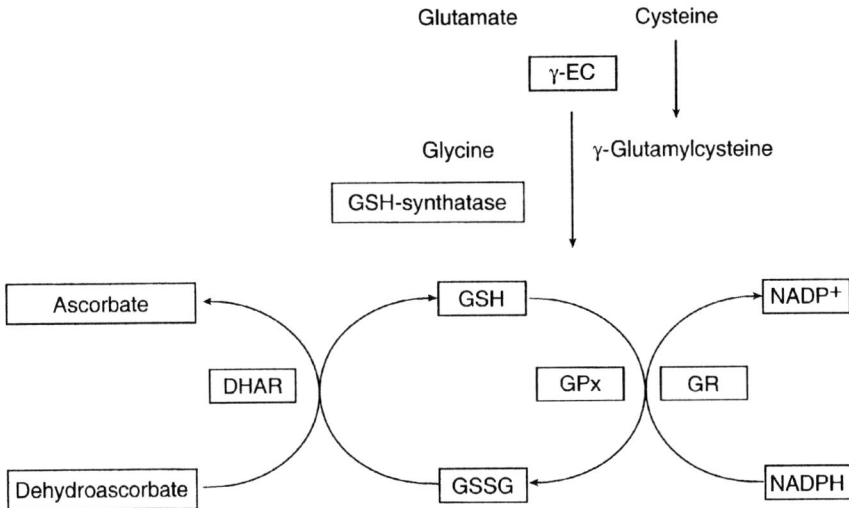

Fig. 8.7   The biosynthesis of glutathione. (GSH: reduced glutathione. GSSG: oxidised
    glutathione. GR: glutathione reductase. GPx: glutathione peroxidase. γ-EC: γ-
    glutamylcysteine synthatase. DHAR: dehydroascorbate reductase.)

severe oxidative stress were evident. Plants that were engineered to contain both
genes were free of these symptoms and were associated with a decline in the
levels of γ-glutamylcysteine. These data suggest that if this intermediate in the
biosynthesis of glutathione is not allowed to accumulate, toxicity symptoms can
be avoided.[31]

Interestingly, the enhancement of glutathione reductase, which catalyses the
reduction of oxidised glutathione (GSSG) to its reduced form (GSH), in one or
more of the cytosol, chloroplasts and mitochondria in cells of transgenic tobacco
or poplar, leads to improved stress tolerance and to a total increase in the foliar
concentration of glutathione in spinach. The link between an enhancement in the
capacity of a plant to reduce the oxidised form of an antioxidant (glutathione is
protective against oxidative damage) and total pool size of that antioxidant is
poorly understood but may also apply to elevation of other antioxidants, such as
ascorbate. Overall redox potential in a cell is a crucial factor in the recognition
of a stressed or normal state which could have a subsequent impact on gene
expression.

8.9   Enhancing micronutrient quality

Plants contain 17 mineral nutrients, 13 vitamins and numerous phytochemicals
that have been shown to have potentially beneficial effects on health. Almost all
human nutrients can be obtained from plant foods; the exceptions are vitamins
B_{12} and D. However, the adequacy of a plant diet in delivering a health benefit

will depend on bioavailability. Many plant beneficial compounds that are associated with the plant cell wall are not easily bioavailable. Any way in which overall levels can be increased will help overcome this difficulty.

8.9.1 Enhancement of vitamin E levels

Vitamin E consists of a mixture of tocopherols (α-, β-, δ- and γ-tocopherol) but α-tocopherol is the most important for health and has the highest vitamin activity. The established relative activity for α-, β-, δ-, and γ-tocopherols are 100%, 50%, 10%, and 3% respectively. In the USA the adult recommended allowance for vitamin E is 8–10 mg (α-tocopherol) based on an avoidance of vitamin deficiency diseases. However, current evidence suggests that an intake of 100–250 mg α-tocopherol is required if long-term disease risks are to be avoided. This is not feasible from unsupplemented diets if general nutritional guidelines are followed, especially since in most plants the ratio of α- to γ-tocopherol is fairly low.

The tocopherol biosynthetic pathway is known but only one gene, encoding the enzyme p-hydroxyphenylpyruvate dioxygenase – HPPDase – is characterised. The genes for HPPDase have been identified from *Daucus carota* and *Arabidopsis thaliana*. In spite of the fact that few genes were available for use in genetic engineering studies, a significant increase in the α-tocopherol levels in plants has been achieved through the over-expression of γ-tocopherol methyltransferase (γ-TMT), the final stage in the biosynthetic pathway.

The fact that many oilseeds contain high levels of γ-tocopherol suggests that the final step of the biosynthetic pathway is rate limited by the activity of γ-TMT (see Fig. 8.8). The successful strategy that was adopted was to focus on the identification of a γ-TMT gene in *Synechocystis* PCC 6803 which, like

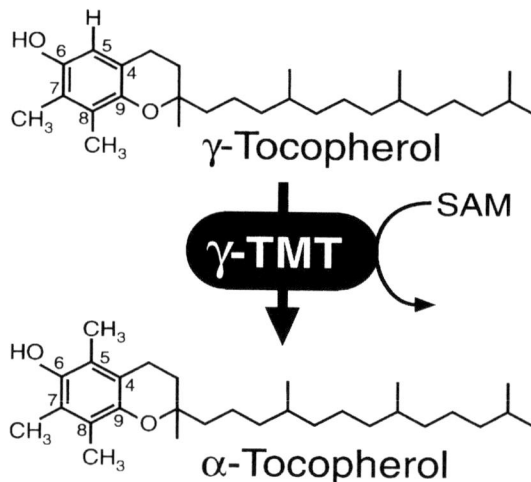

Fig. 8.8   Synthesis of α-tocopherol from γ-tocopherol.

Arabidopsis thaliana, accumulates (R,R,R)-α-tocopherol to an extent greater than 95% of the total tocopherol in the organism.

An *Arabidopsis* gene coding for the HPPDase was used to search the *Synechocystis* genomic database for common identities in a single open reading frame. A gene was located with a 35% homology to the *Arabidopsis* HPPDase gene located in a predicted ten-gene operon. It was hypothesised that related biosynthetic genes might be found within the same operon, given the fact that related biosynthetic genes are frequently located within the same operon in bacteria. The operon contained a candidate open reading frame that predicted a methyl transferase activity. The γ-TMT gene was located through the identification of a close sequence similarity to Δ-(24)-sterol-C-methyltransferase as well as to other structural features common to those of a γ-TMT (e.g. an S-adenosylmethionine binding site).

A null mutant of the gene was created that was shown not to synthesise α-tocopherol but to accumulate the intermediate biosynthetic precursor γ-tocopherol. Further biochemical analysis of the gene product in *E. coli* confirmed that the open reading frame encoded the *Synechocystis* γ-TMT. Expression of the *Synechocystis* gene in *E. coli* showed that the recombinant protein catalysed the methylation of γ-tocopherol to α-tocopherol. Sequence analogy analysis was used to identify the corresponding gene in *Arabidopsis*.

Arabidopsis was transformed by the *Arabidopsis* γ-TMT cDNA driven by the seed-specific carrot DC3-promoter. This resulted in an increase of greater than eightyfold in the levels of α-tocopherol where greater than 90% of the tocopherol content was as the α-isomer compared with the untransformed plant. However, total seed tocopherol levels were unchanged, indicating that γ-TMT plays an important role in determining the composition but not the total content of the seed tocopherol pool.[32] Given the higher potency of α- compared with γ-tocopherol, the possibility exists of increasing their nutritive value of a wide range of commercially important oilseed crops.

The genomics-assisted strategy adopted in this case will be useful in accelerating gene discovery in other secondary metabolic pathways, especially those responsible for the synthesis of nutritionally beneficial phytochemicals. A growing number of sequence databases are available which can be interrogated to discover orthologous pathway genes.

8.9.2 Manipulation of carotenoid levels

The nature of the challenges faced in manipulating plant metabolites is well illustrated through the attempts that have been made to alter carotenoid levels in food plants.

A simplified version of the pathways leading to the synthesis of the carotenoids principally found in food plants is shown in Fig. 8.9.

A crucial enzyme involved in their synthesis is phytoene synthase (PSY 1) which converts geranylgeranylphosphate (GGDP) into phytoene. Inhibition of PSY1 through the use of antisense gene-silencing techniques resulted in a 90%

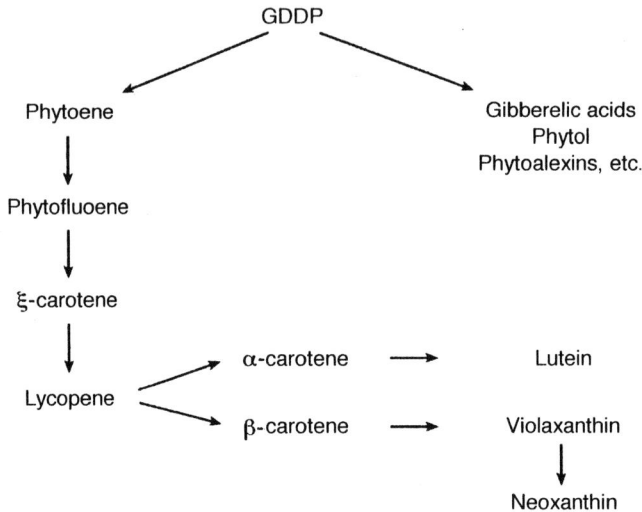

Fig. 8.9   Biosynthesis of carotenoids from GGDP.

reduction in carotenoid levels compared with wild type in the tomato.[33] Over-expression of PSY1 results in dwarfed tomato plants.[34] This has been explained by the increased flow of metabolites into the carotenoid branch of the isoprenoid pathway leading to a reduction in the metabolites available for gibberellin synthesis. The general, isoprenoid pathway is utilised by plants for the synthesis of many important products including sterol, chlorophyll, quinone and phytoalexin production, as well as for the gibberellins. It illustrates the complex interactions that are occurring and the potential disbenefits arising from the manipulation of the level of any one enzyme.

Improvements in the process can be made by ensuring that genes are expressed in a tissue-specific manner through the insertion of specific promoters. This has been achieved for rice where carotenoid levels have been increased significantly through the use of the daffodil *psy* gene.[35] In the case of tomato, a twofold increase in total carotenoid levels occurs using this *psy* transformant which is significantly lower than for rice. In rice the daffodil *psy* cDNA insertion is under the control of an endosperm-specific promoter. The choice of promoter will very much affect the timing and tissue-specific expression of a gene.

It has been possible to induce xanthophyll accumulation in potato tubers that do not normally contain betacarotene.[36] The use of bacterial *psy* genes instead of the daffodil *psy* gene in tomatoes produces a sevenfold increase in betacarotene levels but this is at the expense of the ripening pigment lycopene which is the predominant carotenoid in tomato.

Monsanto has introduced phytoene synthase into rapeseed and has appreciably enhanced levels of betacarotene. Interestingly, a higher level of α-carotene (lutein) is also produced.

This indicates the potential, given the right set of carotenoid biosynthesis genes, with the correct target sequences and promoters, to accumulate carotenoids in other plant tissues/organs/crops that currently contain little or none. This remains a major challenge. Much more needs to be known about the exact regulatory factors that affect carotenoid biosynthesis.

8.9.3 Improvement of iron content of plants

Although plants contain iron, it is invariably in a form that is much less biologically available and utilisable than when it is complexed with protein as in haemoglobin. Consequently regular meat eaters are rarely iron deficient. The challenge to the biotechnologists was how to achieve an improvement in the bioavailability of iron in plants. A lot of attention has been given recently to understanding the processes controlling iron uptake into plants as well as to engineering its uptake.

The nutritional importance of achieving this is unquestionable. It has long been a concern in developed countries that vegan or vegetarian women are at risk of developing anaemia. In the developing world iron-deficient anaemia is a serious problem affecting an estimated 30% of the world's population. As if this was not a sufficient target for the enhancement of levels, it emerges that over-expression of ferritin in tobacco increases the plant's tolerance to oxidative damage and pathogens, opening up the possibility of substantial increases in productivity and environmental benefits.[37]

Simultaneously it has been possible to increase the iron content of rice through the introduction of the soybean ferritin gene into rice through *Agrobacterium*-mediated transformation.[38] The ferritin gene was expressed under the control of a rice seed storage protein glutelin promoter to ensure that ferritin was accumulated in the seed. The protein was found to be located in the endosperm sub-aleurone layer of the seed. The iron content of the transformed seeds was as much as threefold higher than their untransformed counterparts. This would be sufficient to produce 30–50% of the daily adult iron requirement (13–15 mg/day) and in a form that is likely to be bioavailable.

A frequent problem in attempting to introduce foreign proteins is that proteolytic degradation can occur. Ferritin is synthesised from a 32kDa precursor into a 28kDa sub-unit and a 26.5kDa partially degraded sub-unit. Correct assembly of the protein is required for importation of the sub-unit into the plastid as well as for the iron storage function. The stable incorporation of the 28kDa sub-unit was found to occur in these experiments, suggesting that the endosperm tissue is an appropriate tissue for accumulation of foreign ferritin and is protected from the action of plant proteases. Use of a rice-specific promoter appears to have had the advantage not only of conferring endosperm-specific expression of the ferritin gene but also to encourage a higher level of expression than occurs with the cauliflower mosaic virus 35S promoter.

8.10 The effects of food processing

There are not a lot of published data available about the effects of food processing on phytochemicals, other than nutrients. However, it is apparent that, in general, the stronger the processing conditions, the greater the degradation of specific nutrients and phytochemicals. But even under the most severe processing conditions or cooking in the home, some compounds are remarkably stable.

8.10.1 Processing of oils

The initial stages of refining of crude vegetable oils use water or steam to degum, followed by centrifugation. Physical or chemical refining procedures can then be used. Physical methods involve steam treatment to volatilise free fatty acids and bleaching is normally adopted. This removes any carotenoids but without this step the oils are less stable. A compromise has to be adopted to remove materials producing instability and the preservation of some antioxidants. Chemical methods involve saponification with sodium hydroxide, followed by centrifugation.

There are considerable benefits in retaining high levels of antioxidants throughout the processing stages to improve overall product quality and avoid rancidity. However, the processes to produce high quality oils, that is oils acceptable to users, require them to be low in flavour and cloudiness, and light in colour. These demands can lead to oils that are much lower in antioxidant content than the oilseeds from which they are derived.

Given the fact that energy costs of edible oil production are high, and that the nutritional quality is not optimal, other processes, such as membrane separation, are being considered. The preservation of antioxidants in oils is best achieved through the use of stainless steel equipment since metal ions encourage the auto-oxidation of lipids. In addition, air must be removed at temperatures below 100°C before the oil is heated to the final stripping temperature.

Virgin oils are also susceptible to oxidation, even with high antioxidant content. It is essential to keep the peroxide value of these oils low in order to avoid rancidity and the loss of antioxidants since, once oxidation occurs, the process is auto-catalytic. Oil extraction using a two-phase centrifugal decanter yields olive oil with improved quality when compared with those that use the conventional three-phase equipment. The oils produced by the two-phase technology have a higher content of polyphenols, ortho-diphenols, hydroxytyrosol and tocopherols and a higher stability.[39]

8.10.2 Processing of fruits and vegetables

There has not been any systematic examination of the effects of processing on the levels and chemical composition of many bioactive phytochemicals in plant foods. The information that is available is mostly confined to the effects on nutrients, carotenoids and some phenolic components of plant foods. Even so there is incomplete information on the effects of particular processes on the overall nutritive value of fruits and vegetables.

Although the levels of nutrients and phytochemicals can be greatly influenced by agronomic practices, optimal processes for maintaining the content of antioxidant vitamins in fruit and vegetables start from post-harvest handling. Careful attention to temperature in harvesting and minimisation of light and oxygen help reduce loss. Loss of vitamins in fresh vegetables is invariably associated with wilting. The cold storage of vegetables with appropriate humidity helps to preserve vitamin content. Some vegetables, such as broccoli, are more sensitive than others, e.g. green beans, to refrigerated storage. On the other hand, the vitamin content of fresh fruits is not stable for long periods of time in the refrigerator. Inactivation of polyphenol oxidase also helps to maintain antioxidant status.[39]

Modified atmosphere packaging is widely used in fruit and vegetable marketing. While the removal of oxygen and the use of plastics with low gas permeability membranes might be expected to lead to the stability of nutrients, carbon dioxide accumulation occurs, leading to anoxia and loss of quality. Active packaging offers the possibility to overcome these problems from the use of oxygen-scavenging materials such as vitamins C or E into the film. However, this is not happening at the moment. The vitamin A content of sweet potato is maintained after four months' storage if it is stored in an impermeable plastic material with an oxygen scavenger in the packaging material, compared with a retention of only 45% in permeable plastic, 62% in impermeable material with air in the head space, and 73% in vacuum-sealed impermeable plastics.[9]

Dehydration of fruits and vegetables invariably leads to a loss in nutrients other than trace elements due to the greater surface area and exposure to oxygen and light. Betacarotene levels are reasonably stable on processing provided that oxygen is rigidly excluded from the process. A decrease of 30–55% in levels occurs following canning because of the anoxic environment. Freeze-drying does not significantly alter total carotenoid levels. Freezing generally preserves carotenoids, whereas sun or solar drying leads to considerable losses. In developing countries sufficient amounts may remain, however, to provide vitamin A requirements.[40] The problem of vitamin A deficiency is often attributable to the seasonable variations in availability of pro-vitamin A rich foods.

Processing of plant foods rich in phenolic compounds can result in increased levels of some of the phenols after processing. Raspberry juice, prepared by a diffusion extraction process where the juice is held at high temperatures (65°) for a long period, results in an increased content of ellagic acid. Jam making also increases levels of this compound. Anthocyanins appear to survive the jam-making process but conversion to other compounds occurs – probably chalcones – and these compounds are not characterised. These changes are possibly due to the release of ellagic acid from the cell walls by hydrolysis of ellagitanins.[41] However, the changes in phenolic content can vary very widely, depending on the process and compound. Technological processes in juice and wine production can have a marked effect. Skin fermentation of wines results in a higher content of phenols in the product but in general the levels of total phenols in wine are less than found in juices.[42, 43] Very complex changes occur to the anthocyanins when wine is produced. Cooking of onions and tomatoes leads to a marked reduction in the levels of quercitin.[44] The phenolic compounds in olives are transformed depending on the method used in their curing. It is clear that the characterisation of the effects of processing on the concentration of phenolics in plants will need investigating at the level of the individual process and compound since some compounds will increase, others decrease, and a considerable number will be transformed. The biological significance of these changes is going to be extremely complex to unravel. The focus will have to be on those compounds that are consumed in the greatest amounts and dietary studies will be required to determine this.

Apart from effects on the overall levels in foods, processing can affect the chemical composition of the food which may have biological consequences. The carotenoids have been studied in most detail in this regard. Processing can lead to significant losses of epoxicarotenoids (e.g. lutein-5-6-epoxide, neoxanthin and violaxanthin, lutein and to a lesser extent the carotenes where trans to cis isomerisation occurs (e.g. 5-cis-lycopene and 13-cis-β-carotene), as well as to different carotenoid by-products. The extent of these changes is dependent upon the type of vegetable, the method of cooking, and the temperature and time conditions. The higher the temperature and the longer the period of cooking, the greater the change.[45] Heating of carotenoids in the presence of oxygen results in their oxidation to apocarotenals, some of which might still possess biological activity.

New processing techniques, such as high electric pulse fields, or high pressure processing, especially of fruit juices, help to maintain vitamin levels.

8.11 Future trends: the work of NEODIET

The European Commission, under its Food and Agro-Industrial Research programme (FAIR), recognised the important need to improve the nutritional value of food in determining the research priorities for this programme. This was not only from the perspective of providing consumers with potential health benefits but also that of encouraging innovation in industry through the development of new products and processes which would utilise the scientific advances in the field of diet and health. In 1997 they supported a concerted action on the Nutritional Enhancement of Plant Foods in European Trade (NEODIET), in order to give the topic a higher profile throughout Europe, and to bring together research workers in Europe with an interest in this topic.

The overall objectives of the NEODIET concerted action programme are to:

- exchange information in the area of improving the nutritional value of plant foods through the use of genetic modification and food processing technologies; and
- set up a network of collaboration between research scientists in academia and industry who are working both at the EU and national level in this field.

Both the agrochemical and food industries are involved in the project to help stimulate technological development.

8.11.1 Priorities of NEODIET

The steering committee for NEODIET decided that the initial priority areas for the project should be on improving the trace nutrient and potential health protective factors in plants. The particular focus is on those compounds for which there is some evidence that intakes are not presently optimal for health benefits, or where there is some evidence for health benefits, particularly in relation to antioxidant properties. Attention is focused on the following:

- folates
- vitamins C and E
- carotenoids
- glucosinolates
- phytosterols
- flavonoids
- simple phenols
- certain trace elements.

The project has stimulated interest in the topic through the organisation of a series of workshops and meetings to review the latest developments in all of the disciplines that have to be brought together to achieve future progress. These include molecular biologists, biochemists, nutritionists and food technologists. A series of position papers have been produced which have reviewed the current information on all of the priority compounds in the project in terms of the issues raised in this chapter, and which will be a comprehensive overview of the field.[46] The principal purpose, however, is to identify the most important research challenges that will need to be addressed in the future to benefit consumers. In this way it was hoped to encourage future research collaboration throughout Europe. Further information on the project can be found on the website http//:www.ifrn.bbsrc.ac.uk/neodiet/

8.12 References

1 World Health Organization, 'Global prevalence of vitamin A deficiencies', Micronutrient Deficiency Information Systems, Working Paper No. 2, Geneva, WHO 1995.

2   BLOCK, G., PATTERSON, B. and SUBAR, A. 'Fruit, vegetables and cancer prevention: a review of the epidemiological evidence', *Nutr & Cancer*, 1992, **18**, 1–29.

3   SETCHELL, K.D.R., BORRIELLO, S.P., HULME, P. *et al.* 'Non-steroidal estrogens of dietary origin: possible roles in hormone-dependent disease', *Am J Clin Nutr*, 1984, **40**, 569–78.

4   DIPLOCK, A.T. 'Antioxidants and disease prevention', *Mol Aspects Med*, 1994, **15**, 293–376.

5   PAPA, S., SCACCO, S., SCHLIEBS, M., TRAPPE, J. and SEIBEL, P. 'Mitochondrial diseases and ageing', *Mol Aspects Med*, 1996, **17**, 513–58.

6   MECOCCI, P., FANO, G., FULLE, S., MACGARVEY, U. *et al.* 'Age-dependent increases in oxidative damage to DNA, lipids, and proteins in human skeletal muscle', *Free Rad Biol & Med*, 1999, **26**, 303–8.

7   JOHNSON, I.T., WILLIAMSON, G. and MUSK, S.R.R. 'Anticarcinogenic factors in plant foods: a new class of nutrients?', *Nutr Res Rev*, 1994, **7**, 175–204.

8   MULLINEAUX, P.M. and CREISSEN, G.P. 'Opportunities for the genetic manipulation of antioxidants in plant foods', *Trans Biochem Soc*, 1996, **24**, 829–35.

9   SOLOMONS, N.W. and BULUX, J. 'Identification of local carotene-rich foods to combat vitamin A malnutrition', *Eur J Clin Nutrn*, 1997, **51**, S39–S45.

10 AMITOM, 'Role and control of antioxidants in the tomato processing industry', EU FAIR Project (FAIR CT97-3233), http//:www.tomate.org/Antioxidantnetwork.html

11 BURKHARDT, P.K., BEYER, P., WUNN, J. *et al.* 'Transgenic rice (*Oryza sativa*) endosperm expressing daffodil (*Narcissus pseudonarcissus*) phytoene synthase, accumulates phytoene a key intermediate in pro-vitamin A synthesis', *Plant J*, 1997, **11**, 1071–78.

12 GÄRTNER, C., STAHL, W. and SIES, H. 'Increased lycopene bioavailability from tomato paste as compared to fresh tomatoes', *Am J Clin Nutrn*, 1997, **66**, 116–22.

13 ROCK, C.L., LOVALVO, J.L., EMENHISER, C. *et al.* 'Bioavailability of beta-carotene is lower in raw than in processed carrots and spinach in women', *J Nutr*, 1998, **128**, 913–16.

14 LEE, K. and CLYDESDALE, F.M. 'Effect of thermal processing on endogenous and added iron in canned spinach', *J Food Sci*, **46**, 1064–7.

15 AZIZ, A.A., EDWARDS, C.A., LEAN, M.E.J. and CROZIER, A. 'Absorbtion and excretion of conjugated flavonols, including quercitin-4′-O-β-glucoside and isorhamnetin-4′-O-β-glucoside by human volunteers after the consumption of onions', *Free Rad Res*, 1998, **29**, 257–69.

16 MURPHY, D.J. 'Engineering oil production in rapeseed and other oilseed crops', *Trends Biotechnol*, 1996, **14**, 206–13

17 VOELKER, T.A., WORREL, A.C., ANDERSON, L. *et al.* 'Fatty acid biosynthesis redirected to medium chains in transgenic oilseed plants', *Science*, 1992, **257**, 72–3.

18 KROMBOUT, D., BOSSCHIELER, E.B. and DE LEZENNE COULANDER, C. 'The

inverse relationship between fish consumption and 20-year mortality from coronary heart disease', *New Engl J Med*, 1985, **312**, 1205–8.

19 FERNANDES, G. and JOLLY, C.A. 'Nutrition and autoimmune disease', *Nutrn Rev*, 1998, **56**, S161–9.

20 FERNANDES, G., YUMS, E.J. and GOOD, R.A. 'Influence of diet on survival of mice', *Proc Natln Acad Sci*, 1976, **73**, 1279–83.

21 REDDY, A.S. and THOMAS, T.L. 'Expression of a cyanobacterial Δ^6-desaturase gene results in gamma-linolenic acid production in transgenic plants', *Nat Biotechnol*, 1996, **14**, 639–42.

22 MICHAELSON, L.V., LAZARUS, C.M., GRIFFITHS, G. *et al.* 'Isolation of a Δ^5-fatty acid desaturase gene from *Mortierella alpina*', *J Plant Biochem*, 1998, **30**, 19055–9.

23 HOFFMAN, L.M., DONALDSON, D.D. and HERMAN, E.M. 'A modified storage protein is synthesised, processed, and degraded in the seeds of transgenic plants', *Plant Mol Biol*, 1988, **11**, 717–29.

24 PUEYO, J.J., CHRISPEELS, M. and HERMAN, E.M. 'Degradation of transport-competent destabilised phaseolin with a signal for retention in the endoplasmic reticulum occurs in the vacuole', *Planta*, 1995, **19**, 586–96.

25 KJEMTRUP, S., HERMAN, E.M. and CHRISPEELS, M.J. 'Correct post-translational modification and stable vacuolar accumulation of phytohemagglutinin engineered to contain multiple methionine residue', *Eur J Biochem*, 1994, **226**, 385–91.

26 ALTENBACH, S.B., PEARSON, K.W., MEEKER, G. *et al.* 'Enhancement of the methionine content of seed proteins by the expression of a chimeric gene encoding a methionine-rich protein in transgenic plants', *Plant Mol Biol*, 1989, **13**, 513–22.

27 NORDLEE, J.A., TAYLOR, S.L., TOWNSEND, J.A. and BUSH, R.K. 'Identification of a Brazil nut allergen in transgenic soybeans', *N Eng J Med*, 1996, **334**, 688–92.

28 YAMAUCHI, D. and MINAMIKAWA, T. 'Improvement of the nutritional quality of legume seed storage proteins by molecular breeding', *J Plant Res*, 1998, **111**, 1–6.

29 MOLVIG, L., TABE, L.M., EGGUM, B.O., MOORE, A.E., CRAIG, S., SPENCER, D. and HIGGINS, T.J.V. 'Enhanced methionine levels and increased nutritive value of seeds of transgenic lupins (*Lupinus angustifolius*) expressing a sunflower seed albumin gene', *Proc Natl Acad Sci USA*, 1997, **94**, 8393–8.

30 MUNTZ, K. *et al.* 'Genetic engineering of high methionine proteins in grain legumes', in *Sulphur Metabolism in Higher Plants: Molecular, Ecophysiological and Nutritional Aspects*, pp. 71–86, Leiden, Backhuys Publishers, 1997.

31 DOMONEY, C., MULLINEAUX, P. and CASEY, R. 'Nutrition and genetically engineered foods', in *Nutritional Aspects .of Food Processing and Ingredients*, pp. 112–35, Gaithersburg, Aspen Publishers Inc., 1998.

32 SHINTANI, D. and DELLAPENNA, D. 'Elevating the vitamin E content of plants through metabolic engineering', *Science*, 1998, **282**, 2098–100.

33　BROWN, C.R., RAY, J.A., FLETCHER, J.D. *et al.* 'Using antisense RNA to study gene function – inhibition of carotenoid biosynthesis in transgenic tomatoes', *Biotechnology*, 1991, **9**, 635–9.

34　FRAY, D. and GRIERSON, D. 'Molecular genetics of tomato fruit ripening', *Trends Genet*, 1994, **9**, 438–43.

35　BURKHARDT, P.K., BEYER, P., WUNN, J. *et al.* 'Transgenic rice (*Oryza sativa*) endosperm expressing daffodil (*Narcissus pseudonarcissus*) phytoene synthase, accumulates phytoene a key intermediate in pro-vitamin A synthesis', *Plant J*, 1997, **11**, 1071–8.

36　BROWN, C.R., EDWARDS, C.G., YANG, C.P. *et al.* 'Orange flesh trait in potato – inheritance and carotenoid content', *J Am Soc Hort Sci*, 1989, **118**, 145–50.

37　DEAK, M., HORVATH, G.V., DAVLETOVA, G.V. *et al.* 'Plants ectopically expressing the iron-binding protein, ferritin, are tolerant to oxidative damage and pathogens', *Nature Biotechn*, 1999, **17**, 192–6.

38　GOTO, F., YOSHIHARA, T., SHIGEMOTO, N. *et al.* 'Iron fortification of rice seed by the soybean ferritin gene', *Nature Biotechn*, 1999, **17**, 282–6

39　LINDLEY, M.G. 'The impact of food processing on antioxidants in vegetable oils, fruits and vegetables', *Trends in Fd Sci & Tech*, 1998, **9**, 336–40.

40　RODRIGUEZ-AMAYA, D.B. 'Carotenoids and food preparation: the retention of pro-vitamin A carotenoids in prepared, processed and stored foods', USAID, OMNI Project, 1997.

41　ROMMEL, A., WROLSTAD, R.E. 'Ellagic acid content of red raspberry juice as influenced by cultivar, processing, and environmental factors', *J Agric Food Chem*, 1993, **41**, 1951–60.

42　AUW, J.M., BLANC, V., O'KEEFE, S.F., SIMS, C.A. 'Effect of processing on the phenolics and color of Cabernet Sauvignon, Chambourcin, and Noble wines and juices', *Am J Enol Vitic*, 1996, **47**, 279–86.

43　SCHLESIER, K., SHAHRZAD, S., BITSCH, I. and DIETRICH, H. 'Actively anticarcinogenic phenolcarboxylic acids in fruit juices and wines from the same batch of fruit', *Zeitschrift für Ernährungswissenschaft*, 1997, **36**, 79–80.

44　CROZIER, A., LEAN, M.E.J., MCDONALD, M.S. and BLACK, C. 'Quantitative analysis of the flavonoid content of commercial tomatoes, onions, lettuce and celery', *J Ag Food Chem*, 1997, **45**, 590–5.

45　NGUYEN, M.L. and SCHWARTZ, S.J. 'Lycopene stability during food processing', *Proc Soc Exp Biol Med*, 1998, **218**, 101–5.

46　LINDSAY, D.G. and CLIFFORD, M.N. (eds) 'Critical reviews produced within the EU concerted action "Nutritional Enhancement of Plant-based Food in European Trade (NEODIET)" ', *J Sci Food Agric*, 2000, **80**, 793–1197.

9

Developing functional ingredients
A case study

A.-S. Sandberg, Chalmers University of Technology, Gothenburg

9.1 Introduction: the nutritional properties of peas

Legumes include peas, beans, lentils, peanuts and other podded plants that are used as food. Legumes are rich sources of food proteins from plants and have provided a protein source for humans and animals since the earliest of civilisations. Peas (*Pisum sativum*) are known to have been cultivated since 6000 BC in the Near East[1] and at least 4,000 years ago in the New World.[2] Legumes were traditionally an important component of the human diet as protein source and there are numerous traditional recipes in European countries that are based on legumes. Nevertheless, their consumption has declined steadily since the end of World War II, partly due to their image as the so-called 'food for the poor' and partly due to undesirable gastrointestinal effects associated with the consumption of legumes.

Peas are consumed both as fresh immature seeds as well as dry seeds. The latter are mostly consumed as whole seeds after cooking. Pea flour can be used to make a large variety of savouries, e.g. used as the basis for many soups and curries. Recently, the green pea has become an important green vegetable, being consumed as a fresh or processed product, either canned or frozen.

Nowadays there is a consumer trend towards more natural and 'healthy' foods and the food industry is constantly searching for ways to meet the demand for healthy wholefoods and food ingredients. The pea has an image of a traditional, natural foodstuff and pea protein products may fulfil these requirements.

Pea seeds contain high levels of protein and digestible carbohydrates, relatively high concentrations of insoluble dietary fibre and low concentrations of fat. The average starch and crude protein content is about 440 (214–486) and 225 g per kg dry matter respectively.[3, 4]

The average protein content in *Pisum sativum* is reported to be 25% with a wide variation between plants, cultivars and varieties. Selections of a high protein content and high yield in field peas are major goals of plant breeders. Pea protein is a good source of essential amino acids with a high content of lysine and threonine, but like other legumes, it is deficient in sulphur-containing amino acids. The digestibility of pea protein is between 83% and 93% as assessed by rat assays.

Dietary fibre constitutes about 63 g per kg dry matter in whole peas, and the content of total free sugars, *raffinose*, *stachyose* and *verbascose* is about 125; 12, 32 and 19 g per kg dry matter respectively.[5] The range of fat content is 10–24 g per kg dry matter and oleic and linoleic acid are the predominating fatty acids.[3, 6] Peas are good sources of minerals and water-soluble vitamins and are particularly rich in B-group vitamins.

Recently, the nutritional interest for peas and other legumes has increased because of the markedly attenuating effect on blood sugar and insulin response and thereby their potential use for prevention and control of diabetes.[7, 8] The digestibility of starch in legumes is restricted due to intact cell walls,[9] which enclose the starch granules and limit interaction with amylotic enzymes.[10] However, other mechanisms may also be involved; phytic acid polyphenols (tannic acid) and lectins can inhibit α-amylase activity *in vitro*, suggesting that an interaction with starch digestion also could occur *in vivo*.[11] *In vitro* studies have also indicated that the protein matrix in legume products limits the accessibility of starch to amylase.[12] A reduced rate of starch digestion attenuates the blood glucose and insulin response after a meal.

Foods containing carbohydrates which are slow to digest and absorb are of importance in the dietary management of diabetic patients. However, diets characterised by such foods have also been found to improve glucose tolerance in healthy subjects. In fact, dietary carbohydrates that cause a rapid rise in post-prandial insulin levels are extensively discussed as a risk factor for development of metabolic diseases.[13] The goal of diabetes therapy is to achieve normal glycemia and to prevent late complications. The development of vascular complications in diabetes has been related to the metabolic aberrations of uncontrolled diabetes.[14]

A dietary fibre content of 63 g per kg with 34% soluble fibre has been reported in light-hulled peas.[15] Generally, cell wall polysaccharides of seeds from such plants are dominated by pectic substances, cellulose, xyloglucans and glycoproteins.[16] Viscous soluble polysaccharides, such as pectic substances, are considered to have beneficial effects on carbohydrate and lipid metabolism in humans[17–20] by improving glucose tolerance, increasing ileal fat and bile acids excretion and decreasing blood lipids.[21] Pea fibre was shown to lower fasting and post-prandial blood triglyceride concentrations in humans,[22] one of the established risk factors for the development of cardiovascular disease. Except for prevention of non-insulin-dependent diabetes, pea fibre therefore has a potential use in the prevention of cardiovascular disease.

Anti-nutritional factors lower the nutritional value of a food by lowering the digestibility or bioavailability of nutrients. Peas contain a number of anti-nutritive and anti-physiological factors, which may be controlled by suitable processing and breeding programmes. However, the level of anti-nutritional factors is generally lower than in soybeans. The anti-nutritional factors present in pea protein include proteinase inhibitors (e.g. trypsin inhibitors and chymotrypsin inhibitors) and lectins. Non-protein components recognised as anti-nutritional factors in pea include saponins, polyphenols, phytate and raffinose oligosaccharides, although peas generally contain lower amounts of anti-nutritional factors than soy and other grain legumes. All commercial varieties of field peas are considered not to contain polyphenols. The utilisation of peas is restricted due to the presence of these anti-nutritional factors. Trypsin inhibitors decrease the protein digestibility and availability. Lectins are proteins, or glycoproteins, with the unique ability to bind to specific carbohydrate containing molecules on the surface of cells. Lectins have the ability to agglutinate red blood cells[23] and to bind to the intestinal epithelium, resulting in disruption of the brush border[24] atrophy of the microvilli[25] and reduced viability of the epithelial cells,[26] resulting in impaired nutrient transport. Thus, lectins can reduce the uptake of glucose and cause damage to the intestinal mucosal layer, but as these proteins are high in sulphur-containing amino acids (and are of importance for the yield and resistance to plant disease), inactivation of the inhibitors by processing should be preferred to genetic selection of cultivars with low inhibitor levels. Phytate present in peas and their protein products may negatively affect the digestibility of pea proteins. In addition phytate and some of its degradation products form complexes with certain essential dietary minerals (Fe, Zn, Ca), thereby impairing their absorption.[27]

Saponins adhere to proteins and have a bitter taste, generally considered unpleasant. Moreover, saponins may deteriorate the intestinal wall through a detergent effect.[28] Like trypsin inhibitors, selection of these anti-nutritional factors may have an impact on resistance to plant disease. Therefore, development of processing methods that inactivate the anti-nutritional factors post-harvest is preferable. Flatulence is associated with consumption of legume seeds including peas and causes some individuals to avoid these foods. Some indigestible oligosaccharides including raffinose, stachyose and verbascose are responsible for at least some of the flatulence of legume seeds through their fermentation by gut bacteria. Pea protein isolate, prepared by wet processing, contains much less of these oligosaccharides than the concentrated form.[29]

Like other legume proteins, pea proteins may be a potential allergen. The antigenicity of pea proteins is expected to be comparable to that of soy proteins. Experience with soy proteins shows that steam heating does not reduce the antigenicity substantially, whereas other treatments, such as proteolytic cleavage, do. Reports indicate that around 15% of infants who have developed allergy to cow milk protein and switched to soy formula will also be sensitised against soy protein.[30]

One of the most valuable ingredients extracted from pea is its protein fraction, which can be extensively purified as a protein concentrate or a protein isolate. Up until now the major outlet for protein isolate is its use as a functional ingredient, such as an emulsifier, thickener or foaming agent. The pea protein isolate is a valuable protein source, which has a potential to replace soy protein and enhance the nutritional value of foods.

9.2 Improving pea protein

The digestibility of pea protein is between 83% and 93%.[31] Phytic acid present in peas is accumulated in the pea protein fraction and may negatively affect digestibility of the pea protein. Heating may improve the nutritional quality of pea protein materials by increasing protein digestibility or by inactivating anti-nutritional factors such as trypsin inhibitors or lectin. The nutritional quality of pea protein using the protein efficiency ratio (PER) method was found to increase slightly when cooked (boiled 1 h).[32] Although peas generally contain lower quantities of anti-nutritional factors than other grain legumes, trypsin inhibitors are present. Deo et al.[33] demonstrated that cooking destroyed the trypsin inhibitor of all the peas evaluated and an improved digestibility was found. The mode of action of chymotrypsin inhibition was expected to be very similar to that of trypsin inhibitors. The effect of heat treatment on chymotrypsin inhibitors in peas was similar to that for trypsin inhibitors.[34]

Lectins are also heat labile. The activity was completely eliminated by autoclaving of peas at 121°C for five minutes.[35] Removal of 65% of activity after soaking the peas for 18 h was also reported by Bender.[36] Heating can also improve palatability.

Biological food processing techniques increasing the endogenous enzyme activity or adding enzymes can produce an additional and substantial reduction of the anti-nutritional factors. Furthermore, positive effects on carbohydrate and lipid metabolism in humans as a result of fermentation of cereals and legumes have been found. Controlled degradation of phytate by fermentation or by the addition of phytase has been demonstrated to increase the absorption of iron and zinc in meals based on cereals or soy.[37–9]

The pre-digestion of protein and formation of amino acids during fermentation was found to increase the nutritional value of protein and improve the amino acid composition of cereals and legumes. The fermentation process also has the potential to degrade saponins.

Pea protein is a potential allergen.[40] Experience with soy proteins show that steam heating does not reduce this antigenicity substantially, whereas other treatments such as proteolytic cleavage does. Furthermore, it has been suggested that some saponins increase the permeability of intestinal mucosal cells, thereby facilitating the uptake of substances to which the mucosa is normally impermeable.[41] This may lead to uptake of antigens, causing allergic reactions.[42] The fermentation of pea protein might be a possible means of reducing the antigenicity by hydrolysing protein and degrading the saponins.

Fermentation of indigestible oligosaccharides (by gut bacteria) including raffinose, stachyose and verbascose is considered to be responsible for the flatulence associated with pea consumption. These oligosaccharides tend to concentrate in the protein fraction of air-classified pea concentrate.[43] Pea protein isolate, prepared by wet processing, contains much less of these oligosaccharides than pea protein concentrate because some of the carbohydrates are washed away in the effluent.[29] Removal of these compounds can be performed by ultrafiltration, addition of α-galactosidase enzymes or fermentation by microorganisms producing α-galactosidase.

Selection of cultivars with high protein, high amino acid contents, particularly methionine is of great importance. Inactivation of anti-nutritional factors or degradation by processing should be preferred to the genetic selection of cultivars with low content of these factors because they are of importance for the yield and resistance to plant disease. Development of such processing methods, post-harvest, would significantly improve the nutritional quality of pea protein.

9.3 Processing issues in improving pea protein

9.3.1 Standard procedures for preparation of pea protein

One of the most valuable ingredients extracted from pea is its protein fraction. The preparation of pea protein could be an alternative to the well-established versatile soy protein products that dominate the food protein market. Soy protein products are used to extend or replace animal protein such as meat. It is also used as a protein source in infant formulas. Soy milk is used for replacement of cow's milk by vegetarians and persons with intolerance to milk protein. Depending on the low fat content of peas, the need for an oil extraction stage is eliminated and furthermore the relatively low content of anti-nutritive substances compared to soy is an advantage. Pea protein can be prepared in three forms: pea flour, pea protein concentrate and pea isolate. Pea flour is prepared by dry milling of dehulled peas. Pea protein concentrate is usually prepared by dry separation methods, while pea protein isolate is produced by wet processing methods.

Dry process (pea flour, pea protein concentrate)
Pea protein and starches can be efficiently fractionated by dry milling and air classification. By fine grinding, flours containing populations of particles are differentiated by size and density. Air classification of these flours separates the protein (fine fraction) from the starch (coarse fraction).[43] Whole or dehulled peas are, by this dry process, milled to very fine flour. During milling the starch granules remain relatively intact, while the protein matrix is broken down to fine particles. There is, however, a risk for damage of the starch granules during milling. Air classification of the pea flour is performed in a spiral air stream into a fine fraction containing around 75% of the protein, and a coarse fraction containing most of the starch granules. After milling, some starch is still embedded in the protein matrix and some protein bodies still adhere to starch

granules. By repeated milling and air classification, the separation of starch and protein can be improved.[44] It was also found that the percentage protein in air-classified pea fractions positively correlates with the protein content of the original pea flour.[45] Moreover, the percentage of starch recovered in the starch fraction as well as the percentage of protein recovered in the protein fractions both increase with increasing protein content of the pea.[46] Furthermore, air classifying at low speed increases protein content of the protein fractions but also starch fractions with higher levels of protein. Air classification provides a lower cost, effluent-free process for preparing pea protein concentrate, but not as pure fractions as aqueous extraction.

Wet processes (pea protein isolate, pea protein concentrate)
Protein isolates (highly concentrated protein fractions) and protein concentrates from pea can be produced by wet processing. The protein separation is based on solubilisation of protein followed by an isoelectric process or an ultrafiltration process[47] for subsequent recovery. Other processes include 'hydrophobic-out' or 'salting-out'.[31]

Variations of the isoelectric precipitation process and the ultrafiltration process are used commercially. The different steps in the isoelectric process for pea protein isolate are milling of the peas, solubilisation of the proteins in water, alkali, or acid; then centrifugation to remove insoluble components. Then the solubilised proteins are precipitated at their isoelectric pH, and collected by centrifugation, or sieving, and dried as such or neutralised and dried.

The yield of the protein isolate prepared by isoelectric precipitation is influenced by several factors such as particle size of the flour, the kind of solubilising agent, as well as pH of solubilisation and precipitation. Furthermore, the isolate composition is affected by the solubilising and precipitating pH. Isolates precipitated below 5.3 have been found to be lower in protein content and to have higher lipid content than those precipitated at pH 5.3.[48]

Ultrafiltration with non-cellulosic membranes can be used to isolate protein from wet slurries.[47] These membrane systems are stable over a wide range of pH values and elevated temperature and thus offer an alternative to the conventional acid precipitation methods. Ultrafiltration using a hollow fibre system can give protein recoveries of 90–94%. An advantage is that low molecular weight compounds such as oligosaccharides are removed by ultrafiltration.

9.3.2 Possible modifications of the procedure
Possible means to remove anti-nutritional factors in the process for preparation of pea protein include increasing the endogenous enzyme activity by soaking the peas, and fermentation by addition of certain starter cultures or addition of enzymes. This kind of modification can be performed in the wet process for preparation of isolates or the pea flour. Fermentation using lactic acid bacteria, fungi or yeast, is traditionally used in Asian food manufacturing of soybean based products (e.g. soy sauce, miso, tempeh). The effect of fermentation of

peas has so far mainly been studied in relation to protein quality, while systematic studies of the possibility to optimise the reduction of anti-nutritional factors of pea products and, in particular, pea protein for human consumption through biological processing techniques are lacking.

The functional properties of pea proteins suggest that pea proteins have a high potential for use in food products. The type of process used for the preparation of pea concentrate or pea protein isolate affects functional properties of the product. Different combinations of thermal treatment and pH should be evaluated in order to understand the relation between process conditions and functionality.

9.4 Adding improved protein to food products

Effective utilisation of pea proteins in foods for human consumption depends to a large extent on consumer acceptance. Some studies have been conducted on the potentiality of applications of pea products in food; in addition or in substitution to flour (in bread or pasta) or to meat (in patties, hamburgers), in textured products, soups, snacks, and in substitution to milk. The addition of pea products influences the cooking time and texture. As such, modifications of the formulae were sometimes necessary to have acceptable organoleptic properties. Pea protein concentrates have been found useful for producing non-fat dry milk replacements for the baking industry. A non-dairy frozen dessert was developed utilising pea protein isolate with good organoleptic characteristics. In some applications pea proteins could replace soy proteins. It would be of interest to developed tailored pea proteins for specific applications.

Pea materials sometimes have unacceptable flavours but a pea protein isolate with a bland flavour can also be produced. The functional requirements for a plant protein to be useful as a meat extender include good fat and water absorption, emulsification capacity and stability, gelation texturisability and sensory properties.

Pea protein isolate has a high solubility, water and fat binding capacity and emulsifying and foaming capacity to give desired texture and stability. Possible applications are meat and fish products, biscuits and pastry making, desserts, prepared dishes, soups and sauces, dietary, health and baby food. For use of plant protein in infant formulas a high bioavailability of minerals, a high nutritive value of the protein and a low antigenicity are desired.

9.4.1 Cereal and bakery products
The nutritional quality of wheat protein has been improved by addition of pea flour or pea protein concentrate[49] to wheat flour. Replacing 20% of the wheat flour with pea flour gives bread with excellent protein quality. However, at this level of supplementation the bread had decreased in volume and had a relatively poor crumb structure[50, 51] and the acceptance of the supplemented bread was

limited due to poor sensory properties.[52] Also, it was found that addition of pea flour to yeast breads significantly affects the texture. Protein enrichment of pasta product with pea protein has also been performed. Supplemented pasta has a better protein quality, cooks faster and is slightly firmer.[53] The flavour was, however, found to be somewhat inferior to that of unsupplemented wheat pasta. For the application of pea protein in biscuits a series of experiments were first performed to choose process type (creaming or crumbling) and formula (partial substitution of flour or substitution of milk powder). The creaming process was found to be the most suitable process. Colour was found to depend on protein source but was not influenced by fat, sugar and protein content. Biscuits containing milk powder were darker than biscuits made with pea proteins. Hardness was influenced by protein source. Biscuits made with milk proteins were harder than those made with pea protein. A higher percentage of protein also increased hardness, an effect that also was found with increasing sugar content, though not as extensive. Crispiness decreased with high amount of fat and tended to increase with the level of sugar.[54]

9.4.2 Meat products

The requirement for plant proteins to be used as extenders in meat products include good fat and water absorption, emulsification capacity and stability, gelation texturisability and sensory attributes. High solubility is not a determinant of the usefulness of a plant protein in meat systems; in some cases proteins of low solubility are engineered for use in meat systems. The use of pea protein in meat products has mainly been in meat patties,[55] hamburgers and sausages. Sausages extended with pea protein have improved nutritional value compared to unsupplemented products. The optimal sensory concentration was found to be 4–7%; concentrations greater than 10% were found to produce a strong pea flavour.[31]

9.4.3 Milk replacement products

There seems to be some promise in the use of pea protein concentrate as an ingredient for producing non-fat dry milk replacement for the baking industry.[56] Also there have been attempts to produce milk substitutes.[57] Pea milk has a potential use for replacement of cow milk by vegetarians and persons with intolerance and allergy to cow milk and also oral nutritional supplements. Other trials have been carried out to substitute milk powder by pea protein in desserts. The first experiments were made according to a fractional design with five factors: quantity of pea, starch, gum, oil and emulsifier. From the results of the first experiments the most relevant ingredients were then selected, i.e. based upon the quantity of pea protein and starch. These ingredients were then optimised in order to get a dessert close to the commercial form.[54]

9.4.4 Vegetable pâté

The application of pea protein in a vegetable pâté has been investigated. Different quantities of pea protein, gum and starch were tested using a multivate experimental design in order to evaluate the effect of the three factors and to optimise the formula. The main purpose was to get as close as possible to the reference vegetable pâté made with whole egg. Response surface methodology was used to find the optimum formula on physical characteristics with as high an amount of pea protein as possible.

Textural measurements showed only small differences between the reference and the formula. The colour of the vegetable pâté made with pea protein was different from the reference made with whole egg, which also was confirmed in the sensory analysis. Moreover, other characteristics related to appearance (brightness, firmness, straight cut, bubble size) of the pâté were different. For mouth feel the formula was found to be slightly more firm than the reference. Taste of carrot was very close in the samples and the optimal formula was well accepted by the test panel.

The optimisation of vegetable pâté demonstrates, on the one hand, the quality of pea protein as a functional ingredient and, on the other hand, its capability to substitute whole egg. Furthermore, pea protein can reduce the incorporation of other textural agents and has more than 40% less quantity of gum and starch than the reference vegetable pâté.[54, 58]

9.5 Evaluating the functional and sensory properties of improved pea protein in food products

9.5.1 Evaluating nutritional properties

The genetic variation of peas is considerable. As a first step towards producing an improved pea protein a choice of starting material has to be made. The following criteria are important in the selection of pea raw material:

- high level of protein content in the seed and low level in fat content
- high level of limiting amino acids (methionine, cysteine, trypthophan)
- low level of anti-nutritional factors
- availability of the genotype in sufficient quantities
- high yield and resistance to plant disease.

Analysis of relevant nutritional parameters such as protein quality, amino acid composition and a number of anti-nutritional factors including oligosaccharides, phytate, proteinase inhibitors, lectins, saponins and polyphenols therefore has to be performed in raw pea seeds and the pea protein products.

Anti-nutritional factors in different starting materials and from modified process for pea protein products
Analyses of protein isolates from a commercial wet process showed that the contents of oligosaccharides and lectins were effectively reduced during the

processing and no clear relationship was found between saponins and taste. The trypsin inhibitors were found to be partly inactivated by heat treatment. The major important anti-nutrient in protein isolate was determined to be phytate. Determination of the phytate content in protein isolates showed that the phytate accumulated in the protein isolate. Analyses of the oligosaccharide content in protein isolates from selected pea varieties showed that the contents were lower than in the isolates from the standard process (due to an improvement of the cut-off of the ultrafiltration technique).[59]

The saponin content of the pea seeds was determined to be 2–7 mg/g sample. The content of trypsin inhibitors was found to be 50–100 μg/g sample and lectins 1–2.5 mg/g sample.[60]

Analysis of anti-nutritional factors, in vitro *digestibility and antigenicity*
Addition of exogenous phytase reduced the phytate content in pea protein to very low levels. The use of exogenous phytase was tested on pea flour and two different protein isolates from different steps in the process. The optimal conditions for exogenous phytases were 55°C and pH 5.5, and the phytate degradation were virtually complete on all substrates tested.[61] The contents of inositol hexaphosphate (phytate) and its degradation products were analysed in dephytinised pea protein isolates and pea protein infant formula. Dephytinised pea protein isolates contained 0.08 μmol/g of phytate and no detectable amounts of lower inositol phosphates. Dephytinised sample incubated with exogenous phytase for 1 h instead of 2 h, contained 0.5 μmol/g inositol hexaphosphate. Comparison with standard pea protein isolate without enzymatic treatment showed that this sample contained 19.6 μmol/g inositol hexaphosphate. Analysis of pea protein infant formula, produced in the factory scale from dephytinised pea protein isolate, contained only traces of phytate.

The content of proteinase inhibitors (PPI) were much higher in pea flour than in samples incubated at 40% or 70% humidity, both control samples and fermented samples. To investigate the stability of PPI under various conditions a preliminary study was performed. The study showed that only 20% of the original content of PPI were left after 48 h at 37°C and 70% humidity.

Lactic acid fermentation of pea flour was found to decrease the saponin content of pea protein isolate. The most effective saponin reduction (90%) was found in a sample fermented with *Lactobacillus plantarum* for 48 h.

The *in vitro* digestibility was determined by four different methods: reversed phase HPLC, gelfiltration HPLC, sandwich ELISA and SDS-PAGE. The digestibility of dehulled pea seeds, phytase treated pea protein isolate and standard pea protein isolate from the modified process was compared. Analysis by the four methods resulted in a similar outcome for the three investigated products: the pea isolates had an *in vitro* digestibility of 80–90%, whereas the dehulled pea seeds had a much lower digestibility of approximately 40%. The pea protein isolates are thus more digestible than the raw pea.[54]

Bioavailability
The use of pea protein isolate could be an alternative to soy isolate. Soy formulas have been used for a long time period and the nutritional status of infants fed soy formula has been well documented and found to be similar to infants fed cow milk formulas. However, the bioavailability of nutrients, especially minerals, has been reported to be lower than that of milk-based formulas. An important factor contributing to the lower mineral absorption from soy formula is the relatively high concentration of the metal chelator phytic acid, which acts as a dietary inhibitor of the absorption of essential minerals, in particular iron. The negative effect of phytic acid on iron absorption has been shown to be dose dependent.[62] In addition, the soy protein *per se* has recently been demonstrated to inhibit iron absorption.[38] Although the absorption of zinc and calcium may be influenced by the presence of phytic acid, the effect on iron bioavailability is much greater.[27]

The enzymatic degradation of phytate in soy infant formulas was found to improve iron absorption significantly provided that the removal of phytate was virtually complete.[38] The availability of iron and zinc in a dephytinised infant formula based on pea protein was evaluated. Soluble amounts of iron and zinc in the samples were collected during simulated *in vitro* digestion performed in a computer-controlled dynamic gastrointestinal model. Determination of these samples showed that dephytinisation of pea protein increased the amount of iron and zinc potentially available for absorption by 50% and 100%, respectively.[63]

Antigenicity
A substantial part of the antigens found in pea seeds are still antigenic in fermented pea flour. This was reported by Herian *et al.*[64] who found that soy epitopes can be detected in soy protein isolates as well as fermented soy products. On the other hand, some of the pea antigens have been found to be sensitive to the processing procedures. Monoclonal antibodies can be used to identify these antigens as well as more stable antigens. In contrast to the antigens in general, the inhalation allergen cross-reacting proteins Bet v1 homologue and profilin have been found so labile that they are not only undetectable in the processed protein isolates and fermented samples, but also very reduced in pea flour after incubation at 37°C.[40, 54]

9.5.2 Evaluating functional and sensory properties
Research on the functional properties of pea proteins has shown the importance of the preparation treatment of the proteins. Pea proteins are highly soluble at an acidic pH (pH2), and at alkaline pH 7.3 maximum solubility occurs, the minimum solubility being obtained at pH between 4 and 6. The actual solubility of pea proteins at a given pH in the pH region of 5 to 9 can vary widely.

The following functional and sensorial parameters need to be evaluated in improved pea protein:

- Solubility: These properties enable evaluation of the denaturation state of the protein and are good indicators for evaluating the potential applications of proteins. Good solubility can markedly expand potential utilisation of proteins.
- Dispersibility: Oil and water binding capacity. These take an important place in the quality of meat and *charcuterie* products, thanks to the binding effect of their components which reduces the loss of water and fat. Water binding capacity (WBC) is useful in food products such as sausages where there is insufficient water for protein to dissolve, but where the hydrated protein imparts structure and viscosity to the food.
- Foaming properties (*capacity and stability, texture*) These enable the formulation of whipped products. Pea proteins have very high foaming properties in comparison with other vegetable proteins.
- Emulsifying properties (*capacity and stability, texture*) The emulsifying properties of pea protein can contribute towards the formulation of meat or *charcuterie* products, which generally have an emulsified structure.
- Gelatinisation and thickening properties These have an effect on the texture of the different food products.

Such evaluations of pea proteins have been undertaken according to various conditions of use, which are characteristics of the food applications (presence of salt, pH, heat treatment).

The properties of the pea proteins developed by bioprocesses have been compared with those of native pea, soy proteins and meat proteins. The potential use of these ingredients and comparison with other ingredients (e.g. meat, other proteins) should then be determined.

Sensory evaluation
A large range of pea protein products have been tested in a food model (sauce) to evaluate sensory characteristics. Different rates of incorporation were tested. Evaluation by an expert panel assessed the main sensory characteristics of the foods: aspect, flavour, mouth feel, texture.

A study has been carried out to evaluate the effect of different functional properties on the selected pea proteins after treatment at various process conditions.[54] It was observed that thermal treatment had a negative effect on solubility. The solubility decreased in the range from 75°C to 95°C and then increased again at 120°C. A further finding was that heat treatment resulted in increased stability of the emulsions. The visco-elastic properties of the medium were different. After treatment at 80°C for 2 h, the firmness of the medium and the viscosity were higher than samples treated at milder conditions.

Determination of the functional properties of the modified pea protein showed that the reduction of phytate in the pea protein decreased the solubility and emulsifying and rheological properties.

To study effects of functionality, comparisons have been made between processes without pasteurisation or with pasteurisation at different temperatures

(75°C, 85°C, 95°C) or autoclaving at 120°C. Pea protein isolates produced from the variety *Baccara* and processed in a pilot plant system using different heat treatments were to evaluate functional properties. Heating decreased the solubility of the protein and increased the emulsifying stability. The visco-elastic properties of the medium were different: pea protein isolates solidified during heating, remained liquid and exhibited high thickening properties, had different texture compared to lower visco-elastic properties. Gel formation occurred at about 75°C for one of the pea proteins and was therefore selected for food applications.

9.6 Future trends: the work of NUTRIPEA

The following partners are participating in NUTRIPEA (New Technologies for Improved Nutritional and Functional Value of Pea Protein, FAIR CT 95-0193): Chalmers University of Technology, Sweden (co-ordinator), Technical University of Denmark, ETH Zurich, Switzerland, Technical Research Centre of Finland, ADRIA, France, Provital Industries S.A., Belgium, and Semper AB, Sweden.

The general objective of the EU funded project was to use new technologies to develop improved pea protein products, which are devoid of anti-physiological and anti-nutritional factors. The project concerns a novel research field, which will lead to increased knowledge regarding processing and development of products with increased nutrient availability. The nutritional and functional properties of pea proteins suggest a high potential for use in food products. Therefore, the purpose of the project was to design and develop a technical process to prepare improved pea protein products under pilot plant and factory conditions.

The NUTRIPEA program has verified:

- the technical feasibility of a bioprocess to prepare improved pea protein products
- the enhancement of nutritional value of the process within one clinical study
- the legal problems that need to be solved, i.e. development of a phytase 'food grade enzyme' and acceptance of pea protein in European law for infant food
- that pea protein isolate could be a valuable protein source to replace soy protein isolate.

Additional studies and investments are needed to prove the nutritional benefits and safety of pea protein isolate for infant formula including growth tests and studies in children who are intolerant to cow milk.

To reach this main objective the following approach and partial objectives were to be achieved:

- *Task 1* Evaluation of genetic variation. Starting materials and standard pea protein products were evaluated to set nutritional properties regarding digestibility and some anti-nutritional factors. This task generated information for the selection of suitable starting materials for preparation of pea protein products.

- *Task 2* To design and develop a technical process to prepare improved pea protein products under pilot plant conditions with two subtasks:
  - (a) pilot plant preparation of pea products from the varieties in task 1 and application of different modifications of the standard procedure;
  - (b) determination of anti-nutritional factors and antigenicity of pea protein products from the different starting material and from modified process for pea protein products.

The results from these tasks showed that the two anti-nutritional factors, phytate and saponins, were of major importance as the production scheme for pea protein isolate resulted in increased levels of these two anti-nutrients.

- *Task 3* Bioprocessing of pea protein products to use new technologies to develop improved pea protein products including the following three subtasks:
  - (a) preliminary screening of lactic acid bacteria for fermentation processes of pea protein;
  - (b) optimisation of the conditions for bioprocessing of pea protein using solid state fermentation and enzymatic treatment;
  - (c) evaluation of bioprocessed pea protein regarding contents of anti-nutritional factors, antigenicity, microbiological quality, functional and sensory characteristics.

- *Task 4* Development of a modified extraction technique at the pilot plant level. This task involved two different processes: the first was developed to reduce the phytate content and the second generated new functional characteristics.

- *Task 5* Development of test products from pea proteins, infant formulas and pea protein products for adults and evaluation of antigenicity and nutritional and functional value. The abilities of the selected pea proteins developed by food processing were evaluated taking into account technological and sensory aspects. Pea protein infant formulas were produced and evaluated for antigenicity and protein quality in animal models. *In vitro* estimation of iron and zinc bioavailability and iron absorption in humans were also measured.

Determinations of anti-physiological and anti-nutritional factors like oligosaccharides, phytate, proteinase inhibitors, lectins, saponins and tannins have been made in raw pea seeds, pea protein isolates and samples from the production of pea protein isolates. Based on this evaluation, the parameters for the design of a modified process to prepare improved pea protein products were formulated.

The development of pilot plant preparations of pea protein isolates and determination of anti-nutritional factors and antigenicity led to the conclusion that phytate and saponins were the most important anti-nutrients to be reduced, as the production scheme for pea protein isolate resulted in increased levels of both. It was also found that a substantial part of the antigens found in pea seeds were still antigenic in pea protein isolates.

A further task was bioprocessing of pea protein products. The approach of adding exogenous phytase was found to be very effective for reduction of pea protein phytate. Control of the microbiological quality was very important during food processing. Food pathogens and other spoilage organisms such as *Bacillus cereus* originating from peas or the process were found. However, after addition of lactic acid bacteria (LAB) to the soaking water, the growth of spoilage organisms was effectively prevented. Screening of phytase activity of different LAB and fungal strains showed that LAB did not degrade phytate but two food-grade fungi showed phytase activity. Oligosaccharides such as verbascose, stachyose and raffinose were effectively reduced during fermentation with nine selected LAB strains.[54]

The development of a modified extraction technique led to two different modifications of the pilot plant process. The first process was developed in order to reduce the phytate content and the second process was developed to obtain new functionality.

Development of infant pea protein formulas and pea protein products for adults showed that the level of anti-nutritional factors in the final pea protein isolates products were reduced to an acceptable level, i.e. lower than that of soy protein, which is accepted as a protein source in infant feeds. The saponin content of pea protein isolate was compared to soy protein isolate and, although the saponin level in the final pea protein isolate was increased three- to fourfold, this was considerably lower compared to the saponin level in soy protein isolate. This indicated that the pea protein isolate can be regarded as safe for human consumption with regard to saponins. It was also demonstrated that processing steps in the production of pea protein isolates markedly increased the *in vitro* and *in vivo* digestibility of pea protein. Some of the pea antigens were found to be sensitive to the processing procedures but a substantial part of the antigens found in pea seeds were still antigenic in pea protein isolates and fermented pea flour. Evaluation of iron and zinc availability showed a significant increase in the amount of soluble minerals at simulated physiological conditions in a dynamic computer-controlled gastrointestinal model.[63] This was also confirmed in a human study, the iron absorption increasing by more than 50% after phytate removal or addition of ascorbic acid to the pea protein infant formula.[54, 65]

9.6.1 Conclusions

Bioprocessing of pea protein using addition of exogenous phytase was found to be very effective for the reduction of pea protein phytate. Evaluation of iron and zinc availability also showed a significant increase in the amounts of soluble minerals at simulated physiological conditions.[63] Iron absorption increased by more than 50% after phytate removal or addition of ascorbic acid to pea protein infant formulas. Determination of iron absorption using adult women indicated relatively high fractional iron absorption from the bioprocessed pea protein formula, as compared to earlier data on iron absorption from soy formulas in adults.[65] Infant formula based on pea protein could therefore be an alternative to soy isolates.

Control of microbiological quality is very important during food processing. Food pathogens and other spoilage organisms could be controlled by the addition of LAB to the soaking water. This indicates promising possibilities for further developments and up-scaling of the microbicidic soaking and its application in the industrial process.

Screening of phytase activity of different LAB and fungal strains showed that LAB did not degrade phytate but two food-grade fungi exhibited activity. Oligosaccharides such as verbascose, stachyose and raffinose were effectively reduced during fermentation with nine of the selected LAB strains.

Determination of anti-nutritional factors like proteinase inhibitors, lectins, saponins and tannins were made in raw pea seeds, pea protein isolates and samples from the production of pea protein isolates. The same anti-nutritional factors were likewise quantified in soy flour and soy protein isolates and the amounts determined in soy and pea were compared. The level of anti-nutritional factors in the final pea protein isolates products was reduced to an acceptable value. It was also demonstrated that processing steps in the production of pea protein isolates markedly increased the *in vitro* and *in vivo* digestibility of pea protein. Some of the pea antigens were found to be sensitive to the processing procedures but a substantial part of the antigens found in pea seeds are still antigenic in pea protein isolates and fermented pea flour.

Even with high nutritional properties, pea protein products can only be used if they enable the formulation of foods with high sensory and technological qualities. The study showed that pea protein has a high potential for incorporation into different products like vegetable pâté, drinks, desserts and biscuits.

9.7 Sources of further information and advice: Ongoing EU projects and networks in the field

LINK Legume Interactive Network (Concerted Action FAIR-CT-98-3923)
A multidisciplinary scientific network for the benefit of grain legume integrated chain to meet the protein demand of the European end-use industry.
Coordinators: Frédéric Muel, Anne Schneider

COST 916
Bioactive plant cell wall components in nutrition and health.
Coordinator: R. Amadò

PROFETAS
Protein foods, environment, technology and society.
Coordinators: P. Vellinga, W.M.F. Jongen

EUROPROTEINS 93–96
Development of plant protein-rich products by plant breeding and biotechnology for application in human and animal nutrition.
Coordinator: K. Cherrière
With the following outline and main objectives:

- ruminants: to optimise technological treatments to protect proteins against excessive degradation in the rumen;
- poultry: to determine physical and biological criteria responsible for potential decrease in egg weight and of punctual occurrence in dirty eggs.

Increased utilisation of peas in food and feed products by improvement of the protein quality by enzymatic modification.
Coordinator: L. Sijtsma
With the following outline and main objectives:

- improved utilisation of pea proteins
- improvement of the quality of pea protein
- design of a model for quality prediction.

TRANSLEG
Coordination of a joint approach on grain legume transformation (methods and objectives) to develop commercial applications.
Coordinator: H.-J. Jacobsen
With the following outline and main objectives:

- to establish a network of experts in the European Union sharing the know-how of grain legume transformation
- to coordinate a ring test to define a widely applicable transformation protocol, to discuss with end-users, such as commercial breeders, about their needs, constraints and priorities regarding commercial applications of transgenic grain legumes
- to prepare joint research projects on several specific gene transfers.

UNCLE
Understanding nitrogen and carbohydrate metabolism for legume engineering.
Coordinator: U. Wobus
With the following outline and main objectives:

- to analyse the capacity of selected legume seeds (pea and faba bean) to accumulate storage products (seed sink capacity)
- to analyse the relationship between carbohydrate and storage protein/nitrogen metabolism at the level of gene expression
- to isolate promoters for temporally and spatially regulated gene expression in seeds
- to use these promoters, in combination with existing and new gene sequences, to specifically change sink capacity and/or storage product composition in

legume seeds, as a prerequisite for quality improvement and engineering into seeds of exogenous high-added-value components

NUTRIPEA

New technologies for improved nutritional and functional value of pea protein.
Coordinator: A.-S. Sandberg
With the following outline and main objectives:

- to use new technologies to develop improved pea protein products that are devoid of anti-physiological and anti-nutritional factors
- to design and develop a technical process to prepare improved pea protein products under pilot plant and factory conditions
- to evaluate the functional and sensory properties of improved pea protein products added to a variety of foods for human consumption
- to screen *in vitro* and in animal models the nutritional properties and antigenicity of the protein products
- to develop an infant formula based on the improved pea protein products and to evaluate antigenicity and protein quality in animals and iron absorption in infants.

CABINET

Carbohydrate biotechnology network for grain legumes.
Coordinator: C. Hedley
With the following outline and main objective:

- multidisciplinary approach on legume carbohydrates.

PRELEG

Pathogen-resistant grain legumes using gene transfer methods.
Coordinator: G. Ramsay
With the following outline and main objectives:

- selected methods for transformation of grain legumes are developed for routine use to permit the regeneration of the numbers of transformants required
- effects of each type of gene on selected major pathogens of grain legumes *in vivo* are explored, using ELISA quantification of pathogen multiplication.

AMINOPIG

Amino acid true availability in pig.
Coordinator: M. Sève
With the following outline and main objectives:

- to improve scientific knowledge of protein utilisation in pigs
- to understand better amino acid digestibility, effect of dietary factors on endogenous amino acid losses, metabolic expense for endogenous losses, etc.

LUPINE
Creation of varieties and technologies for increasing production and utilisation of high quality proteins from white lupin in Europe.
Coordinator: C. Huyghe
With the following outline and main objectives:

- to provide improved genotypes of winter type and determinated lupins
- to improve cropping management techniques
- to introduce new technologies (physical and enzymatic treatments) to enhance the use value.

PHASELIEU
Improvement of sustainable *Phaseolus* production in Europe for human consumption.
Coordinator: A. De Ron
With the following outline and main objectives:

- to establish an EU network of experts on *Phaseolus* for analysing and exploiting the potential of *Phaseolus* for European agriculture
- to improve the management of genetic resources, their characterisation and exploitation
- to identify the biotic and abiotic stresses or constraints and to enhance the farming systems
- to enhance the seed quality
- to develop biotechnology's tools for *Phaseolus*.

FRYMED
Yield stability and resistance of faba bean to major pathogens in western Mediterranean basin.
Coordinator: G. Caubel
With the following outline and main objectives:

- to assess the genetic variability in faba bean germplasm for resistance to diseases
- to characterise the pathogen populations for testing resistance
- to evaluate resistant genotypes in the Maghreb region
- to develop a simple technological package including resistant cultivars.

FYSAME
Nitrogen fixation and yield of grain legume in saline Mediterranean zones.
Coordinator: J.-J. Drevon
With the following outline and main objectives:

- to select chickpea and common bean and their adapted *Rhizobium* strains for symbiotic nitrogen fixation tolerance to NaCl salinity
- to assess the yield of selected symbioses in Northern Africa and Southern Europe

- to progress understanding of biochemical mechanisms

EU – PEA INGREDIENT
Exploitation of the unique genetic variability of peas in the production of food and non-food ingredients.
Coordinator: H. Nijhuis

- novel pea genotypes
- fractionation of pea components
- food and non-food uses
- starch.

9.8 References

1 ZOHARY, D. and HOPF, M. 'Domestication of pulses in the old world', *Science,* 1973, **182**, 887–94.

2 BRESSANI, R. and ELIAS, L.G. 'Legumes foods'. In A.M. Altschul (ed.), pp. 230–97, *New Protein Foods*, New York, Academic Press, 1974.

3 ADSULE, R.N., LAWANDE, K.M. and KADAM, S.S. 'Pea'. In D.K. Salunkhe and S.S. Kadam (eds), pp. 215–51, *Handbook of World Food Legumes: Nutritional Chemistry, Processing Technology, and Utilization*, Boca Raton, FL, CRC Press, 1989.

4 KADAM, S.S., DESPHANDE, S.S. and JAMBHALE, N.D. 'Seed structure and composition'. In D.K. Salunkhe and S.S. Kadam (eds), pp. 23–50, *Handbook of World Food Legumes: Nutritional Chemistry, Processing Technology, and Utilization*, Boca Raton, FL, CRC Press, 1989.

5 KUO, T.M., VAN MIDDLESWORTH, J.F. and WOLF, W.J. 'Content of raffinose oligosaccharides and sucrose in various plant seeds', *J Agric Food Chem,* 1988, **36**, 32–6.

6 SALUNKHE, D.K., SATHE, S.K. and REDDY, N.R. 'Lipids'. In D.K. Salunkhe and S.S. Kadam (eds), pp. 99–116, *Handbook of World Food Legumes: Nutritional Chemistry, Processing Technology and Utilization*, Boca Raton, FL, CRC Press, 1989.

7 JENKINS, D.J.A., WOLEVER, T.M.S., TAYLOR, R.H., BARKER, H.M. and FIELDEN, M. 'Exceptionally low blood glucose response to dried beans: comparison with other carbohydate foods', *Br Med J,* 1980, **281**, 578–80.

8 JENKINS, D.J.A., WOLEVER, T.M.S., JENKINS, A.L. *et al.* 'The glycaemic index of foods tested in diabetic patients: a new basis for carbohydrate exchange favouring the use of legumes', *Diabetologia,* 1983, **24**, 257–64.

9 WÜRSCH, P., DEL VEDOVO, S. and KOELLREUTER, B. 'Cell structure and starch nature as key determinants of the digestion rate of starch in legumes', *Am J Clin Nutr,* 1986, **43**, 25–9.

10 ENGLYST, H.N. and CUMMINGS, J.H. 'Non-starch polysaccharides (dietary fiber) and resistant starch'. In I. Furda and C. Brine (eds), pp. 205–25, *New*

Developments in Dietary Fiber, New York, Plenum Press, 1990.

11 BJÖRCK, I. 'Starch: nutritional aspects'. In A.-C. Eliasson (ed.), pp. 505–53, *Carbohydrates in Food*, New York, Marcel Dekker, 1996.

12 TOVAR, J., BJÖRCK, I.M. and ASP, N.-G. 'Starch content and alfa-amylosis rate in precooked legume flours', *J Agric Food Chem*, 1990, **38**, 1818–23.

13 DUCIMETIERE, P., ESCHWEGE, E., PAPOZ, L., RICHARD, J.L., CLAUDE, J.R. and ROSSELIN, G. 'Relationship of plasma insulin levels to the incidence of myocardial infarction and coronary heart disease mortality in a middle-aged population', *Diabetologia*, 1980, **19**, 205–10.

14 WYLIE-ROSETT, J. and RIFLEIN, H. 'The history of nutrition and diabetes'. In L. Jovanovic and C.M. Peterson (eds), pp. 1–13, *Nutrition and Diabetes*, New York, Alan R. Liss Inc., 1985.

15 SCHAKEL, S., SIEVERT, Y. and BUZZARD, I. 'Dietary fiber values for common foods'. In G. Spiller (ed.), *Handbook of Dietary Fiber in Human Nutrition*, 2nd edn, Boca Raton, FL, CRC Press, 1992.

16 SELVENDRAN, R.R., STEVENS, B.J.H. and DUPONT, M.S. 'Dietary fiber: chemistry, analysis and properties', *Adv Food Res*, 1987, **31**, 117–209.

17 SANDBERG, A.-S., AHDERINNE, R., ANDERSSON, H., HALLGREN, B. and HULTÉN, L. 'The effect of citrus pectin on the absorption of nutrients in the small intestine', *Hum Nutr: Clin Nutr*, 1983, **37C**, 171–83.

18 BOSAEUS, I., ANDERSSON, H., CARLSSON, N.-G. and SANDBERG, A.-S. 'Effect of wheat bran and pectin on bile salt excretion in ileostomy patients', *Hum Nutr: Clin Nutr*, 1986, **40C**, 429–40.

19 JENKINS, D., WOLEVER, T., RAO, V. *et al.* 'Effect on blood lipids of very high intakes of fiber in diets low in saturated fat and cholesterol', *N Engl J Med*, 1993, **329**, 21–6.

20 TRUSWELL, A.S. and BEYNEN, A.C. 'Dietary fibre and plasma lipids: potential for prevention and treatment of hyperlipidaemias'. In T.F. Schweizer and C.A. Edwards (eds), pp. 295–332, *Dietary Fibre – A Component of Food: Nutritional Function in Health and Disease*, London, Springer-Verlag, 1992.

21 JENKINS, D., WOLEVER, T. COLLIER, G. *et al.* 'Metabolic effects of a low-glycemic-index diet', *Am J Clin Nutr*, 1987, **46**, 968–75.

22 SANDSTRÖM, B., TROND HANSEN, L. and SÖRENSEN, A. 'Pea fiber lowers fasting and postprandial blood triglyceride concentrations in humans', *J Nutr*, 1994, **124**, 2386–96.

23 LIENER, I. 'Control of antinutritional and toxic factors in oilseeds and legumes'. In E. Lusas, D. Erickson and W. Nip (eds), pp. 344–71, *Food Uses of Whole Oil and Protein Seeds*, Campaign, American Oil Chemists' Society, 1989.

24 PUSZTAI, A., EWEN, S., GRANT, G. *et al.* 'Relationship between survival and binding of plant lectins during small intestinal passage and their effectiveness as growth factors', *Digestion*, 1990, **46**, (Supp. 2), 308–16.

25 JINDAHL, S., SONI, G. and SINGH, R. 'Biochemical and histopathological studies in albino rats fed on soybean lectin', *Nutr Rep Int*, 1984, **29**, 95–106.

26 ISHIGURO, M., NAKASHIMA, H., TANABE, S. and SAKAKIBARA, R. 'Interaction of toxic lectin with epithelial cells of rat small intestine *in vitro*', *Chem Pharm Bull Tokyo*, 1992, **40**, 441–5.

27 ROSSANDER-HULTHÉN, L., SANDBERG, A.-S. and SANDSTRÖM, B. 'The effect of dietary fibre on mineral absorption and utilization'. In T. Schweizer and C.A. Edwards (eds), pp. 197–216, *Dietary Fibre – A Component of Food: Nutritional Function in Health and Disease*, London, Springer-Verlag, 1992.

28 PRICE, K. and FENWICK, G. 'Soyasaponin I, a compound possessing undesirable taste characteristics isolated from the dried pea *(Pisum sativum L.)*', *J Sci Food Agric*, 1984, **35**, 887–92.

29 GUEGUEN, J. 'Solubility of faba bean *(Vicia faba L)* and pea *(Pisum sativum L.)*', *Lebensm Wiss u Technol*, 1980, **13**, 156–63.

30 ZEIGER, R.S., SAMPSON, H., BOCK, S. *et al.* 'Soy allergy in infants and children with IgE-associated cow's milk allergy', *J Pediatr*, 1999, **134**, 614–22.

31 OWUSU-ANSAH, Y.J. and MCCURDY, S.M. 'Pea proteins: a review of chemistry, technology of production, and utilization', *Food Rev Int*, 1991, 7, 103–34.

32 JAMES, K. and HOVE, E. 'The ineffectiveness of supplementary cystine in legume-based rat diets', *J Nutr*, 1980, **110**, 1736–44.

33 DEO, S., SAVAGE, G. and JERMYN, W. 'The effect of cooking on the nutritional quality of New Zealand grown peas', International Food Legume Research Conference on Pea, Lentil, Faba Bean and Chickpea, Washington, DC, Spokane, 1986.

34 GRIFFITHS, D. 'The trypsin and chymotrypsin inhibitor activities of various pea *(Pisum spp.)* and field bean *(Vicia faba)* cultivars', *J Sci Food Agr*, 1984, **35**, 481–6.

35 TANNOUS, R. and ULLAH, M. 'Effects of autoclaving on nutritional factors in legume seeds', *Trop Agric*, 1969, **46**, 123–9.

36 BENDER, A. 'Haemagglutinins (lectins) in beans', *Food Chem*, 1983, **11**, 309–20.

37 SANDBERG, A.-S. 'The effect of food processing on phytate hydrolysis and availability of iron and zinc. Nutritional and Toxicological Consequences of Food Processing. AIN Symposium, Washington 1990', *Adv Exp Med Biol*, 1991, **289**, 499–508.

38 HURRELL, R., JUILLERAT, M.-A., REDDY, M., LYNCH, S., DASSENKO, S. and COOK, J. 'Soy protein, phytate, and iron absorption in humans', *Am J Clin Nutr*, 1992, **56**, 573–8.

39 BRUNE, M., ROSSANDER-HULTHÉN, L., HALLBERG, L., GLEERUP, A., SANDBERG, A.-S. 'Human iron absorption from bread: inhibiting effects of cereal fiber, phytate and inositol phosphates with different numbers of phosphate groups', *J Nutr*, 1992, **122**, 442–9.

40 BARKHOLT, V., JÖRGENSEN, P., SÖRENSEN, D. *et al.* 'Protein modification by fermentation: effect of fermentation on the potential allergenicity of pea', *Allergy*, 1998, **53**, 106–8.

41 JOHNSON, I., GEE, J., PRICE, K., CURL, C., FENWICK, G. 'Influence of saponins on

gut permeability and active nutrient transport *in vitro*', *J Nutr,* 1986, **116**, 2270–7.

42 GEE, J., PRICE, K., RIDOUT, C., WORTLEY, G., HURRELL, R. and JOHNSON, I. 'Saponins of quinoa (*Chenopodium quinoia*): effects of processing on their abundance in quinoa products and their biological effects on intestinal mucosal tissue', *J Sci Food Agric,* 1993, **63**, 201–9.

43 VOSE, J., BASTERRECHEA, M., GORIN, P., FINLAYSON, A. and YOUNGS, C. 'Air classification of field peas and horsebean flours: chemical studies of starch and protein fractions', *Cereal Chem,* 1976, **53**, 928–36.

44 REICHERT, R.D. and YOUNGS, C.G. 'Nature of the residual protein associated with starch fractions from air-classified field peas', *Cereal Chem,* 1978, **55**, 469–80.

45 TYLER, R.T., YOUNGS, C.G. and SOSULSKI, F.W. 'Air classification of legumes. I. Separation efficiency yield, and composition of the starch and protein fractions', *Cereal Chem,* 1981, **58**, 144–8.

46 REICHERT, R.D. 'Air classification of peas (*Pisum sativum*) varying widely in protein content', *J Food Sci,* 1982, **47**, 1263–7.

47 VOSE, J.R. 'Production and functionality of starches and protein isolates from legume seeds (field peas and horse beans)', *Cereal Chem,* 1980, **57**, 406–10.

48 GUEGUEN, J. 'Legume seed protein extraction, processing, and end-product characteristics'. In C.E. Bodwell and L. Petiti (eds), p. 267–303, *Plant Proteins for Human Food*, The Hague, Martinus Nijhoff/Dr W. Junk, 1983.

49 FLEMING, S.E. and SOSULSKI, F.W. 'Nutritive value of bread fortified with concentrated plant proteins and lysine', *Cereal Chem,* 1977, **54**, 1238–48.

50 FLEMING, S.E. and SOSULSKI, F.W. 'Breadmaking properties of four concentrated plant proteins', *Cereal Chem,* 1977, **54**, 1124–40.

51 JEFFERS, H.C., RUBENTHALER, G.L., FINNEY, P.L., ANDERSON, P.D. and BRUINS-MA, B.L. 'Pea: a highly functional fortifier in wheat flour blends', *Bakers Dig,* 1978, **52**, 36.

52 SOSULSKI, F.W. and FLEMING, S.E. 'Sensory evaluation of bread prepared from composite flours', *Bakers Dig,* 1979, **53**, 20–5.

53 NIELSEN, M A, SUMNER, A.K. and WHALLEY, L.L. 'Fortification of pasta with pea flour and air-classified pea protein concentrate', *Cereal Chem,* 1980, **57**, 203–6.

54 EU, New Technologies for Improved Nutritional and Functional Value of Pea Protein: FAIR CT 95-0193, NUTRIPEA C1004-95, Report 1999.

55 WATTERS, K.H. and HEATON, R.K. 'Quality characteristics of ground beef patties extended with moist-heated and unheated seed meals', *J Am Oil Chem Soc,* **56**, 86–90A, 1979.

56 PATEL, P.R., YOUNGS, C.G. and GRANT, D.R. 'Preparation and properties of spray-dried pea protein concentrate-cheese whey blends', *Cereal Chem,* 1981, **58**, 249–55.

57 SOSULSKI, F.W. CHAKRABORTY, P. and HUMBERT, E.S. 'Legume-based imitation and blended milk products', *Can Inst Food Sci Technol J,* 1978, **3**, 117–23.

58 DULAU, I. and THEBAUDIN, J.-Y. 'Functional properties of leguminous protein: applications in food', *Grain Legumes,* 1998, **20**, 15–11.

59 FREDRIKSON, M., BIOT, P., CARLSSON, N.-G., ALMINGER-LARSSON, M. and SANDBERG, A.-S. 'Production of high quality pea protein isolate, with low content of oligosaccharides and phytate'. *In progress,* 2000.

60 SØRENSEN, A.D., HANSEN, A.B., SØRENSEN, S., BARKHOLT, V. and FRØKIÆR, H. 'Influence of industrial processing of peas on the content of antinutritional factors and the *in vitro* digestibility', 3rd European Conference on Grain Legumes, Valladolid, 1998, pp. 348–9.

61 FREDRIKSON, M., ALMINGER-LARSSON, M., SANDBERG, A.-S. 'Phytate content and phytate degradation by endogenous phytase in pea (*Pisum sativum*)', *In progress,* 2000.

62 HALLBERG, L., BRUNE, M. and ROSSANDER, L. 'Iron absorption in man: ascorbic acid and dose-dependent inhibition by phytate', *Am J Clin Nutr,* 1989, **49**, 140–4.

63 FREDRIKSON, M., ALMINGER, M., SANDBERG, A.-S. 'Improved *in vitro* availability of zinc and iron from dephytinized pea protein formulas'. *In progress,* 2000.

64 HERIAN, A.M., TAYLOR, S.L. and BUSH, R.K. 'Allergenic reactivity of various soybean products as determined by RAST inhibition', *J Food Sci,* 1993, **58**, 385–8.

65 DAVIDSSON, L., DIMITRIOU, T., WALCZYK, T. and HURRELL, R.F. 'Iron absorption from experimental infant formulas based on pea protein isolate: the effect of phytic acid and ascorbic acid'. *In progress,* 2000.

10

Functional fats and spreads

E.A.M. de Deckere and P.M. Verschuren, Unilever Research, Vlaardingen

10.1 Introduction

The first attempt to provide a substitute for butter, margarine, was developed to feed soldiers and labourers in France during the reign of Napoleon III in order to fight better and work harder. Margarine can be seen as a forerunner of modern functional foods. Because butter contains vitamin A, margarine was enriched in vitamin A in addition to vitamin D, and became an important source of these vitamins in Western countries. In these countries there is no vitamin A deficiency, but world-wide vitamin A deficiency is still an important issue. Recently, the use of margarine as a product for increasing vitamin A intake was studied in the Philippines, demonstrating the importance of enriched foods in combating nutrient deficiency.[1]

In the 1950s it became clear that dietary saturated fatty acids were positively related to plasma cholesterol concentration and the incidence of coronary heart disease (CHD). Replacement of saturated fatty acids by polyunsaturated fatty acids (mainly linoleic acid) reduced blood cholesterol and consequently the incidence of CHD. As early as the 1960s, Unilever developed a margarine rich in linoleic acid marketed as a food to lower blood cholesterol. This can be seen as a functional food in the sense used nowadays. While there are many definitions, for the purposes of this chapter a functional food is defined as:

> a food that contains a functional ingredient (a nutrient or non-nutrient)
> in order to improve the state of health and well-being and/or to reduce
> the risk of disease beyond that of nutritional deficiency.

There remains some debate as to whether a product can be considered a functional food when a nutrient is added to a food product to avoid deficiency, as in the case of vitamins A and D added to margarine. In many population groups there is, however, an imbalance in nutrient and non-nutrient (e.g. fibre) intake which can be corrected by functional foods with a positive impact on health and the risk of disease. Target groups for functional foods range from the whole population to the elderly, people with increased risk of a chronic disease, or with a chronic disease. There are a number of spreads and fats with functional ingredients already on the market. The claims used are content and intake claims such as 'fits into a cholesterol-lowering diet' or 'fits into a healthy lifestyle'. A claim such as 'this product helps to reduce risk of disease' is currently not allowed in European countries or the USA.

This chapter concentrates on functional ingredients that can be present in fats and spreads. Spreads range from zero fat spreads (3% fat content) to full fat spreads such as margarine (80% fat content). Spreads are a particularly suitable vehicle for functional ingredients, because they are eaten daily. Full fat spreads, in addition to fats, could be vehicles for fatty functional ingredients whereas low fat spreads could be vehicles for water-soluble functional ingredients.

10.2 Functional ingredients and chronic diseases: applications in fats and spreads

A number of nutrients and non-nutrients have the potential to be applied as functional ingredients in fats and spreads. This chapter discusses mainly the use of spreads because spreads can be used for fat-soluble and water-soluble ingredients. It goes without saying that fats can be used for fat-soluble functional ingredients. The most important potential functional ingredients with their (putative) mode of action in preventing or alleviating chronic diseases are listed in Table 10.1. The scientific background to each ingredient and its application in spreads (and fats where applicable) are discussed below.

10.3 Fatty acids

10.3.1 Introduction
A number of fatty acids (Fig. 10.1) have the potential to be used as functional ingredients, because their intake has been found to be positively related to health. In the USA, and in most other countries, health claims for specific fatty acids are not allowed on packaged foods. The nutritional label must list the amounts of total fat and saturated fats per serving, whereas the listing of monounsaturated and polyunsaturated fats is voluntary.

10.3.2 Linoleic acid
Numerous studies have shown the plasma cholesterol-lowering capacity of linoleic acid and it has become an established functional ingredient in this

Table 10.1   Nutrients and non-nutrients suitable for use in fats and spreads to lower the risk of chronic disease

Chronic disease	Functional ingredient/ functional food	Mechanism/ purported mechanism
Coronary heart disease	Linoleic acid	Lowering blood cholesterol
	Conjugated linoleic acid	Reducing atherosclerosis
	α-Linolenic acid	?
	VLC n-3 polyunsaturated fatty acids*	Lowering blood triglycerides, reducing arrhythmias
	Phytosterols	Lowering blood cholesterol
	Antioxidants (vitamin E, carotenes, polyphenols, ubiquinone)	Lowering LDL oxidation, reducing atherosclerotic progression
Obesity	Low fat or low energy spreads (modified triglycerides, coagel, sucrose polyester, inulin)	Reduction fat mass
	Conjugated linoleic acid	Reduction fat mass
Hypertriglyceridaemia (e.g. in diabetes type II)	VLC n-3 polyunsaturated fatty acids	Lowering blood triglycerides
Chronic inflammatory diseases	γ-Linolenic acid	Reducing eicosanoid production
	Stearidonic acid	Reducing eicosanoid production
	VLC n-3 polyunsaturated fatty acids	Reducing eicosanoid production
Cancer	Vitamin E	Scavenging radicals
Cataract	Vitamin E	Scavenging radicals
Osteoporosis	Calcium (+ vitamin D)	Increasing bone mass
Large intestine ailments	Inulin	Stimulation of fermentation, increasing stool mass

Note:
* VLC: very long chain (fish oil n-3 fatty acids)

respect. As early as the 1950s, it became clear that replacing saturated fatty acids with linoleic acid in the diet could decrease plasma cholesterol concentration and thus mortality from CHD. Early research resulted in the prediction equations of Keys and Hegsted published in 1957 and 1965, respectively, relating changes in plasma total cholesterol concentration to changes in the amounts of dietary fatty acids. The prediction equation has been analysed again on basis of more recent studies[2, 3]. The conclusions do not differ from the original ones: saturated fatty acids elevate serum cholesterol, polyunsaturated fatty acids (linoleic acid) actively lower serum cholesterol, and monounsaturated fatty acids (oleic acid) have little or no effect (Fig. 10.2).[4]

On the basis of the inverse relationships between linoleic acid intake and plasma cholesterol concentration, and the link between plasma cholesterol concentration and the incidence of CHD, advisory agencies in Western countries

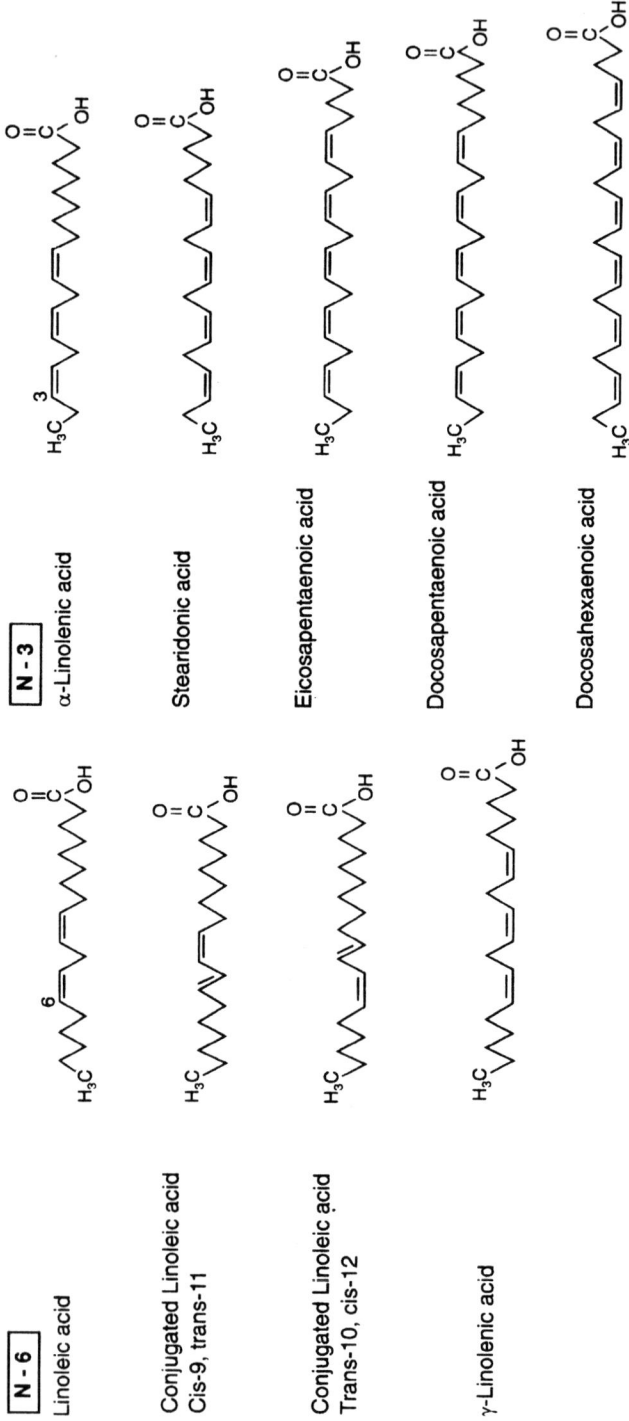

N - 6

Linoleic acid

Conjugated Linoleic acid
Cis-9, trans-11

Conjugated Linoleic acid
Trans-10, cis-12

γ-Linolenic acid

N - 3

α-Linolenic acid

Stearidonic acid

Eicosapentaenoic acid

Docosapentaenoic acid

Docosahexaenoic acid

Fig. 10.1 N-6 and n-3 polyunsaturated fatty acids with (potential) health benefits. N-6 and n-3 denote the first double bond from the methyl end (−CH₃) of the molecule. Humans can only insert double bonds into unsaturated fatty acid molecules between the last double bond counting from the methyl end and the carboxyl group, resulting in n-6 and n-3 families of fatty acids.

$$\Delta SC = 2.10\Delta S - 1.16\Delta P + 0.067\Delta C$$

ΔSC is the change (+ or −) in the serum total cholesterol concentration (in mg/dL; divide by 38.7 for mmol/L),

ΔS and ΔP are the changes in the percentages of dietary energy of saturated and polyunsaturated fatty acids, respectively,

ΔC is the change in the amount of dietary cholesterol (in kg/J).

Replacing 1% of energy of saturated fatty acids ($\Delta S = -1$) with 1% of energy of polyunsaturated fatty acids ($\Delta P = +1$), at unchanged dietary cholesterol, decreases the serum total cholesterol concentration by 3.26 mg/dL (0.084 mmol/L).

A reduction in serum cholesterol concentration by 0.6 mmol/L decreases relative risk of CHD by 50% at age of 40 falling to 20% at age of 70.[4]

Fig. 10.2   Prediction equation for effect of dietary fatty acids on plasma cholesterol concentration[2]

have long recommended increasing linoleic acid intake to 4–10% of energy intake.[5, 6] When intakes of saturated fatty acids and cholesterol are relatively high, an intake of 10% of energy intake as linoleic acid is recommended. Such recommendations have contributed to a substantial decrease in the incidence of CHD in the last few decades. In the USA, for example, the incidence of CHD decreased by 53% between 1950 and 1992.[7] Some authorities caution against the intake of higher amounts of linoleic acid and recommend lowering the dietary ratio of n-6 fatty acids (primarily linoleic acid) over n-3 fatty acids (α-linolenic acid and fish oil polyunsaturated fatty acids). However, there is no solid evidence that high intakes of linoleic acid have adverse effects in humans. Some recent dietary guidelines for the prevention of CHD recommended a reduction in total fat intake without recommending an increase in linoleic acid intake.[7] However, there is no solid evidence from clinical trials that solely a reduction in fat intake lowers the risk of CHD. Replacing saturated fatty acids by polyunsaturated fatty acids remains the best advice with respect to dietary fats and risk of CHD.[6, 8] Spreads high in linoleic acid are now widely available, and are used by a substantial proportion of the population in the developed world, making linoleic acid one of the most important current functional ingredients.

10.3.3 α-Linolenic acid

α-Linolenic acid (like linoleic acid) is an essential fatty acid. To avoid deficiency, the minimal intake should be 0.2–0.3% of energy intake (approximately 0.5–0.75 g/day for an adult person). The recommended daily intake is 1–2 g.[9] In the body, α-linolenic acid is converted into docosapentaenoic acid (DPA, C22:5 n-3) and docosahexaenoic acid (DHA, C22:6 n-3) which are incorporated into the phospholipids of cell membranes, particularly in the brain and retina. An intermediate fatty acid is eicosapentaenoic acid (EPA, C20:5 n-3). A few epidemiological studies[10, 11] suggest that people who have α-linolenic acid intakes below the recommended intake have an increased risk of CHD. Recent studies, however, show that α-linolenic acid does not affect the parameters of thrombotic risk.[12, 13] α-Linolenic acid and linoleic acid are desaturated and elongated by the same enzymes and suppress each other's metabolism. However, increasing α-linolenic acid intake (e.g. to 10 g/day or more) hardly affects phospholipid arachidonic acid levels in plasma and cell membranes.[14] Moreover, DHA levels are not affected, showing that the average habitual intake of α-linolenic acid is sufficient to meet the body's requirement for DHA. Only very high intakes of α-linolenic acid (>30 g/day) decrease blood triglycerides.[15] α-Linolenic acid may be as effective as linoleic acid in lowering LDL cholesterol.

Increased intakes of α-linolenic acid may affect some physiological processes, because EPA is formed from α-linolenic acid and incorporated into cell membrane phospholipids. EPA is an inhibitor of eicosanoid synthesis and is released from phospholipids at the same time as arachidonic acid (from which the eicosanoids are formed). Inflammatory and immunological processes can be affected in this way.

Although the mean intakes of α-linolenic acid in Western countries may well be within the range of the recommended intake, more than a quarter of the population may have a daily intake below 1 g and these people might have an increased risk of CHD.[10, 11, 16] The intake of α-linolenic acid of this population group can easily be increased to the recommended level by spreads containing 5% α-linolenic acid. A number of advisory bodies recommend increasing the intake of α-linolenic acid in order to lower the dietary ratio of linoleic acid over α-linolenic acid (e.g. to 5:1) without increasing fat intake. However, solid underpinning of this recommendation is lacking.

α-Linolenic acid is present in significant amounts in soybean, canola, linseed and perilla seed oil. It can give off-flavours and its use in spreads needs protection by antioxidants. In most spreads on the European market low amounts of α-linolenic acid are present. Linolenic acid isomers, including trans isomers, are also present, probably due to partial hydrogenation or deodorisation during processing of the rapeseed and soybean oils used.[16] In view of the significance of trans fatty acids, the presence of trans fatty acid isomers should be minimised.

10.3.4   Fish oil n-3 polyunsaturated fatty acids

Fish oil n-3 polyunsaturated fatty acids (fish oil PUFAs) comprise EPA, DPA, and DHA (see section 10.3.3). Numerous studies have shown beneficial effects in CHD, in particular a reduction in the risk of fatal CHD, and in inflammatory and immunological diseases.[9, 17–19] The hallmark effect of fish oil PUFAs, however, is the decrease in plasma triglyceride concentration.[15] A high plasma triglyceride concentration is a recognised independent risk factor of CHD.[20] Intakes of fish oil PUFAs up to 3 g/day are safe according to the US Food and Drug Administration,[21] but intake of vitamin E should increase accordingly.[22] Fish oil PUFAs are poorly stored in adipose tissue.

High blood pressure is a risk factor of CHD and stroke. A prolonged 5 mmHg lower level of diastolic blood pressure is associated with a 35–40% lower risk of stroke.[23] The elderly still suffer the largest majority of blood pressure-related cerebrovascular disease. Two studies have shown a clinically relevant reduction in blood pressure through daily consumption of 3 g of fish oil PUFAs.[24, 25] Some studies suggest that fish oil PUFAs in combination with other dietary measures can reduce blood pressure.

Generally, the average intake of fish oil PUFAs in developed countries is low (about 120 mg/day), but this has risen more recently due to an increase in the consumption of poultry fed on fish meal feed.[26] Average daily intakes of habitual fish consumers were found to be between 0.5 g (less than two servings a week) and 1.6 g (more than four servings a week).[27] On average, a decrease in plasma triglycerides by 25% can be obtained by an intake of 3–4 g fish PUFAs daily.[15] For primary prevention of CHD a daily intake of 2–3 g is desirable.[18] Recently, a study in Italy[19] showed that a daily intake of 1 g fish oil PUFAs decreased risk of cardiovascular death by 17% in a group of patients who had a first myocardial infarction. For a daily intake of 3 g fish oil PUFAs at a spread consumption of 25 g/day the spread should contain 15 g fish oil PUFAs per 100 g fat, which means that the spreads should be made predominantly of fish oil. However, those spreads containing fish oil that are (or have been) on the market contain only a small amount of fish oil, insufficient for triglyceride-lowering or cardiovascular health claims (see section 10.4).

10.3.5 γ-Linolenic acid

γ-Linolenic acid (GLA) (C18:3 n-6) is present in plant seed oils of evening primrose (about 8% of total fatty acids), blackcurrant (18%), and borage (22%). In humans it is converted into dihomo-γ-linolenic acid (DGLA) and incorporated into phospholipids of cell membranes. On stimulation of cells, DGLA is released and converted into prostaglandin E1 which exerts anti-inflammatory activity. DGLA can also be converted (by 15-lipoxygenase) into a metabolite which can inhibit the synthesis of leukotrienes from arachidonic acid as a result of which inflammatory reactions might also be mitigated. Furthermore, DGLA can also be converted into arachidonic acid and in cases in which the activity of Δ6 desaturase is decreased, like in atopic eczema and diabetes,[28] DGLA may increase the synthesis of arachidonic acid. In *in vitro* studies and animal models a great number of effects of GLA have been reported, but in human studies limited beneficial effects have been found so far.

GLA-containing oils are available as encapsulated supplements. At the moment, natural sources of GLA are limited, but these can be increased readily. GLA might be applied in a number of chronic inflammatory diseases like rheumatoid arthritis in which approximately 3 g/day GLA may improve clinical symptoms slightly.[29, 30] GLA has not yet been approved for the treatment of any disease, but might be used as an adjunctive therapy. The regulatory status has been summarised by Kulow.[31] GLA is more prone to oxidation than linoleic acid and has to be protected by extra vitamin E.

10.3.6 Conjugated linoleic acid

Conjugated linoleic acid (CLA) refers to isomers of linoleic acid with several positional and geometric conjugated double bond configurations.[32] Mainly the cis-9, trans-11 CLA isomer (80–90% of total isomers) is present in small amounts in dairy products and meat (approximately 5 mg/g fat). Beneficial effects of mixtures of CLA isomers (mainly cis-9, trans-11 CLA and trans-10, cis-12 CLA; 0.5–1.0 g/100 g diet) have been found in a number of animal models of cholesterol metabolism and atherosclerosis,[33, 34] carcinogenesis,[32, 35] and body fat regulation.[36] A recent clinical trial showed that a mixture of CLA isomers (4 g/day) decreased body fat in humans by 3%.[37] However, it has been shown that trans-10, cis-12 CLA, and not cis-9, trans-11 CLA, affected lipid metabolism and body fat in animals.[34, 36] Consequently, the 'natural' occurring CLA isomer (cis-9, trans-11) might be ineffective as far as these parameters are concerned. Some studies suggest that CLA, like fish oil PUFAs, can increase the level of antioxidant enzymes in cells.[38] Toxicological studies so far did not show harmful effects of CLA.[39]

CLA can be synthesised from pure linoleic acid, sunflower seed oil or safflower oil by alkalic isomerisation. Approximately 90% of linoleic acid can be converted into equal amounts of cis-9, trans-11 CLA and trans-10, cis-12 CLA.[40] Although only one isomer might be effective there are no physiological reasons to make preparations enriched in the active isomer at the moment. CLA isomers can be incorporated into triglycerides by interesterification and used for the production of spreads. Oxidisability of CLA might be greater than that of linoleic acid, but the results are equivocal.[41, 42]

CLA is already on the market as a supplement, e.g. for body builders to increase lean body mass. However, this effect has not been scientifically proven.

10.3.7 Stearidonic acid

Stearidonic acid (C18:4 n-3) is present in a few plant seed oils.[43] It is a desaturation product of α-linolenic acid. It may have anti-inflammatory properties due to inhibition of leukotriene B4 synthesis.[44] Leukotriene B4 synthesis is also inhibited by EPA (fish oil PUFAs), but stearidonic acid is of plant origin and contains one double bond less and is therefore less prone to oxidation. Only a few studies have been published.

10.4 Spreads containing fish oil

Spreads containing unhardened fish oil have been on the market in Denmark, the UK and Ireland for more than a decade (a number were already withdrawn). The amount of fish oil varies (varied) between 5% and 25% of total fat. In addition to a fish oil PUFA content claim they carry (carried) claims such as '... may help to maintain a healthy heart'. A few studies have been published in which fish oil-containing spreads were used which show that spreads are a useful vehicle and that approximately 1 g fish oil PUFAs daily is sufficient to increase plasma levels of fish oil PUFAs markedly and to lower plasma triglyceride concentrations.[45, 46]

Adding fish oil to spreads reduces oxidative stability, resulting in the formation of off-flavours and a decreased shelf life. This is still a major problem and understanding of the oxidation process of fish oil PUFAs will help the manufacturing of fish oil PUFA spreads. Antioxidants can inhibit oxidation of the fish oil PUFAs. Oxidation comprises initiation, propagation and termination reactions followed by the formation of volatile compounds from the hydroperoxides formed which give the off-flavour. In addition to heat and light, metal ions are involved in the initiation reaction and sequestration of these ions generally will inhibit oxidation. Also, antioxidants can inhibit the initiation reaction. In the propagation reaction oxygen is involved and replacing oxygen with nitrogen will improve shelf life of the spread. However, oxygen has to be removed completely, because traces of oxygen are sufficient to maintain the oxidation process. Termination reactions can be inhibited by antioxidants. Furthermore, antioxidants can inhibit the formation of volatile compounds from hydroperoxides. Both sequestrants and antioxidants are needed and the spreads with fish oil PUFAs contain EDTA and citric acid as sequestrants, propylgallate and tocopherol as antioxidants and ascorbylpalmitate as oxygen scavenger. Sequestrants are more important than antioxidants, because they reduce more effectively oxidation of fish oil PUFAs than antioxidants. The fish for the production of oil should be of good quality and processed as soon as possible. The raw fish oil should be refined and stored under optimal conditions, avoiding oxidation. Nevertheless, when exposed to air off-flavours develop rather quickly. Oxidative stability may be increased by removing metal ions completely from the oil. However, removing metal ions is no common practice and they are bound by chelators (compounds which tightly bind metal ions). Furthermore, because the other ingredients of the spread will also contain metal ions, it might be less useful to remove metal ions completely from the oil. Oxidative stability may also be improved by using liposomes.[47] These liposomes consist of a lipid bilayer in which triglyceride-containing fish oil PUFAs together with fat-soluble antioxidants are incorporated.

10.5 Modified fats and oils

10.5.1 Interesterification (rearrangement)
Since the 1920s glyceride interesterification has been used in the production of spreads with specific physical properties. For a number of decades interesterification has also been used for the production of triglycerides with specific compositions and nutritional properties.[48] Interesterification offers the possibility to distribute randomly the fatty acids over the glyceride molecule (randomised oil; chemical interesterification) or to incorporate other fatty acids into the triglyceride molecule (both by chemical and enzymatic

interesterification). Randomisation of an oil or fat can affect the metabolism of fatty acids, because in most oils and fats PUFAs are in the sn-2 position. Fatty acids in the sn-2 position are absorbed as monoglyceride and absorption is generally somewhat greater than that of fatty acids in the other two positions. For instance, exchanging linoleic acid in the sn-2 position for a saturated fatty acid can improve fat absorption, because linoleic acid is more easily absorbed than saturated fatty acids. In enzymatic esterification regiospecific lipases can exchange fatty acids in the sn-1,-3 positions. Furthermore, lipases have also been described which can incorporate some fatty acids preferentially or less readily.

10.5.2 Medium chain triglycerides

Medium chain triglycerides are modified lipids. Spreads containing medium chain triglycerides have been on the market for half a century. The product quality does not differ from that of common spreads. Medium chain triglycerides consist of C8:0 and C10:0 fatty acids obtained from, for example, coconut and palm kernel oil. They are used in the treatment of lipid disorders or in cases in which a dense source of easily metabolisable energy is required.[49] They might have a beneficial effect on glycemic control in diabetics, but the results are conflicting.[50] They might also be used for weight reduction in obesity due to the lower energy content and greater thermogenesis, in comparison with long chain triglycerides,[51] but the findings are still equivocal.[52] In each case they are poorly stored in adipose tissue. Furthermore, in comparison with the longer chain saturated fatty acids (C12:0, C14:0, C16:0), they do not increase plasma total cholesterol.[53]

10.5.3 Structured triglycerides

More recently, structured triglycerides containing various combinations of fatty acids can be made.[49, 54] They offer possibilities for functional foods and can easily be incorporated into spreads or other fat-containing products. They may be used to improve intestinal absorption of fatty acids in infants and critically ill patients. They can also be used in enteral and parenteral nutrition. Numerous clinical trials with structured triglycerides have been done. For instance, structured triglycerides containing medium chain fatty acids and fish oil PUFAs have been tested in patients. The medium chain fatty acids are more rapidly absorbed, cleared from the blood and oxidised than the long chain fatty acids, whereas fish oil PUFAs can decrease inflammatory responses.

Structured triglycerides can also be used to decrease energy intake. A structured triglyceride containing medium chain fatty acids and behenic acid (C22:0) is on the market and present in some snacks, but not in spreads. The energy content is about 5 kcal/g due to the lower energy content of the medium chain fatty acids (8.3 kcal/g) and the poor absorption of behenic acid. Sources of medium chain fatty acids are coconut and palm kernel oil, whereas peanut oil and fully hydrogenated high erucic rapeseed and fish oil are sources of behenic acid.

10.5.4 Fatty acid modification of crops

Traditionally, breeding and gene modification give possibilities to change fatty acid composition of vegetable oils or to change or increase minor constituents such as tocopherols and phytosterols.[48] Under way are the developments of a rapeseed oil containing lauric acid (medium chain triglycerides) and EPA,[55] and of vegetable oils free of saturated fatty acids.

10.5.5 Miscellaneous

There are several new technologies to produce triglycerides with special fatty acid compositions. A major development is with EPA and DHA. Already available are fish oils enriched in EPA and DHA (hydrolysis of fish oil, separation of fatty acids by molecular distillation, re-esterification of the EPA and DHA-enriched FA fractions), EPA and DHA containing triglycerides produced by microalgae and bacteria,[56] and microencapsulated (EPA and DHA-enriched) fish oils (oil drops surrounded by a layer of starch).[57] Generally, production costs are high, but research is under way to reduce costs. The triglycerides can be incorporated into spreads using standard technologies, but the development of spreads with microencapsulated ingredients, in particular liposomes, is a promising new area.[58]

10.6 Phytosterols

10.6.1 Phytosterols and plasma cholesterol lowering

At the beginning of the 1950s the plasma cholesterol-lowering potential of phytosterols or plant sterols was studied in humans.[59] Since then, numerous studies have shown that this potential is due to inhibition of cholesterol absorption. Phytosterols are minor constituents of crude vegetable oils and most oils contains 0.1–0.5% (by weight of oil) phytosterols. Some oils such as rice bran, oat and wheatgerm oil contain amounts up to 4%. The main phytosterol in vegetable oils is β-sitosterol (a 4-desmethylsterol) which is present as free sterol and esterified with fatty acids.[60] Rice bran oil contains also 4,4'-dimethylsterols esterified to ferulic acid and the plasma cholesterol-lowering potential of rice bran oil has been ascribed partly to these compounds.[61] A recent study, however, showed that these compounds (as oryzanol) were much less effective than phytosterols from soybean oil (mainly β-sitosterol).[62] Crude maize (corn) oil is also relatively rich in phytosterols (approximately 0.9%). In studies by Keys et al.[63] it was found that diets rich in maize oil showed a cholesterol-lowering effect which could only partially be explained by the fatty acid compositions. The greater hypocholesterolaemic effect of maize oil compared to that of sunflower seed oil in spite of its lower linoleic acid content was coined the 'maize oil aberration'. It was confirmed recently[64] and indicates that amounts of phytosterols slightly less than 1 g per day can lower the plasma cholesterol concentration. However, for an appreciable reduction in plasma cholesterol

(10–15%) the daily phytosterol (β-sitosterol) intake should be 1–3 g. The habitual diet (adults) delivers approximately 250 mg phytosterols per day. So, products have to be supplemented with phytosterols in order to achieve a significant cholesterol reduction.

10.6.2 Phytosterol esters

The solubility of free plant sterols in oils is about 2–3% (by weight of oil) at body temperature which is too low for application in cholesterol-lowering spreads. When phytosterols are not solubilised, the cholesterol-lowering potential is much less. The solubility of fatty acid esters of phytosterols is much greater (>15%) and they can easily be incorporated into spreads. The esters have to be hydrolysed by pancreatic cholesterol esterase in the small intestine for phytosterols to be effective as inhibitors of cholesterol absorption. The cholesterol-lowering efficacy of free β-sitosterol and of sitosterol esterified to oleate or linolate may be similar.[65, 66] However, the efficacy of saturated fatty acid esters might be less than that of oleate esters due to the lower rate of hydrolysis in the small intestine.

10.6.3 Phytosterol-containing spreads

Recently, phytosterol-containing spreads with a cholesterol-lowering claim were launched in several European countries, the USA, Australia and New Zealand. Beforehand, these spreads were extensively tested in human clinical trials for their cholesterol-lowering capacity. Spread supplemented with soybean sterols (11% phytosterol equivalents/100 g spread) partly (65%) esterified with fatty acids from sunflowerseed oil were studied by Weststrate and co-workers. At a daily intake of 30 g spread (3.3 g phytosterol equivalents/day) plasma total cholesterol and LDL cholesterol decreased by 8% and 13%, respectively. The plasma cholesterol concentrations were decreased both in normo- and mildly cholesterolaemic subjects. Furthermore, similar effects were found for sitosterol and sitostanol.[62] Also, lower intakes of partly esterified and non-esterified soybean sterols (0.8, 1.6 g/day) decreased LDL cholesterol by 6.0–8.5%.[67, 68]

Miettinen and co-workers have extensively investigated the cholesterol-lowering effect of spreads supplemented with sitostanyl fatty acid ester. They used β-sitosterol extracted from tall oil (from wood pulp) in which the double bond at the position C5–C6 in the molecule was hydrogenated (hydrogenation gives sitostanol) and which was esterified with fatty acids by chemical interesterification with fatty acid methyl esters from rapeseed oil.[69] In a study with hypercholesterolaemic subjects a spread supplemented with sitostanyl ester (9 g sitostanol equivalents/100 g margarine) was tested.[70] The intake of sitostanol was approximately 1.8 g or 2.6 g per day. After 12 months, serum total cholesterol and LDL cholesterol concentrations had been decreased in the low and high sitostanol groups, in comparison with the control group, by 11% and

13% and by 14% and 17%, respectively. No significant change in HDL cholesterol occurred.

10.6.4 Safety

Intestinal absorption of β-sitosterol is approximately 5% of intake. It is excreted by the liver into the bile. A tenfold increase in the intake of β-sitosterol increased the plasma level by less than a factor of two.[62] Sitostanol is not or hardly absorbed. Recently, various safety evaluations of phytosterols have been published.[71, 72] No adverse effects were found. However, in humans phytosterol- and phytostanol-containing spreads can decrease the plasma carotene concentration if the daily intake of phytosterols is higher than 1.6 g.[62, 67]

10.7 Antioxidants

10.7.1 Introduction

Antioxidants may reduce the risk of CHD and cancer.[73] With respect to CHD, it has been hypothesised that oxidation of LDL in the vessel wall plays a key role in atherogenesis. Furthermore, oxidative processes may also be involved in the progression phase of the atherosclerotic plaque.[74] Antioxidants occur abundantly in fruits and vegetables, but also vegetable oils contain antioxidants, in particular vitamin E. In addition, red palm oil contains also carotenoids (up to 0.2%) and extra virgin olive oil (unrefined) contains polyphenols.

10.7.2 Vitamin E

Vitamin E comprises tocopherols and tocotrienols of which α-tocopherol is by far the most important constituent (90% of the vitamin E present in human tissues, e.g. in LDL particles in which vitamin E is the most abundant antioxidant present). Epidemiological studies and primary and secondary prevention trials have shown that vitamin E intake is inversely associated with the risk of CHD.[19, 75–79] Epidemiological data suggest that 40–60 mg vitamin E daily is effective while clinical trials suggest that vitamin E is effective from 100 mg (100 mg of dl-alpha-tocopherol acetate) daily. This latter is ten times the recommended dietary allowance (RDA). The RDA, however, is defined as the amount to prevent nutrient deficiency and does not take into account possible reductions in the risk of a disease by a nutrient.

Vitamin E supplements may decrease risk of cataract, but vitamin E does not protect against age-related degeneration of the macular of the eye. Epidemiological studies on vitamin E and cancer are inconsistent and there is no proof that vitamin E can protect against neurological disorders and inflammatory disorders like rheumatoid arthritis. However, vitamin E supplements may reduce pain in rheumatoid arthritis. A number of aspects of the immune system decline with age. Several studies in the elderly have shown that vitamin E supplementation can counteract these age-related declines in immune parameters.[80]

Of all antioxidants vitamin E has the strongest evidence to reduce risk of CHD and by this vitamin E-rich spread may also contribute to a lower risk of CHD. The principal sources of vitamin E are vegetable oils, and spreads made from vegetable oils are therefore the main dietary sources of vitamin E. Generally, it is recommended that spreads contain 0.6 g vitamin E per gram of linoleic acid. Higher levels are necessary for spreads containing α-linolenic acid and fish oil PUFAs. The contribution of spreads, dressings and oils to vitamin E intake is approximately 50%. Spreads are a good vehicle for fat-soluble antioxidants, because for a number of these antioxidants, fat is needed for an efficient absorption. Spreads enriched in vitamin E (31 mg/day) and α- and β-carotene (3–5 mg/day) increased vitamin E and α- and β-carotene concentrations in plasma and LDL particles.[81] The increase in resistance to oxidation of LDL particles *ex vivo* (outside the body), however, was marginal. Higher intakes of vitamin E (100 mg/day or more) can significantly increase the resistance of LDL to *ex vivo* oxidation.

Several spreads are on the markets with content claims: 'enriched in vitamin E', 'supplies 100% of the RDA', etc.

10.7.3 Tocotrienols
Crude palm and rice bran oil are rich in tocotrienols (300–1,200 mg/kg oil). Some authors have suggested that tocotrienols can lower blood cholesterol concentrations,[82] but there is no proof in humans.[83]

10.7.4 Carotenoids
The major dietary carotenoids are α- and β-carotene, β-cryptoxanthin, lycopene, lutein and zeaxanthin. Although epidemiological data suggest that β-carotene has a role in CHD prevention,[84] clinical trials have repeatedly shown that high dose supplements of β-carotene are ineffective in CHD.[85,86] With respect to cancer, epidemiological studies have shown that β-carotene may lower risk of lung cancer.[87] Also, a great number of animal studies have shown that carotenoids including β-carotene exert anti-carcinogenic activity. However, intervention studies in humans do not support the use of β-carotene supplements for reducing the risk of cancer.[88–90] In fact, in habitual heavy smokers β-carotene supplement increased lung cancer risk.[91] In the intervention studies relatively high amounts of β-carotene were used. Because carotenoids can also exert pro-oxidant activity in biological systems, it is not clear whether lower amounts, as suggested by epidemiological studies, might be effective. An anti-cancer effect has not been found for vitamin A, which is synthesised from β-carotene. However, pre-cancerous lesions may be reduced by retinoids.[90]

Lycopene may have more promise than β-carotene. Intake of lycopene is largely from tomatoes. It is absorbed and found in several tissues. Lycopene has potent antioxidant properties, particularly in quenching singlet oxygen. Intact lycopene is regenerated by a series of rotational and vibrational interactions with surrounding molecules. Many observational studies have shown that consumption of tomatoes and tomato products and blood lycopene levels are inversely related with the risk of numerous cancers, particularly with prostate, lung and stomach cancer. Lycopene may account for this effect, but this has not yet been proven.[92]

β-Carotene and lycopene are fat-soluble compounds and might be applied in spreads. However, they colour spreads orange or red, which limits their application. This should not be a drawback. Encapsulation of β-carotene and lycopene into liposomes may reduce colouring. Red palm oil is rich in carotenoids and can be used for the production of spreads in countries where vitamin A is a health problem.

10.7.5 Polyphenols
It is suggested that polyphenols may contribute to the lower incidence of CHD in the Mediterranean area. Polyphenols are non-nutrient antioxidants which are present in (extra) virgin olive oil (up to 0.08%), but not in refined olive oil, and give a bitter and pungent taste to the oil. Polyphenols from virgin olive oil inhibited the oxidation of LDL particles *ex vivo*.[93, 94] However, their effectiveness as an antioxidant in the body remains to be established.

10.7.6 Ubiquinol/ubiquinone (coenzyme Q)
Ubiquinol is a fat-soluble antioxidant synthesised by the body. The ability to synthesise ubiquinol decreases with age. Dietary intake of ubiquinone is about 2 mg/day. Dietary supplements of ubiquinone are on the market as an antioxidant and its use as an antioxidant in fat containing (food) products has been patented.[95] Its structure is very similar to that of vitamin K. It is present in cell membranes where it complements the antioxidant activity of vitamin E and in mitochondria where it has a role in oxidative phosphorylation. It is already used to treat various cardiovascular disorders because it improves mitochondrial function.[96] Like vitamin E it is also present in LDL particles (but in much lower levels than vitamin E) and may contribute to the resistance of LDL particles to oxidation.[97] Approximately half of the ubiquinol in plasma is present in LDL particles and an increase in intake (100 mg/day) increases ubiquinol in LDL particles.

10.8 Low (zero) fat spreads

10.8.1 Use of low fat spreads in obesity
A few lipid-based fat substitutes have been developed[49] which can be applied in low (zero) fat spreads. Low fat spreads can help in reducing fat and energy

intake in obese people. World-wide, 7% of the adult population may be obese.[98] In Western countries like the USA obesity among youth already ranges from 11% to 24%.[99] Obesity is a risk factor of diabetes,[100] cardiovascular diseases,[101] and cancer, in particular of breast and colon cancer.[102] Obesity is a main cause of hypertension which is a risk factor of nephropathy and retinopathy in diabetes. It is also a risk factor of stroke. Decreasing and prevention of obesity has become a major public health target. A varied diet, restricted energy intake and modest exercise, the so-called healthy lifestyle, can help in the maintenance of appropriate body weight (for height). Epidemiological data consistently support the role of dietary fat in obesity.[103] Reduced and low fat spreads help consumers in making their choice of food products for restricted dietary fat intake. In the USA health claims on low (saturated) fat content is authorised. Low fat spreads might lead to a decrease in vitamin E intake.[104] Therefore, low fat spreads must be enriched in vitamin E.

10.8.2 Coagel
A zero fat spread (less than 4% fat) has been on the American market since 1997. The spread is based on a coagel phase consisting of a network of saturated monoglyceride crystals. The crystalline coagel state has a fat-like consistency and can consist of 95% water.[105]

10.8.3 Sucrose polyester
Low fat spreads can also be made by using sucrose polyester (SPE) which is a fatty acyl ester of sucrose with six to eight fatty acid moieties. SPE has fat-like properties (physical and organoleptic), can also be used for frying, is not hydrolysed in the gastrointestinal tract by lipases due to steric hindrance, and is completely excreted in the faeces.[49, 106] It can help in reducing fat and energy intake, but the effect on body weight is equivocal.[107, 108] It is already on the market as a non-energetic fat substitute and present in a number of low fat snacks, but use in other foods like spreads is not allowed by the Food and Drug Administration (USA). A number of studies with SPE-containing spreads have been published. At high intakes (30 g SPE/day) SPE-containing spreads decreased plasma total cholesterol and triacylglycerol.[109]

SPE evokes a persistent lipophilic phase in the intestine by which the absorption of lipophilic substances such as cholesterol is decreased.[110] This is also the reason that SPE decreases plasma vitamin E and β-carotene.[111] The plasma concentrations of vitamin D and K, which are also fat-soluble vitamins, are not affected by SPE. Another problem of SPE is anal leakage (oil loss via the anus). This may be prevented by increasing the number of saturated fatty acids in the polyester molecule.

10.8.4 Other lipid-based fat substitutes

Other carbohydrate polyesters are those of sorbitol, trehalose, raffinose and stachyose and alkyl glycoside polyesters like methyl glucoside polyester.[49] They are also non-digestible but, compared to SPE, they are in an early stage of development and therefore not discussed here.

10.9 Inulin

Inulin, which is a dietary fibre of low viscosity and present in the habitual diet, has been investigated as a potential functional ingredient for a number of years.[112] It is marketed as a fat replacer and used as such successfully in spreads and dressings. Inulin is a fructan with 2–60 fructose units linked via a $\beta(1-2)$ bond, is partly soluble in water (10% at 20°C) and has a sweetening power of 15% of that of sucrose. It is not digested, but is almost quantitatively and exclusively fermented by colonic bifidobacteria yielding short chain fatty acids which are taken up as a result of which the metabolisable energy content of inulin is approximately 6.3 kJ/g. In addition, inulin may decrease lipid apparent digestibility by 1–2%.[113] Due to the fermentation of inulin the pH in the large intestine decreases by which growth of pathogens is inhibited. Furthermore, the microbial biomass increases by which the concentration of carcinogenic compounds (such as deoxycholic acid) in the large intestine can be decreased. These possible beneficial effects are accompanied by discomfort from flatulence and increased motility of the colon. Inulin at high intakes (20 g/day) might also decrease plasma triglycerides and cholesterol and might improve glucose tolerance in diabetics. However, these results are conflicting.[114] Furthermore, by lowering fat intake inulin-containing spreads may also lower risk of colorectal cancer.[115] In summary, inulin may be used in the maintenance of gastrointestinal health, but due to lack of an increase in viscosity of intestinal contents it may have no or only small effects on plasma lipids and glucose.

When mixed with water inulin gives an opaque gel consisting of a mixture of a network of small inulin crystallites. Such a gel has a fatty spread-like consistency as a result of which inulin can replace fat in reduced fat (medium fat) or in low fat (<4% fat) spreads. By using other ingredients the melting behaviour and the mouth feel of inulin-based spreads can be varied.

10.10 Calcium

Adequately high life-long intake of calcium can reduce risk of osteoporosis at old age and therefore calcium is considered to be a functional ingredient.[116] In the elderly, calcium supplementation (in combination with vitamin D) may reduce bone loss and fracture incidence.[117] Both in elderly and hypertensives, increased consumption of calcium may lower blood pressure. Recently, a number of calcium supplemented foods, including spreads, came on the market. A spread enriched in vitamin D and calcium is on the market in the Netherlands with the following content claim: 'intake of 25 g spread daily supplies 15% of the RDA of calcium'.

10.11   Conclusions

In addition to the existing role as a vehicle of vitamins, spreads (and fats) offer excellent opportunities for the incorporation of functional ingredients. In fact, they are already used as such. Both fat-soluble and water-soluble functional ingredients can be applied in spreads, which is, for some ingredients, a real technological challenge. Although many positive effects of the applicable functional ingredients have been described, most of the beneficial effects are awaiting proof.

10.12   References

1 SOLON, E.S., SOLON, M.S., MEHANSHO, H. *et al.* 'Evaluation of the effect of vitamin A-fortified margarine on the vitamin A status of preschool Filipino children', *Eur J Clin Nutr*, 1996, **50**, 720–3.

2 HEGSTED, D.M., AUSMAN, L.M., JOHNSON, J.A., DALLAL, G.E. 'Dietary fat and serum lipids: an evaluation of the experimental data', *Am J Clin Nutr*, 1993, **57**, 875–83.

3 HEGSTED, D.M. and KRITCHEVSKY, D. 'Diet and serum lipid concentrations: where are we?' *Am J Clin Nutr*, 1997, **65**, 1893–6.

4 LAW, M.R., WALD, N.J. and THOMPSON, S.G. 'By how much and how quickly does reduction in serum cholesterol concentration lower risk of ischaemic heart disease?' *BMJ*, 1994, **308**, 367–72.

5 FAO/WHO Experts Consultation on Fats and Oils 'Experts' recommendation on fats and oils in human nutrition', *Fd Nutr Agric*, 1994, **11**, 2–6.

6 HEYDEN, S. 'Polyunsaturated and monounsaturated fatty acids in the diet to prevent coronary heart disease via cholesterol reduction', *Ann Nutr Metab*, 1994, **38**, 117–22.

7 KRITCHEVSKY, D. 'History of recommendations to the public about dietary fat', *J Nutr*, 1998, **128** (supp.), 449S–52S.

8 OLIVER, M.F. 'It is more important to increase the intake of unsaturated fats than to decrease the intake of saturated fats: evidence from clinical trials relating to ischemic heart disease', *Am J Clin Nutr*, 1997, **66**, (supp.), 980S–6S.

9 DE DECKERE, E.A.M., KORVER, O., VERSCHUREN, P.M. and KATAN, M.B. 'Health aspects of fish and n-3 polyunsaturated fatty acids from plant and marine origin', *Eur J Clin Nutr*, 1998, **52**, 749–53.

10 ASCHERIO, A., RIMM, E.B., GIOVANNUCCI, E.L., SPIEGELMAN, D., STAMPFER, M.

and WILLETT, W.C. 'Dietary fat and risk of coronary heart disease in men: cohort follow-up study in the United States', *BMJ*, 1996, **313**, 84–90.

11 HU, F.B., STAMPFER, M.J., MANSON, J.E., RIMM, E.B., WOLK, A., COLDITZ, G.A., HENNEKENS, C.H. WILLETT, W.C. 'Dietary intake of alpha-linolenic acid and risk of fatal ischemic heart disease among women', *Am J Clin Nutr*, 1999, **69**, 890–7.

12 LI, D., SINCLAIR, A., WILSON, A., NAKKOTE, S., KELLY, F., ABEDIN, L., MANN, N. and TURNER, A. 'Effect of dietary alpha-linolenic acid on thrombotic risk factors in vegetarian men', *Am J Clin Nutr,* 1999, **69**, 872–82.

13 WENSING, A.G.C.L., MENSINK, R.P. and HORNSTRA, G. 'Effects of dietary n-3 polyunsaturated fatty acids from plant and marine origin on platelet aggregation in healthy elderly subjects', *Brit J Nutr*, 1999, **82**, 183–91.

14 MANTZIORIS, E., JAMES, M.J., GIBSON, R.A. and CLELAND, L.G. 'Differences exist in the relationships between dietary linoleic and α-linolenic acids and their respective long-chain metabolites', *Am J Clin Nutr*, 1995, **61**, 320–4.

15 HARRIS, W.S. 'N-3 fatty acids and serum lipoproteins: human studies', *Am J Clin Nutr*, 1997, **65**, S1645–54.

16 HULSHOF, K.F., VAN ERP-BAART, M.A., ANTTOLAINEN, M. *et al.* 'Intake of fatty acids in western Europe with emphasis on trans fatty acids: the TRANSFAIR Study', *Eur J Clin Nutr*, 1999, **53**, 143–57.

17 ENDRES, S., DE CATERINA, R., SCHMIDT, E.B. and KRISTENSEN, S.D. 'n-3 Polyunsaturated fatty acids: update', *Eur J Clin Invest*, 1995, **25**, 629–38.

18 CONNOR, W.E. and CONNOR, S.L. 'Are fish oils beneficial in the prevention and treatment of coronary artery disease?' *Am J Clin Nutr*, 1997, **66** (supp.), 1020S–31S.

19 GISSI Prevenzione Investigators 'Dietary supplementation with n-3 polyunsaturated fatty acids and vitamin E after myocardial infarction: results of the GISSI-Prevenzione trial', *Lancet*, 1999, **354**, 447–55.

20 AUSTIN, M.A., HOKANSON, J.E. and EDWARDS, K.L. 'Hypertriglyceridemia as a cardiovascular risk factor', *Am J Cardiol*, 1998, **81**, 7B–12B.

21 Food and Drug Administration (FDA) 'Substances affirmed as generally recognized as safe: menhaden oil', *Federal Register*, 1997, **62**, 30751–7.

22 SANDERS, T.A.B. and HINDS, A. 'The influence of the fish oil diet high in docosahexaenoic acid on plasma lipoprotein and vitamin E concentrations and haemostatic function in healthy male volunteers', *Br J Nutr*, 1992, **68**, 163–7.

23 CHALMERS, J., MACMAHON, S., MANCIA, G., WHITWORTH, J., BEILIN, L., HANSSON, L., NEIL, B., RODGERS, A., NI MHURCHU, C. and CLARK, T. '1999 World Health Organization – International Society of Hypertension Guidelines for the management of hypertension. Guidelines sub-committee', *Clin Exp Hypertens*, 1999, **21**, 1009–60.

24 APPEL, L.J., MILLER, E.R., SEIDLER, A.J. and WHELTON, P.K. 'Does supplementation of diet with fish oil reduce blood pressure? A meta-analysis of controlled clinical trials', *Arch Intern Med*, 1993, **153**, 429–38.

25 MORRIS, M.C., SACKS, F. and ROSNER, B. 'Does fish oil lower blood pressure?

A meta-analysis of controlled trials', *Circulation*, 1993, **88**, 523–33.

26 RAPER, N.R., CRONIN, F.J. and EXLER, J. 'Omega-3 fatty acid content of the US food supply', *J Am Coll Nutr*, 1992, **11**, 304–8.

27 BØNAA, K.H., BJERVE, K.S. and NORDØY, A. 'Habitual fish consumption, plasma phospholipid fatty acids, and serum lipids: the Tromso Study', *Am J Clin Nutr*, 1992, **55**, 1126–34.

28 HORROBIN, D.F. 'Fatty acid metabolism in health and disease: the role of delta-6-desaturase', *Am J Clin Nutr*, 1993, **57** (supp.), 732S–6S.

29 ROTHMAN, D., DELUCA, P. and ZURIER, R.B. 'Botanical lipids: effects on inflammation, immune responses, and rheumatoid arthritis', *Semin Arthritis Rheum*, 1995, **25**, 87–96.

30 KREMER, J.M. 'Effects of modulation of inflammatory and immune parameters in patients with rheumatic and inflammatory disease receiving dietary supplementation of n-3 and n-6 fatty acids', *Lipids*, 1996, **31**, S243–7.

31 KULOW, F.C. 'Global regulatory status of γ-linolenic acid'. In Y.-S. Huang and D.E. Mills (eds), pp. 304–10, *γ-Linolenic Acid: Metabolism and its Roles in Nutrition and Medicine*, Champaign, IL, AOCS Press, 1996.

32 PARIZA, M.W. 'Dietary fat and cancer risk: evidence and research needs', *Ann Rev Nutr*, 1988, **8**, 167–83.

33 LEE, K.N., KRITCHEVSKY, D. and PARIZA, M.W. 'Conjugated linoleic acid and atherosclerosis in rabbits', *Atherosclerosis*, 1994, **108**, 19–25.

34 DE DECKERE, E.A.M., VAN AMELSVOORT, J.M.M., MCNEILL, G.P. and JONES, P. 'Effects of conjugated linoleic acid (CLA) isomers on lipid levels and peroxisome proliferation in the hamster', *Brit J Nutr*, 1999, **82**, 309–17.

35 IP, C., SCIMECA, J.A. and THOMPSON, H. 'Effect of timing and duration of dietary conjugated linoleic acid on mammary cancer prevention', *Nutr Cancer*, 1995, **24**, 241–7.

36 PARK, Y., STORKSON, J.M., ALBRIGHT, K.J., LIU, K.J. and PARIZA, M.W. 'Evidence that the trans-10,cis-12 isomer of conjugated linoleic acid induces body composition changes in mice', *Lipids*, 1999, **34**, 235–41.

37 VESSBY, B. and SMEDMAN, A. 'Conjugated linoleic acid (CLA) reduces the body fat content in humans', *Chem Phys Lipids*, 1999, **101**, 152.

38 FARQUHARSON, A., WU, H.C., GRANT, I., GRAF, B., CHOUNG, J.J., EREMIN, O., HEYS, S. and WAHLE, K. 'Possible mechanisms for the putative antiatherogenic and antitumorigenic effects of conjugated polyenoic fatty acids', *Lipids*, 1999, **34**, (supp.), S343.

39 SCIMECA, J.J. 'Toxicological evaluation of dietary conjugated linoleic acid in male Fischer 344 rats', *Food Chem Toxicol*, 1998, **36**, 391–5.

40 IP, C., CHIN, S.F., SCIMECA, J.A. and PARIZA, M.W. 'Mammary cancer prevention by conjugated dienoic derivative of linoleic acid', *Cancer Res*, 1991, **51**, 6118–24.

41 ZHANG, A. and CHEN, Z.Y. 'Oxidative stability of conjugated linoleic acids relative to other polyunsaturated fatty acids', *J Am Oil Chem Soc*, 1997, **74**, 1611–13.

42 JIANG, J. and KAMAL-ELDIN, A. 'Comparing methylene blue-photosensitized oxidation of methyl-conjugated linoleate and methyl linoleate', *J Agr Food Chem*, 1998, **46**, 923–7.

43 WOLF, R.B., KLEIMAN, R. and ENGLAND, R.E. 'New sources of γ-linolenic acid', *J Am Oil Chem Soc*, 1983, **60**, 1885–60.

44 GUICHARDANT, M., TRAITLER, H., SPIELMANN, D., SPRECHER, H. and FINOT, P.A. 'Stearidonic acid, an inhibitor of the 5-lipoxygenase pathway: a comparison with timnodonic and dihomogammalinolenic acid', *Lipids*, 1993, **28**, 321–4.

45 ROCHE, H. and GIBNEY, M.J. 'The effect of consumption of fish oil-enriched spreadable fats on platelet phospholipid fatty acid composition in human volunteers', *Int J Vitam Nutr Res*, 1994, **64**, 237–42.

46 SØRENSEN, N.S., MARCHMANN, P., HOY, C.E., VAN DUYVENVOORDE, W. and PRINCEN, H.M. 'Effect of fish-oil-enriched margarine on plasma lipids, low-density-lipoprotein particle composition, size, and susceptibility to oxidation', *Am J Clin Nutr*, 1998, **68**, 235–41.

47 HAYNES, L.C., LEVINE, H. and FINLEY, J.W. 'Method and liposome composition for the stabilization of oxidizable substances', US Patent No. 5.139.803 (1992).

48 WILLIS, W.M., LENCKI, R.W. and MARANGONI, A.G. 'Lipid modification strategies in the production of nutritionally functional fats and oils', *Crit Rev Food Sci Nutr*, 1998, **38**, 639–74.

49 AKOH, C.C. 'Lipid-based fat substitutes', *Crit Rev Food Sci Nutr*, 1995, **35**, 405–30.

50 YOST, T.J., ERSKINE, J.M., GREGG, T.S., PODLECKI, D.L., BRASS, E.P. and ECKEL, R.H. 'Dietary substitution of medium chain triglycerides in subjects with non-insulin-dependent diabetes mellitus in an ambulatory setting: impact on glycemic control and insulin-mediated glucose metabolism', *J Am Coll Nutr*, 1994, **13**, 615–22.

51 PAPAMANDJARIS, A.A., MACDOUGALL, D.E. and JONES, P.J. 'Medium chain fatty acid metabolism and energy expenditure: obesity treatment implications', *Life Sci*, 1998, **62**, 1203–15.

52 BACH, A.C., INGENBLEEK, Y. and FREU, A. 'The usefulness of dietary medium-chain triglycerides in body weight control: fact or fancy?' *J Lipid Res*, 1996, **37**, 708–26.

53 DIETSCHY, J.M. 'Dietary fatty acids and the regulation of plasma low density lipoprotein cholesterol concentrations', *J Nutr*, 1998, **128**, (supp.), 444S–8S.

54 BELL, S.J., BRADLEY, D., FORSE, R.A. and BISTRIAN, B.R. 'The new dietary fats in health and disease', *J Am Diet Assoc*, 1997, **97**, 280–6.

55 KNAUF, V.C. and FACCIOTTI, D. 'Genetic engineering of foods to reduce the risk of heart disease and cancer', In J.B. Longenecker (ed.) *Nutrition and Biotechnology in Heart Disease and Cancer*, New York, Plenum Press, 1995.

56 MEDINA, A.R., GRIMA, E.M., GIMENEZ, A.G. and GONZALEZ, M.J.I. 'Downstream

processing of algal polyunsaturated fatty acids', *Biotechnol Adv*, 1998, **16**, 517–80.

57 HEINZELMANN, K. and FRANKE, K. 'Using freezing and drying techniques of emulsions for the microencapsulation of fish oil to improve oxidation stability', *Colloid Surface B*, 1999, **12**, 223–9.

58 GIBBS, B.F., KERMASHA, S., ALLI, I. and MULLIGAN, C.N. 'Encapsulation in the food industry: a review', *Int J Fd Sci Nutr*, 1999, **50**, 213–24.

59 POLLAK, O.J. 'Reduction of blood cholesterol in man', *Circulation*, 1953, **7**, 702–6.

60 KOCHHAR, S.P. 'Influence of processing on sterols of edible vegetable oils', *Prog Lipid Res*, 1983, **22**, 161–88.

61 DE DECKERE, E.A.M. and KORVER, K. 'Minor constituents of rice bran oil as functional foods', *Nutr Rev*, 1996, **54**, S120–6.

62 WESTSTRATE. J.A. and MEIJER, G.W. 'Plant sterol-enriched margarines and reduction of plasma total- and LDL-cholesterol concentrations in normocholesterolaemic and mildly hypercholesterolaemic subjects', *Eur J Clin Nutr*, 1998, **52**, 334–43.

63 KEYS, A., ANDERSON, J.T. and GRANDE, F. '"Essential" fatty acids, degree of unsaturation and effect of corn (maize) oil on the serum cholesterol level in man', *Lancet*, 1957, **i**, 66–8.

64 HOWELL, T.J., MACDOUGALL, D.E. and JONES, P.J. 'Phytosterols partially explain differences in cholesterol metabolism caused by corn or olive oil feeding', *J Lipid Res,* 1998, **39**, 892–900.

65 MATTSON, F.H., VOLPENHEIM, F.A. and ERICKSON, B.A. 'Effect of plant sterol esters on the absorption of dietary cholesterol', *J Nutr*, 1977, **107**, 1139–46.

66 MATTSON, F.H., GRUNDY, S.M. and CROUSE, J.R. 'Optimizing the effect of plant sterols on cholesterol absorption in man', *Am J Clin Nutr*, 1982, **35**, 697–700.

67 HENDRIKS, H.F., WESTSTRATE, J.A. and MEIJER, G.W. 'Spreads enriched with three different levels of vegetable oil sterols and the degree of cholesterol lowering in normocholesterolaemic and mildly hypercholesterolaemic subjects', *Eur J Clin Nutr*, 1999, **53**, 319–27.

68 SIERKSMA, A., WESTSTRATE, J.A. and MEIJER, G.W. 'Spreads enriched with plant sterols, either esterified 4,4-dimethylsterols or free 4-desmethylsterols, and plasma total- and LDL-cholesterol concentrations', *Brit J Nutr*, 1999, **82**, 273–82.

69 MIETTINEN, T., VANHANEN, H. and WESTER, I. 'A substance for lowering high cholesterol level in serum and a method for preparing the same', Patent WO 92/19640 (1992).

70 MIETTINEN, T.A., PUSKA, P., GYLLING, H., VANHANEN, H. and VARTIAINEN, E. 'Reduction of serum cholesterol with sitostanol-ester margarine in a mildly hypercholesterolemic population', *N Eng J Med*, 1995, **333**, 1308–12.

71 WAALKENS-BERENDSEN, D.H., WOLTERBEEK, A.P., WIJNANDS, M.V., RICHOLD, M. and HEPBURN, P.A. 'Safety evaluation of phytosterol esters. Part 3. Two-generation reproduction study in rats with phytosterol esters – a novel

functional food', *Food Chem Toxicol*, 1999, **37**, 683–96.

72 WHITTAKER, M.H., FRANKOS, V.H., WOLTERBEEK, A.P. and WAALKENS-BERENDSEN, D.H. 'Two-generation reproductive toxicity study of plant stanol esters in rats', *Regul Toxicol Pharmacol*, 1999, **29**, 196–204.

73 DIPLOCK, A.T., CHARLEUX, J.L., CROZIER-WILLI, G., KOK, F.J., RICE-EVANS, C., ROBERFROID, M., STAHL, W. and VIÑA-RIBET, J. 'Functional food science and defence against reactive oxidative species', *Br J Nutr*, 1998, **80**, (supp. 1), S77–S112.

74 CHAN, A.C. 'Vitamin E and atherosclerosis', *J Nutr*, 1998, **128**, 1593–6.

75 ABBEY, M. 'The importance of vitamin E in reducing cardiovascular risk', *Nutr Rev*, 1995, **53** (supp.), S28–S32.

76 STAMPFER, M.J. and RIMM, E.B. 'Epidemiologic evidence for vitamin E in prevention of cardiovascular disease', *Am J Clin Nutr*, 1995, **62** (supp.), 1365S–9S.

77 KUSHI, L.H., FROST, C., COLLINS, R., APPLEBY, P. and PETO, R. 'Dietary antioxidant vitamins and death from coronary heart disease in postmenopausal women', *N Engl J Med*, 1996, **334**, 1156–62.

78 KUSHI, L.H. 'Vitamin E and heart disease: a case study', *Am J Clin Nutr*, 1999, **69**, 1322S–9S.

79 TRIBBLE, D.L. 'AHA Science Advisory. Antioxidant consumption and risk of coronary heart disease: emphasis on vitamin C, vitamin E, and beta-carotene: A statement for healthcare professionals from the American Heart Association', *Circulation*, 1999, **99**, 591–5.

80 PALLAST, E.G., SCHOUTEN, E.G., DE WAART, F.G., FONK, H.C., DOEKES, G., VON BLOMBERG, B.M. and KOK, F.J. 'Effect of 50- and 100-mg vitamin E supplements on cellular immune function in noninstitutionalized elderly persons', *Am J Clin Nutr*, 1999, **69**, 1273–81.

81 VAN HET HOF, K.H., TIJBURG, L.B., DE BOER, H.S., WISEMAN, S.A. and WESTSTRATE, J.A. 'Antioxidant fortified margarine increases the antioxidant status', *Eur J Clin Nutr*, 1998, **52**, 292–9.

82 QURESHI, N. and QURESHI, A.A. 'Tocotrienols: novel hypocholesterolemic agents with antioxidant properties', In L. Packer and J. Fuchs (eds), pp. 247–67, *Vitamin E in Health and Disease*, New York, Marcel Dekker, 1993.

83 MENSINK, R.P., VAN HOUWELINGEN, A.C., KROMHOUT, D. and HORNSTRA, G. 'A vitamin E concentrate rich in tocotrienols had no effect on serum lipids, lipoproteins, or platelet function in men with mildly elevated serum lipid concentrations', *Am J Clin Nutr*, 1999, **69**, 213–19.

84 KOHLMEIER, L. and HASTINGS, S.B. 'Epidemiologic evidence of a role of carotenoids in cardiovascular disease prevention', *Am J Clin Nutr*, 1995, **62** (supp.), 1370S–6S.

85 OLSSON, A.G. and YUAN, X.M. 'Antioxidants in the prevention of atherosclerosis', *Curr Opin Lipidol*, 1996, **7**, 374–80.

86 REXRODE, K.M. and MANSON, J.E. 'Antioxidants and coronary heart disease: observational studies', *J Cardiovasc Risk*, 1996, **3**, 363–7.

87 VAN POPPEL, G. and GOLDBOHM, R.A. 'Epidemiologic evidence for beta-carotene and cancer prevention', *Am J Clin Nutr*, 1995, **62** (supp.), 1393S–1402S.

88 HENNEKENS, C.H., BURING, J.E., MANSON, J.E. *et al.* 'Lack of effect of long-term supplementation with beta carotene on the incidence of malignant neoplasms and cardiovascular disease', *N Engl J Med*, 1996, **334**, 1145–9.

89 OMENN, G.S., GOODMAN, G.E., THORNQUIST, M.D. *et al.* 'Effects of a combination of beta carotene and vitamin A on lung cancer and cardiovascular disease', *N Engl J Med*, 1996, **334**, 1150–5.

90 YOUNG, K.J. and LEE, P.N. 'Intervention studies on cancer', *Eur J Cancer Prev*, 1999, **8**, 91–103.

91 ALBANES, D., HEINONEN, O.P., TAYLOR, P.R. *et al.* 'Alpha-tocopherol and beta-carotene supplements and lung cancer incidence in the alpha-tocopherol, beta-carotene cancer prevention study: effects of base-line characteristics and study compliance', *J Natl Cancer Inst*, 1996, **88**, 1560–70.

92 GIOVANNUCCI, E. 'Tomatoes, tomato-based products, lycopene, and cancer: review of the epidemiologic literature', *J Natl Cancer Inst*, 1999, **91**, 317–31.

93 WISEMAN, S.A., MATHOT, J.N., DE FOUW, N.J. and TIJBURG, L.B. 'Dietary non-tocopherol antioxidants present in extra virgin olive oil increase the resistance of low density lipoproteins to oxidation in rabbits', *Atherosclerosis*, 1996, **120**, 15–23.

94 GALLI, C. and VISIOLI, F. 'Antioxidant and other activities of phenolics in olives/olive oil, typical components of the Mediterranean diet', *Lipids*, 1999, **34** (supp.), S23–6.

95 BRACCO, U., LÖLIGER, J. and SAUCY, F. 'Protection d'un produit alimentaire, cosmétique ou pharmaceutique de l'oxydation', European Patent Office, 1991, EP 0 424 679 A2.

96 GREENBERG, S. and FRISHMAN, W.H. 'Co-enzyme Q10: a new drug for cardiovascular disease', *J Clin Pharmacol*, 1990, **30**, 596–608.

97 THOMAS, S.R., NEUZIL, J. and STOCKER, R. 'Inhibition of LDL oxidation by ubiquinol-10. A protective mechanism for coenzyme Q in atherogenesis?' *Mol Aspects Med*, 1997, **18** (supp.), S85–S103.

98 SEIDELL, J.C. 'Obesity: a growing problem', *Acta Paediatr*, 1999, **88** (supp.), 46–50.

99 TROIANO, R.P. and FLEGAL, K.M. 'Overweight prevalence among youth in the United States: why so many different numbers?' *Int J Obes Relat Metab Disord*, 1999, **23** (supp. 2), S22–7.

100 LEBOVITZ, H.E. 'Type 2 diabetes: an overview', *Clin Chem*, 1999, **45**, 1339–45.

101 ABATE, N. 'Obesity as a risk factor for cardiovascular disease', *Am J Med*, 1999, **107**, 12S–13S.

102 CARROLL, K.K. 'Obesity as a risk factor for certain types of cancer', *Lipids*, 1998, **33**, 1055–9.

103 RAVUSSIN, E. and TATARANNI, P.A. 'Dietary fat and human obesity', *J Am Diet Assoc*, 1997, **97** (supp.), S42–6.

104 ADAM, O., LEMMEN, C., KLESS, T., ADAM, P., DENZLINGER, C. and HAILER, S. 'Low fat diet decreases alpha-tocopherol levels, and stimulates LDL oxidation and eicosanoid biosynthesis in man', *Eur J Med Res*, 1995, **1**, 65–71.

105 HEERTJE, I., ROIJERS, E.C. and HENDRICKX, H.A.C.M. 'Liquid crystalline phases in the structuring of food products', *Food Sci Technol*, 1998, **31**, 387–96.

106 JANDACEK, R.J. 'The development of olestra, a noncaloric substitute for dietary fat', *J Chem Educ*, 1991, **68**, 476–9.

107 ROLLS, B.J., PIRRAGLIA, P.A., JONES, M.B. and PETERS, J.C. 'Effects of olestra, a noncaloric fat substitute, on daily energy and fat intakes in lean men', *Am J Clin Nutr*, 1992, **56**, 84–92.

108 DE GRAAF, C., HULSHOF, T., WESTSTRATE, J.A. and HAUTVAST, J.G. 'Nonabsorbable fat (sucrose polyester) and the regulation of energy intake and body weight', *Am J Physiol*, 1996, **270**, R1386–93.

109 GRUNDY, S.M., ANASTASIA, J.V., KESANIEMI, Y.A. and ABRAMS, J. 'Influence of sucrose polyester on plasma lipoproteins, and cholesterol metabolism in obese patients with and without diabetes mellitus', *Am J Clin Nutr*, 1986, **44**, 620–9.

110 JANDACEK, R.J., RAMIREZ, M.M. and CROUSE, J.R. 'Effects of partial replacement of dietary fat by olestra on dietary cholesterol absorption in man', *Metabolism*, 1990, **39**, 848–52.

111 WESTSTRATE, J.A. and VAN HET HOF, K.H. 'Sucrose polyester and plasma carotenoid concentrations in healthy subjects', *Am J Clin Nutr*, 1995, **62**, 591–7.

112 ROBERFROID, M.B. and DELZENNE, N.M. 'Dietary fructans', *Ann Rev Nutr*, 1998, **18**, 117–43.

113 CASTIGLIA-DELAVAUD, C., VERDIER, E., BESLE, J.M., VERNET, J., BOIRIE, Y., BEAUFRERE, B., DE BAYNAST, R. and VERMOREL, M. 'Net energy value of non-starch polysaccharide isolates (sugarbeet fibre and commercial inulin) and their impact on nutrient digestive utilization in healthy human subjects', *Br J Nutr*, 1998, **80**, 343–52.

114 WILLIAMS, C.M. 'Effects of inulin on lipid parameters in humans', *J Nutr*, 1999, **129**, 1471S–3S.

115 REDDY, B.S. 'Nutritional factors and colon cancer', *Crit Rev Fd Sci Nutr*, 1995, **35**, 175–90.

116 CASHMAN, K.D. and FLYNN, A. 'Optimal nutrition: calcium, magnesium and phosphorus', *Proc Nutr Soc*, 1999, **58**, 477–87.

117 DAWSOM-HUGHES, B., HARRIS, S.S., KRALL, E.A. and DALLAL, G.E. 'Effect of calcium and vitamin D supplementation on bone density in men and women 65 years of age or older', *N Engl J Med*, 1997, **337**, 670–6.

11

Functional confectionery

E.F. Pickford and N.J. Jardine, Nestlé Product Technology Centre, York

11.1 Introduction

Since the age of the Pharaohs and before, functional confectionery has been benefiting humankind. It is a time-served remedy for many of the minor ills that befall us. History casts sweet confections in a highly complimentary light, and in this context sweet sugar as a health-giving spice.

The absolute origins of both confectionery itself and its functional utilisation are lost in the mists of time. But the historical record and hieroglyphic evidence certainly date it from the time of the Ancient Egyptians.[1] Imagine a sweet confection for curing intestinal worms – by 3400 BC our forebears had formulated such a remedy, as testified by a manuscript in a tomb at Thebes. What were the active ingredients? Fenugreek seeds and other herbs, all bound together with honey. Another delight for the Ancient Egyptian palate were breath-freshening lozenges – date flour and honey, tastefully holding together copious quantities of active ingredients such as herbs and incense. These have more than an echo at the present time in widely available confectionery products.

Sugar (sucrose) has long been thought of as a curative in its own right, its health-giving and enhancing properties being handed down through several early cultures. This view of sugar entered Europe from the eighth century onwards through Arabic colonisation of Spain. Sugar, derived at that time from sugar cane grown in the Mediterranean basin, was looked on as a spice with health-giving properties. It reached Europe around AD 1100, but at that time it was affordable only by the very rich. Pharmacopoeias from around this date based on Islamic knowledge mention many other properties of sucrose which make it useful in confectionery-like medicinal preparations.[2] It was known even at that time that sucrose can act as a preservative, a solvent, to give body, a stabiliser, mask unpleasant flavours, as a binder for tablets, excipient, coating agent, diluent, sweetener, oil-sugar base and as a cough lozenge base.

Over the succeeding centuries, this knowledge was applied and expanded in Europe by confectioners and apothecaries. The latter play an important part in this story because they influenced the development of a number of modern confectioneries, sugar-coated pills and lozenges, for example. However, the actual origins of both these are ancient: lozenges can be traced to ancient Egypt and pills to Roman times.

From a historical perspective, the current interest in functional foods can be viewed as rekindling an interest that humans have had in the specific properties of what they eat. Many ingredients of the diet have traditionally been endowed with health-promoting properties, in particular spices and herbs. Modern nutrition has a radically different perspective, with its emphasis on macro- and micronutrients. This has obscured the fact that foods may contain other constituents of value to our health and well-being. However, there has been an increasing interest in the physiological properties of phytochemicals and this is now a thriving area of research.[3]

In previous ages, new foods were of interest for their health-giving potential. An example of this is the many new foods brought from the New World in the sixteenth century, cocoa being one of those foods. Various medical properties were soon ascribed to cocoa, admittedly not well justified according to our present-day standards. It even had a reputation as an aphrodisiac which lingers to this day. Cocoa has, however, never entirely lost its health-giving image. At the present time it is of interest for its content of phytochemicals, being rich in polyphenolic antioxidants which has prompted the launch in Japan of chocolate rich in polyphenols.

11.1.1 The aims and scope of this chapter

This chapter will examine the current status of functional confectionery and will outline some of the steps in its development. It will give an overview of confectionery techniques and how they can be applied to functional confectionery, and also some of the problems that have to be faced in manufacture. Marketing is also a crucial issue which will be addressed in general terms.

It is important at the outset to define what is meant by confectionery. For the purposes of this chapter we will include sugar confectionery, chocolate confectionery, countlines (confectionery bars whether chocolate covered or not) and chewing gum. We will exclude flour confections like biscuits and cakes which are in a different market sector. In this text, candy will be used as a term for sugar confectionery excluding chewing gum. The analogous British term is 'sweets' but this term can be misunderstood.

'Functional' as applied to confectionery will be defined fairly broadly to mean confectionery with an added health benefit. Clearly there are already well-known functional confectioneries on the market in the form of medicated candy. These products contain specific curative ingredients. There are also products occupying small niches in the market containing active ingredients aimed at specific consumers, for example sportspeople. However, there have also been considerable developments recently in other, more mass market areas such as low calorie, low fat and sugar free. These products are all designed to provide benefits to distinguish them from standard products, even if specific health claims are not made. A reasonably broad definition of functional confectionery will permit an interesting overview of how the market is developing in the early years of this millennium.

11.2 Types of functional confectionery

Functional confectionery can be defined as 'a confectionery item that has undergone the addition, removal or replacement of standard confectionery ingredients with an ingredient that fulfils a specific physiological function or offers a potential health benefit'.

The market for functional confectionery is still in its infancy with only a few well-developed sectors. The earliest types of modern functional candies were throat soothers and breath fresheners. These were followed onto the market by candies designed to cure a variety of ills such as travel sickness and hangovers or improve oral health, or confectioneries to assist weight control as well as fortified products. At the present time there are many products being launched whose aims vary from meal replacement (e.g. breakfast bars), performance enhancement whether mental or physical through to a variety of health protective actions (see Table 11.1).

11.3 The current market in functional confectionery

Apart from a few of the older established products, these products are at the stage of fighting for establishment on the market. There are consequently few quantified data available to market analysts, and information tends to be fragmentary. The following survey, largely using data compiled by the Leatherhead Food Research Association,[4] can only give a very partial snapshot of developments in some of the most visible markets.

11.3.1 Country-by-country survey of functional confectionery

Table 11.2 displays the key varieties of functional confectionery and their market value in different countries.

Table 11.1   Categories of functional ingredients and their proposed physiological properties

Ingredient	Proposed physiological properties
Vitamins and minerals	Various: required by the body in small amounts to perform essential functions and are thought to contribute to prevention of certain conditions, e.g. calcium fortification for osteoporosis, zinc and vitamin C to relieve cold symptoms and the addition of antioxidants for defence against free radicals
Fibre (soluble and insoluble)	Soluble: delay gastric emptying, decrease serum cholesterol levels and control the rate at which glucose is released into the blood. Insoluble: increase faecal transit time and weight to relieve constipation and delay glucose absorption.
Plant extracts, e.g. Ginseng Guarana *Gingko biloba*	Various: Relieve fatigue and stress Increase alertness Increase blood flow to the brain and proposed to aid mental functioning
Prebiotics	Non-digestible oligosaccharides that 'feed' our gut flora and improve our immune system and relieve constipation
Probiotics Phytochemicals	Strengthen the immune system Prevention of cancer, heart disease, maintenance of good vision and healthy skin

Table 11.2   Main functional confectionery varieties by country and value, 1998[4]

Country	Chewing gum (sugar free) $(US)m	Sugar-free sweets $(US)m	Other types* $(US)
Australia	57	8	Medicated 64m
France	135	72	Fortified sweets 3.5m
Germany	392	298	Cough sweets 104m Fortified sweets 56m Herbal 38m
Italy	158	150	
Japan	306	320	
Scandinavia	284	165	
Spain	138	26	
United Kingdom	227	67	Low calorie chocolate 43m Fortified sweets 10m
United States	856	160	

Source: Pettit 1999.
* May overlap with chewing gum or sugar-free gum.

11.3.2 United States

This is the biggest single market for confectionery, even if annual per capita consumption at 12.2 Kg/head is less than in some countries.[5] It is also one of the most diverse markets.

The market for sugar-free candy is small in comparison to sugar-free chewing gum, but it appears to be growing quite fast. It is quite competitive with many different brands, and promotional activity is likely to assist future growth in this sector.

The low calorie/low fat chocolate confectionery market has seen major developments in recent years, with offerings from major manufacturers, for example, M&M Mars' Milky Way Lite and Hershey's Sweet Escapes. Other manufacturers have also introduced new products into this sector.

The confectionery market contains a wide variety of niche products. Confectionery aimed at sports is an example: in recent years PowerBar, 'athletic energy food', has become particularly widespread. Fruit chews containing creatine are aimed at the same market: there is good evidence that creatine enhances muscular performance. Exotic ingredients are also becoming more widely used, for example, Balance+ bars which contain ginseng and *Gingko biloba*.

Another recent development is the introduction of fortified products in a confectionery format aimed at children, for example gummi bears with vitamins, zinc-enriched lollipops to relieve cold symptoms, and candies containing phytochemicals.

The market for chewing gum in the USA is now very mature. Per capita consumption is around 80% higher than in European countries like UK and Germany. Sugar-free gum accounts for around 38% of the total gum market. This level of penetration is much less than in most European countries. Nevertheless, sugar-free gum accounts for 73% of the total sugar-free confectionery market.

A variety of gums of a more overtly functional nature have been launched in the USA, including dentally protective and fortified gums. A gum containing zinc, menthol and other ingredients has been marketed with the promise that it reduces the symptoms of the common cold. Also to be found is a gum that claims to aid learning, memory and concentration. It contains phosphatidyl serine, and another containing caffeine to increase alertness.

The future development of the functional market in the USA will depend on the regulatory environment. Since 1990, health claims on products have been allowed, but so far only nine types of claim have been authorised by the FDA,[6] and these model claims have the disincentive of being too laborious for good communication to consumers. It is possible that functional foods could be marketed under 1994 legislation covering dietary supplements, having a potential advantage that claims could focus on 'wellness' rather than having to focus on links to disease as in the health claims legislation. However, there is a good deal of uncertainty as to how the legislation will be applied in practice.[7] Restrictions and uncertainty in the regulatory environment will impede the development of functional foods including confectionery.

11.3.3 Germany

Confectionery consumption in Germany is high at 15 kg per capita. It is a mature market with low volume growth.

Sugar-free confectionery has achieved 25% penetration of the sugar confectionery market. Of this, 54% is cough sweets, 41% is mints and 5% is fruit/refreshing sweets. On the other hand, low calorie chocolate products represent only a very small market. Sugar-free chocolate is aimed at the diabetic market (about 500 tonnes/annum), but are not generally reduced in fat or calories.

The market for fortified confectionery is the largest in Europe, and accounts for over 7% of sugar confectionery sales. Most of these products are sugar free. Addition of antioxidant vitamins is popular. Various 'energy' brands have been launched or relaunched recently. None of these products make health claims but many German consumers are well informed about the potential benefits of healthy ingredients.

Herbal candies are also a growing market, currently claiming 5% of the sugar confectionery market.

Sugar-free chewing gum accounts for 71% of market value of chewing gum. Almost half sugar-free gum is sold on a dental-care platform. Some gums now also have added nutrients.

The regulatory framework for functional confectionery in Germany is governed by EU legislation. Under this legislation, medicinal claims or even implied claims that a product can prevent, treat or cure a medical condition are prohibited unless the product holds a medical licence. Nutritional claims can be made but require statutory nutritional labelling. Health claims on the other hand are highly restricted under this legislation. It is also worth pointing out in passing that because EU legislation has to be absorbed into national legislation with often very different traditions, this can lead to differences in detail of how the directives are enacted.

11.3.4 Japan

Japan is a country with a low confectionery consumption – 3.5 kg/capita in 1997. It is, however, a dynamically changing market in comparison to most of the others mentioned in this brief survey, with some very active product development. Functional foods have been part of the Japanese food scene for nearly two decades, so it should not be surprising that similar thinking should influence confectionery. The Japanese have a more positive attitude to connections between food and health than do many Western cultures. The FOSHU (food for specific health use) framework was established by the government to control health claims on food. Its success is an indication of the Japanese consumers' interest in food products that have naturally occurring ingredients which may promote health.

Sugar-free candies have been launched by most major manufacturers in Japan, and these account for around 15% of the sugar confectionery market. Many recent launches have used xylitol as the sweetener.

Chewing gum has low penetration in Japanese markets, but within this limited market there has been high growth in sugar-free gum, which has been fuelled by the approval of xylitol in Japan.

A number of interesting products have been launched in the chocolate sector. Sugar-free chocolate – Zero Sugarless – was developed, using a technology that also removed the lactose from milk. It is 20% lower in calories than conventional milk chocolate. Lactitol is the sugar substitute. Tooth Friendly chocolate has also been launched, using trehalose as the sugar replacer. Chocolate claimed to be rich in polyphenols is also available. There is much current interest in polyphenols as compounds found widely in plants which may be important in the health-protective qualities of plant foods. Much research has been done in Japan on the biological properties of such compounds found in tea. Similar compounds are found in cocoa, and quite a lot is already known about the major polyphenol (epicatechin) in cocoa as it is widespread in the plant kingdom.[8] Different again is Chocolite, which is calorie reduced containing royal jelly, collagen and vitamins B and C.

The above gives an indication of the breadth of the functional chocolate market in Japan. The sugar confectionery sector is, if anything, even more innovative. There is a large variety of fortified products on the market, and various products containing novel ingredients. Recent examples include sugar-coated wine gums with collagen and vitamin C, and candies promoted for their antioxidant properties which contain green tea extracts. However, many products are launched in the Japanese confectionery market but disappear equally quickly if success is not forthcoming.

11.3.5 Scandinavia

Total confectionery consumption in Sweden, Denmark, Norway and Finland averages 12 kg per head.

Sugar-free sweets are popular in this region, achieving 45% of the market in Sweden, for example. Fortified confectionery is so far quite rare, and there are few functional chocolate brands, one of the few being the Lo bar low calorie countline.

In Scandinavia, sugar-free chewing gum has achieved great success, claiming 84–98% of total chewing gum sales, depending on the country. This is due to the development of xylitol by the Finnish manufacturer Xyrofin. The dental profession endorsed the non-cariogenic status of this sweetener, and the public clearly followed this lead. A number of products are directly targeted at the dental aspect. A number of other functional chewing gum products exist to combat allergies, suppress appetite or protect against colds and influenza.

11.3.6 United Kingdom

The UK is one of the big markets for confectionery with per capita consumption at an annual 15 kg. In volume terms, chocolate confectionery claims the major share at 65%.

As elsewhere, there have been major developments in the sugar-free market. Sales of sugar-free chewing gum doubled between 1993 and 1998, and now account for 73% of the market. Some is sold on an overtly dental health basis. Others are marketed as clearing nasal congestion. Despite rapid growth in sugar-free candy, it still accounts for only 2.7% of the value of the sugar confectionery market. Much of the activity was in the mint market, where sugar-free mints tripled in value between 1993 and 1998 with a variety of new introductions stimulated by the introduction of a sugar-free version of Nestlé's Polo mints.

Vitamin- and mineral-enriched sugar confectionery products are beginning to appear in the UK market. This is especially the case in the medicated sector. There are many medicated confectionery products, and the line between such confectionery and over-the-counter medication is blurred. Many medicated brands are also sugar free.

The chocolate market has seen some interesting developments in recent years. Traditionally the main target for modified chocolate has been diabetic chocolate where the sucrose has been substituted by alternative sweeteners, commonly sorbitol or fructose. This has now fallen out of favour following changes in views of how diabetes should be treated dietetically. On the other hand, there have been a number of introductions of low calorie/fat reduced products, mostly countlines. These products aim to provide indulgence while having less calories and fat than standard products. This market is at an early stage of development, however, as they accounted for less than 2% by value of the chocolate sector in 1998, but the growth has been considerable as it was only 0.2% in 1992.

Sports confectionery is another small niche in the UK market, with a variety of products sold in specialist outlets. Most sports products aim to give a boost to energy or performance.

The regulatory environment in the UK is, as outlined for Germany, governed by EU directives. It is worth noting, however, that such directives are often enacted so as to bring local food legislation into line with the EU framework. It is not surprising therefore if interpretations of directives differ in points of detail from country to country. This can also permit local initiatives to take place, and a pertinent example is the UK's Joint Health Claims Initiative.[9] This has taken a unique approach in bringing together law enforcement officers, the food industry and consumer groups who have agreed a code of practice on health claims on food. Following this success, an administration body will be set up to oversee implementation of the code, including the adjudication of which health claims are allowable. If successful, the initiative should clarify development and marketing issues for manufacturers of functional foods, while protecting the consumer from unwarranted claims. Success may also stimulate a wider adoption of such an approach, as the issues being faced are relevant to many other countries.

11.3.7 Italy

Less confectionery is consumed in southern Europe, and this is exemplified by Italy where per capita consumption is less than 5 kg. There is some growth in the market, in chocolate confectionery. This, however, masks developments in the sugar confectionery sector with an increasing share going to sugar-free sweets, growing from 20% in 1993 to 25% in 1998, the sector as a whole growing by 36% in that time, although growth now seems to have plateaued. Fortified confectionery accounts for about 1% of the sugar confectionery market, most of this being sugar free.

As elsewhere in Europe, the chewing gum market is showing a strong trend towards sugar free, although penetration is behind some other markets at 53% in 1998 (40% in 1993).

There appears to be no market for functional chocolate confectionery.

11.3.8 France

The total confectionery market in France is again relatively small at 6 kg per capita. Chewing gum holds 12% of market by value, with sugar-free gum achieving 57% penetration.

Sugar-free candy accounts for 14% by value of the sugar confectionery market, mostly in the pocket confectionery sector. Indeed, sugar-free lines lead in this sector (Ricola with herbal sweets, with Kiss Cool second).

Low calorie and sugar-free chocolate has been on the French market for some years but has failed to make much growth – sales now appear to be in decline. Low calorie chocolate confectionery is confined to block chocolates, unlike in other countries where countlines are the favoured vehicle for such concepts.

Vitaminised confectionery is mostly found in the bagged sugar confectionery sector but it remains small at about 1% of sales. Herbal sweets appear to be more established and more popular.

Choline has been used in a number of confectionery products, notably Carré Mémoire and Barres Mémoire, on the premise that it aids concentration and memory. Prebiotics and probiotics have also found their way into French confectionery in the form of fructo-oligosaccharides (Barre Chocolat Orange) and *Lactobacillus acidophilus* in NutraFruit fruit gums.

11.3.9 Spain

The Spanish confectionery market is small by European standards with a consumption of 4.5 kg per capita. It also differs in that, in volume terms at least, the sugar confectionery market is much greater than for chocolate.

The sugar-free market has been stimulated by the EU directive of 1996 which regulates and authorises the use of intense sweeteners and sugar substitutes. New products have been launched, and old ones relaunched with new formulations to take advantage of better ingredients. Many sugar-free products have functional aspirations, being either in the medicated or in the breath-freshener sectors.

Important brands in the former target cough sweets, while there are vitamin/mineral fortified products as well as herb confectionery.

The chewing gum market is also quite small, but the sugar-free segment is growing fast, accounting for 74% of the market in 1997. A number of chewing gums have now been launched onto the market which are branded on a dental care basis as well as others with ginseng or added vitamin C.

11.3.10 Australia

The total confectionery market in Australia is 10 kg per capita. Chewing gum holds 7% of the market, with sugar-free gum achieving 67% penetration of the gum market. Medicated confectionery holds 5% of the market while the fortified confectionery market is small in comparison but growing. Sugar-free confectionery is a small sector at about 2%, but is showing high growth at 82% per annum.

11.4 The development and manufacture of functional confectionery products

The survey in the previous section gives a good indication of well-established areas of functional confectionery, e.g. throat soothers, and also where some of the leading edge developments are taking place. We have also indicated the generally restrictive regulatory environment in many traditional countries. One exception is Japan with its FOSHU framework.

The regulatory hurdle is but one that has to be faced in the development of a functional confectionery product. It is, however, an important one to be considered early in the development phase as it can determine whether the product concept is potentially viable. The consumer attitude to a product concept also needs to be researched at an early stage. Is the concept understood, and does it fit well with delivery via a confectionery product? Another question is how the functional ingredient can be incorporated into confectionery, and also how much needs to be incorporated if a claim is to be made regarding efficacy. Even at this early stage some thought needs to be given to retail aspects – major retailers or niche outlets – and to how the product will be priced. Keeping qualities also need to be defined. Confectionery is generally designed for a long shelf life (compared to many foods), but this may not be the case when functional ingredients are incorporated. Other aspects which must not be forgotten at the concept-generation stage of product development are regulatory and safety issues. The point is that a concept needs to be well thought through to define the scope of practical development.

We will return to these questions in more detail later. In this section we examine the practical aspects of functional confectionery development, starting with a survey of the ingredients commonly used in confectionery.

11.4.1 Overview of ingredients in sugar, chocolate and baked confectionery

Sugars and sugar syrups

Sugars are carbohydrates and are used in confectionery to fulfil a variety of roles including provision of sweetness, flavour, colour, bulk, texture and preservation.

The term 'sugar' is often used to describe the key confectionery ingredient, sucrose. Different forms of sucrose can be produced which have different confectionery applications such as granulated sugar, icing sugar, caster sugar and brown sugar.

Syrups, such as glucose syrup (corn syrup) are produced through the hydrolysis of starch. They offer specific functions such as preventing or controlling crystallisation (graining) or act as humectants, as in the case of invert syrup. Invert syrup is the product of the breakdown of sucrose into dextrose and fructose. Invert sugar syrups contain nearly equal proportion of these two sugars. Spray-dried glucose syrup, dextrose monohydrate, dextrose anhydrous and maltodextrin are products derived from glucose syrup which have a wide range of uses. The ultimate choice depends upon the desired function, for example, to absorb fats and oils. Honey, another syrup, is essentially used for flavour purposes in confectionery, as are treacle, molasses and golden syrup.[10]

Fats and oils

A variety of edible fats and oils are used in confectionery products. For example, milk fat, cocoa butter, and oils of palm kernel, groundnut, coconut and soya. Many of these can undergo hydrogenation to produce fats of varying hardness. Vegetable fats are used in great quantities for manufacture of caramels, fudges, pralines, truffles, pastes, biscuits, biscuit fillings and as cocoa butter equivalents in chocolate.

Milk and milk products

Milk fat, butter and butter fat are used commonly in products such as caramels, pralines, toffee and fudge to provide colour, flavour and texture. Condensed milk and whey are an alternative means of introducing milk solids into confectionery. Dried milk powders will often be used as substitutes for sweetened condensed milks. Whole milk can be incorporated into milk chocolate via the crumb method of chocolate manufacture.

Gelling agents, whipping agents, gums and glazes

Starch from wheat, tapioca, potato and maize is used in sugar confectionery as a basic gelling ingredient along with gelatin, pectins and agar agar. Whipping agents help to hold air in a product. This is an essential feature of marshmallows, some chocolate centres and frappés. The common whipping agents are egg albumen, gelatine, casein and soya protein. Gums, often used as extenders for pectin and agar agar, include locust bean gum (carob gum) and guar gum. They are useful in starch gels to prevent cracking and shrinking. Common glazes, particularly for panned sweets or dragées, are shellac, beeswax and carnuba wax.

Miscellaneous ingredients

Nuts, such as almonds, brazil, cashew, hazelnuts, coconut, peanut or walnuts, along with dried fruits, such as cherries, dates, sultanas, currants and raisins, all add colour, flavour and textural interest to confectionery. For many years, fruit juices, purées and pulps have been used to confer flavour, colour and 'natural fruit' into confectionery. They can also be used for centre fillings, high boiled sweets and fondant cremes or to enhance sales appeal in products. Flavourings for confectionery encompass a multitude of ingredients. These include essential oils and essences, such as vanillin, and wide ranges of natural, nature identical and synthetic flavours. Colours are available in both a synthetic and purely natural form. Common acids for confectionery products are citric, tartaric, malic, acetic, benzoic and sorbic. Some act as preservatives as well as having acidulant properties, while others are used solely to lift or complement any fruit flavours that are present.[10]

11.4.2 Chocolate recipes

Dark chocolate commonly consists of sugar, cocoa solids, cocoa butter, anti-blooming agents, lecithin (or other emulsifiers) and flavours. Milk chocolate is composed of sugar, milk solids, milk fat, cocoa solids, cocoa butter, lecithin (emulsifiers) and flavours. 'White' chocolate uses all of the conventional ingredients of chocolate except for non-fat cocoa solids. Compound coatings are used as economical replacements for chocolate, with cocoa butter being completely or partially substituted by less expensive hard fats of other origin.

Regional variation in ingredients, such as the milk flavour, cocoa bean roasting, cocoa blending and manufacturers' variation in recipes and processes, give rise to many different flavours and textures of the finished chocolate. Recipes can also be manipulated to produce types of chocolate-like products with individual tastes, for example the Nestlé product 'Caramac'.[11]

Recently low calorie and sugar-free 'chocolates' have been produced by replacing the sugar with combinations of appropriate sugar alcohols and bulking agents. Successful fat replacement in other types of food products has involved increasing the water content of the product. However, the scope for doing this in confectionery is limited as in these products the moisture content must be strictly controlled and small changes, especially in chocolate, can affect the organoleptic properties and shelf life significantly. Fat substitution can be equally problematic. For example, cocoa butter has very specific properties that are difficult to replace. Such fat replacers for chocolate often present processing difficulties or they may not mimic the sensory characteristics of chocolate. The development of partially digested fats and low calorie fats has been a fast-developing field. Some might prove to have a useful role in chocolate products, but as yet they are not approved for use in confectionery.

The Japanese company Meiji, launched 'Chocolate Kouka', a 'high in polyphenol' chocolate, positioned as a chocolate with additional health benefits attributed to the natural antioxidant activity of cocoa phytochemicals. Not only can chocolate act as a carrier for functional ingredients but it might itself already possess an inherent health benefit.[8]

11.4.3 Sugar confectionery techniques and their application in functional confectionery development

Sugar confectionery is an ideal vehicle for certain functional ingredients. It is portable, convenient and many functional concepts are technically feasible.

High boilings

Boiled sweets consist of mixtures of sucrose and glucose syrup which are cooked to such a high temperature that the mass has the following characteristics:

- Non-crystalline, clear and glassy in appearance.
- Moisture content is 1–3% with an equilibrium relative humidity (ERH) below 30%.
- During cooking, some of the sucrose is 'inverted', that is, hydrolysed to its constituent glucose and fructose.[12]

Flavour, acid and colour are added to satisfy the consumer taste. If a functional high boil is to be produced, any added ingredients must not disturb these three key characteristics of a high boil. Also, the processing methods may determine the type of functional high boil that can be produced. Some functional ingredients may not withstand high boiling temperatures, or conversely their addition to the mass might result in a higher boiling point. They may also be less soluble or produce a mass that takes a longer time to cool. High boils remain in the mouth for a considerable length of time so functional ingredients must not cause roughness or drying of the mouth.

Low boilings

Low boiled confectionery can be chewed. If you produce a chew from a glucose/sucrose blend there must be a balance between the crystalline phase of the chew, the non-crystalline phase and any gelatine or fat that is added. This results in a sweet with an appropriate 'chew' that is not too sticky. 'Chewability', in part, depends upon the extent of crystallisation that occurs and this, in turn, is affected by the final moisture content of the sweet. An ideal moisture content is between 6% and 10% of the final sweet. Too little moisture and the chew will become very hard, while too much moisture will give a sticky sweet. Again, added functional ingredients must comply with these characteristics. For example, when producing a sugar-free chew, the sugar substitutes do not crystallise like sucrose so seeding crystals must be added.

Caramels, toffees and fudge

The basic ingredients of caramels, toffees and fudge are sugar, glucose syrup, milk protein, fat, salt and water. This mix is concentrated to a high total solids content. Caramels usually have more moisture than toffees. Fudge is simply a toffee that has had 'grain' (i.e. sugar crystallisation) introduced, usually by adding fondant, or by mechanically inducing grain into the cooked batch. All three can act as a vehicle for functional ingredients. Fudge is an ideal vehicle for functional ingredients that have a rough texture. Recipes can easily be manipulated to include, for example, prebiotics, vitamins and minerals. Difficulties can be encountered when the product is to be sugar free as this requires the use of a low lactose/lactose-free milk or whey powder. These ingredients can be expensive and often the total lactose content is not low enough to constitute a sugar-free claim. Colour may also need to be added since such products do not provide the same extent of Maillard browning.

Gums and jellies

Gums and jellies are hydrocolloid candies which means they gel and thicken but also stabilise. Various hydrocolloids can produce candies with very different eating characteristics. For example, agar agar gives a short breaking jelly with good clarity, whereas gum acacia will produce a long-lasting, chewy sweet.[12] Functional ingredients for inclusion within hydrocolloids should be carefully selected so that they do not disrupt the colloidal characteristics that produce the correct texture, clarity and gelling properties. The following points need to be considered.

- *Total solids content* Recipes require modification so that the addition of functional ingredients results in a solids content that is appropriate for the hydrocolloid in question. Otherwise mould growth, convex sweet backs, crystallisation or drying out/stickiness may occur.
- *Thermal stability of functional ingredients* Added ingredients, in some cases, may be required to withstand very high temperatures. For example, a starch-based confection must be typically at 90°C to ensure depositing without gelation.
- *Good solubility of functional ingredients* Undissolved functional ingredients may produce a cloudy or grainy sweet.
- *pH* The pH of some hydrocolloid systems are critical in determining the final set. Acid is the last addition as it has a major effect on gel strength. The acid stability of functional ingredients should be determined. Functional ingredients themselves might also affect pH and cause degradation of a product. For example, agar will degrade below pH 5.[13] Pectins gel very quickly which should be borne in mind if functional ingredients are added at the end of production.

Marshmallow and nougat

The two most important ingredients for marshmallow are air and moisture. Marshmallow contains one of the highest moisture contents of any confection. Gelatine and egg albumen are the most common whipping/gelation agents used. It is possible to produce a gelatin-free marshmallow but it has a slightly different texture to a gelatin marshmallow. Recipe modification to incorporate functional ingredients should account for the following:

- a minimum total solids content of 75%
- a final moisture content of around 20%
- solubility and heat stability of added functional ingredients should be noted.

Nougat appears in various different forms around the world. It is basically a high-boiled syrup, containing fat, which is added to a frappé of either egg albumen, gelatine or Hyfoama. Nougat can be used as a vehicle for a variety of functional ingredients. For example, it is possible to create reduced sugar nougat through recipe manipulation and sucrose-alternative bulking agents. If functional ingredients are rough in texture, the 'grain' of the nougat can be used to mask this.

Fondants, cremes and crystallised confectionery
Fondants and cremes are sugar confectionery products that contain mixed sugars in a solid and crystalline phase. When producing a functional fondant or creme:

- The particle size of functional ingredients in a fondant creme should be less than 25 μm. They can be slightly larger for a standard fondant, but no bigger than 35 μm.
- Final ERH of a fondant should be 75–80% and for cremes 80–85%.

Tablets, lozenges and extruded pastes
Tablets, such as Polo, combine base material with binding, lubricant and flavourings. These are held under pressure and form a hard, cohesive sweet with low moisture. Incorporating functional ingredients into a pressed tablet is relatively straightforward. The ingredients must be in a free-flowing powder form and capable of being compressed together. If added ingredients have a tendency to pick up moisture, careful packaging will be required.

Lozenges are sugar doughs that are flavoured, rolled, cut to shape and then dried to remove most of the added water. Functional ingredients in the form of fine powders are most suited to this confection.

Panned confections
The technique of panning can be traced back via apothecaries to ancient times. It presumably originated in the need to cover the bitter taste of ingredients. Panning remains a useful strategy to this day and is still a common method for drug delivery.[13]

Panned confections, or dragées, consist of small centres that are coated in a 'shell'. Usually the shell is made from sugar or chocolate, but it is possible to pan centres with various different coatings. 'Smarties' are an example of a panned confection. Panning involves placing the centres into a large revolving drum; as the centres tumble around in the drum a 'charge' of liquid coating is added. Once the centres are covered, and the coating has solidified, another 'charge' can be added and the layers of the coating slowly build up. Once the layers are complete, the sweets can be polished. It is possible to pan a 'functional coating' to the outside of a centre. Alternatively, functional ingredients can be concentrated into the panned centre. During panning it is possible that functional ingredients might adhere to the inside of the pan and should be accounted for when calculating the 'dosage'. Re-work for functional panned confections is easier to manage if functional ingredients are concentrated into the centre rather than the shell.

Chewing gum

Chewing gum is sold as panned pieces or in a stick form. It is made from a mix of natural and synthetic gums, a crystalline sweetener, a liquid sweetener, flavouring materials and texture modifiers. In developed markets, sugar-free chewing gum, however, is now often the norm rather than the exception and is developing a strong connection among consumers as 'good for teeth'. This opens the door for chewing gum to become an acceptable vehicle for functional ingredients, and such ingredients are being increasingly seen in certain markets.

11.4.4 Cereal components of confectionery

Cereal components within confectionery can provide a textural/taste contrast within a product. Cereals (e.g. corn flakes, rice krispies) must be used in low-moisture confections otherwise they lose crispness and deteriorate in flavour. Biscuit components of confectionery are also prone to becoming soft. Higher fat biscuits or biscuit protected by a fatty layer will retard or prevent moisture transfer. Wafers are a specialised type of biscuit formed from a batter and baked between pairs of heated metal plates. The batter is usually very simple, containing a low proportion of sugar and fat.[14] Cereals in confectionery are becoming increasingly important as a result of their healthy image and the proposed health effects attributed to particular cereal types such as oats. Recently, cereals in confectionery are being associated with the use of seeds such as sunflower and linseeds. Many of these seeds have proposed health benefits that can be used to add value to a functional product.

11.4.5 Formulating a functional confectionery recipe

Formulating a functional confectionery product begins at the same point as standard confectionery development: the generation of a recipe for a good-tasting product. Where functional confectionery is concerned, the steps might progress as follows:

1. *Choose a suitable confectionery 'vehicle'*
    This will be defined to some extent by the product concept. Some concepts will fit better with sugar confectionery, others with bars or may be dictated by practical considerations. The cost of added functional ingredients can be quite expensive, so keeping the manufacturing method as simple as possible is desirable.
2. *Where to incorporate the functional ingredients in the product*
    This will depend upon the amount of functional ingredients needed, the

nature of the ingredients, such as powder or liquid, fine particles or large particles; whether or not they will be affected by certain processing conditions, for example, high temperatures or shearing action. How they behave in a moist or fat-based medium must also be considered and whether the functional ingredients will interact with other ingredients in the recipe.

3. *Manipulation of ingredients*
   Any ingredients that are excluded or reduced to make room for functional ingredients should not result in deterioration of product taste, shelf life or quality.

4. *Masking agents*
   The recipe may require the addition of masking agents to disguise any undesirable tastes from the functional ingredients.

5. *How the functional ingredients affect critical parameters of the end product*
   Moisture content, total solids, ERH, pH, gel strength, viscosity, texture or crystallisation will all need to be considered here.

Ingredients often have a dual function within a recipe, and this must be taken into account. Consider prebiotics, for example. These are oligosaccharides of particular current interest for their potentially beneficial effects on gut health. However, they also function as bulking sucrose substitutes. Generally, the larger the molecular weight of the oligosaccharide, the weaker its intensity of sweetness. The sweetness of highly purified oligosaccharides is less than half that of sucrose, therefore the use of an intense sweetener may need to be considered.

11.4.6 Bench development

Bench development begins with certain unknowns. Recipe manipulation is often straightforward as long as the confectionery format is capable of allowing a proportion of its ingredients to be substituted by functional ingredients. Surprises usually occur as a result of the interaction of functional ingredients with the standard confectionery ingredients. Sometimes this can be predicted.

A common uncertainty is how the product will taste once the functional ingredients have been added. Some can be masked quite successfully with flavours alone, others may have 'backtastes' that require disguising with specific masking agents. Some functional ingredients will also alter the texture of a product, for example, functional fibres. It is often wise to select a textured product, such as a wafer bar or biscuit, if such substances are to be incorporated. Alternatively, fibre content can be increased using other methods such as the incorporation of fruit fibres into a paste or baked confection.

11.4.7 Stability of functional ingredients

Functional ingredients may affect or be affected by certain aspects of processing, for example, high temperatures or shearing action. They may also react differently in a moist or fat-based medium. As discussed previously, other ingredients present in the recipe might affect the action or stability of the functional ingredients.

Some functional ingredients could affect critical parameters of the finished product, such as moisture content, total solids, ERH, pH, gel strength, viscosity, texture or crystallisation. Conversely, one or more of these factors might affect the action or stability of the functional ingredients themselves.

Concerning the area of vitamin and mineral addition to products, industry understanding is more advanced. In the light of their long experience, suppliers are very good at advising necessary 'overages' for products to ensure that the required amount is within the product at the end of processing and throughout shelf life.

11.4.8 Stability and shelf life: laboratory techniques to analyse quantities of new functional ingredients within a product

To produce a credible and consistently high quality product, analytical methods must be used to determine the levels of functional ingredients present within a product at the point of manufacturing and throughout the shelf life. For many active ingredients, assays exist that are relatively straightforward to apply to a confectionery product. However, some are less developed, such as those for many of the plant extracts. They may require considerable time, effort and money to develop.

Methods are generally available for the majority of vitamins, some determined analytically by HPLC, for example, vitamins A and E, or more classical techniques such as for vitamin C. Others require microbiological assay (vitamin B_6 and B_{12}). Generally, analysis in chocolate is more difficult than sugar confectionery (this is true for virtually all analytes, not just vitamins). Due to the number of other compounds present in chocolate, the analyte of interest must be separated. The extraction and clean-up from chocolate is generally challenging. Vitamin testing in general is quite difficult and as vitamins can degrade easily, care has to be taken in analysis. Reliable results can be hard to find.

Most minerals can be analysed relatively easily at trace levels in both chocolate and sugar confectionery using atomic absorption/emission spectroscopy. Classical techniques are also employed for phosphorus. There are a number of different methods available for total dietary fibre analysis, none of which are particularly easy but most of which are used routinely around the world. The most favoured is the AOAC method.

Prebiotics (oligosaccharides and inulin) can be determined using ion chromatography/HPLC. Analysis/interpretation is difficult and costly. Probiotic counts can be determined by bioassay, but are quite difficult to test for. Fatty acid analysis – in particular the fish oils for DHA – is performed by profiling fatty acids using capillary GC-FID. It is a relatively easy, widely available technique. Polyphenols can be analysed by HPLC/GC. Some methods are routinely available for other 'classes' of these types of compounds, e.g. alkaloids.

Protein content is very simple and cheap to analyse and widely available – either by Kjeldahl classic titration method, or more modern combustion techniques. Amino acids are also relatively easy to analyse, either using a specific amino acid analyser, HPLC or capillary electrophoresis, but costs are much higher than for protein.

11.4.9 Processing constraints

When a product undergoes scale-up from the bench to a pilot plant or factory environment, various difficulties can be encountered, some of which are exacerbated by the presence of functional ingredients. For example, some functional ingredients may cause product discoloration during large-scale factory production that did not occur during small-scale kitchen trials. Also, a mechanism for accurately 'dosing' product must be possible within the factory. This is simple if all ingredients exist as a pre-mix and can be dosed at a simple production stage or mixed with other standard ingredients. Dosing is more difficult if the nature of the functional ingredients means that they can only be added at a particular stage due to being heat or pH sensitive, for example. It may also be difficult to incorporate re-work into a product that contains many different functional ingredients while at the same time ensuring that dosage levels of the functional ingredients in each finished product remains constant. Processing techniques should aim to avoid the use of re-work but for reasons of cost it may not be possible to avoid its use completely.

When a finished product comes off the manufacturing line, it may be necessary to subject it to analytical tests to ensure that the levels of active ingredients are to specification. Assays must be developed that are reliable, low cost, quick and as simple to perform as possible. Any delays or inaccuracies in assays could result in potential loss of product and expensive functional ingredients.

Some functional ingredients have the potential to taint production lines. This could pose a problem where products are made on shared product lines. There is a risk of carrying taint over to standard products and a thorough clean-down must be scheduled into production runs. Alternatively, single lines can be allocated to producing the functional product for restricted time period.

11.4.10 Safety considerations for production workers

Many new functional ingredients will not have been used in a production environment before. Production workers will become exposed to high levels of new ingredients. The health and safety aspects of this must be considered and a thorough HACCP and quality analysis would be necessary for all new functional ingredients used.

11.5   Marketing and retailing functional confectionery

In our country survey we looked at 'traditional' functional confectionery as well as giving indications as to areas of current interest that may be about to open up. Other chapters in this book have discussed various areas of functional food science that are attracting attention at the present time. A challenge for manufacturers who want to introduce new products is to decide on the many opportunities that exist. Which of the vast number of potential concepts will the consumer accept?

There are a whole host of functional ingredients currently available to add to confectionery products. The selection will depend upon the product's proposition to the consumer. Current popular ingredients are vitamins, minerals, prebiotics and probiotics, sugar replacers, plant extracts and essential fatty acids.

The development of functional confectionery is still very much in its infancy and there are certain issues to address before products can be launched. These begin during concept and bench development and can become more complex as we progress to production. Practical experience concludes that functional confectionery concepts should be kept simple, limiting the number of functional ingredients. Too many functional ingredients may not only complicate manufacturing processes, but also add complexity to the product message for the consumer.

A product entering an established part of the market, for example cough sweets or throat soothers, will face competition from products that in some cases may have been established for decades. Unless a point of differentiation can be devised, the new product is unlikely to thrive against well-distributed competition.

11.5.1   Defining the concept for a product

From the above it will be clear that it is important to choose a concept that the consumer can identify with, but that sticking with already successful concepts to produce 'me too' products is all too likely to result in an 'also ran' product. This means that it is often necessary to devise new concepts for functional confectionery. At its simplest, this can be done by examining successful concepts from other food sectors. An example where this has been successful is the recent growth in the 'lite' and fat-reduced confectionery in the USA which has seen the introduction of both new products (e.g. Sweet Escapes) and variants of existing products (Milky Way Lite).

This success has been the outcome of considerable market activity across the food industry in the USA. The concept itself has been launched on the back of high profile health campaigns, which ensured that the consumer understood the basic premise behind the products. The promise of health gains to some extent has offset the organoleptic losses that these products often entail. The lesson is that for mainstream variants it is necessary to have concepts that are broadly understood and accepted by the consumer. In other countries where campaigns about fat and health have been more muted, for example the UK, fat-reduced foods are less widely distributed, and the concept has struggled to reach mainstream confectionery products.

Consumer understanding is therefore one key to success. The less consumers understand a product's underlying concepts, the more likely it is that only a niche market can be aimed at. In marketing parlance, such products are aimed at the innovators in society. The hope is then that these innovators will influence a larger group, the early adopters, to buy the product. These opinion formers can then influence a wider public to accept the product. Launching products may be an act of faith that the consumer will come to understand the proposition behind them. As far as functional concepts are concerned, many will need to be explained to the consumer and in many cases the manufacturer will have to aim initially at a small niche market, and at the start such products will only be found in specialist retail outlets.

Advertising a concept is one way round this dilemma, but immediate success is not guaranteed, and a long-term campaign may be necessary. In any case, advertising is unlikely to succeed, and indeed may be regarded with some cynicism by consumers, in the absence of understanding. Take for example the case of probiotics. Such products have been more successful in markets that accept the health-giving properties of yoghurts and fermented milk products, but they have struggled to some extent in markets like the UK where there is less acceptance of the concept. Unfamiliar concepts therefore need to be explained to consumers. While advertising may be seen as the first resort by marketing-led companies, it is becoming increasingly apparent that communication of new concepts to consumers needs to be patiently done, using the media as a means to explain the underlying scientific concepts.[15] It is also necessary to have backing of the scientific community. This not only reassures consumers, adding credibility to the product, but also can assist in allaying criticism which new ideas can attract.

That science can be used to advantage is clear. Chewing gum (sugar free) is increasingly sold on a dental health proposition. Some advertisements for these products indicate the scientific basis for the claims quite explicitly.

We have seen therefore that choosing an appropriate concept is difficult. A lot depends on the culture of the market into which the product is to be launched, and there are a host of factors that will influence consumer acceptance of a concept. We have already mentioned consumer understanding as key to this. This will vary from market to market. For example, herbal confectionery is likely to be more successful in markets where herbal products are already popular or herbal health remedies are well accepted. Nations can also be very different in their health preoccupations, and this will be an important factor in the acceptance of a product's proposition. Medical and health traditions in many countries may differ markedly from much standard Western medical thinking, and this may profoundly influence consumer choice.

11.5.2 Confectionery as a vehicle for functional concepts

Another issue that has to be confronted during concept development is the type of product that should be developed. While there are many functional products that are based on confectionery models, it is likely that this will work for only certain types of product. It is true that confectionery can offer the convenience, taste acceptability and affordability that many current supplements cannot. As such, confectionery-type concepts may be technically very acceptable vehicles for some functional ingredients, especially those that do not taste very nice, where confectionery techniques can be used to cover up such unpalatable aspects. However, this may work against such products on a number of grounds. First, products that taste too good may be viewed by consumers as too indulgent, and not serious for the purpose for which they were intended. Although 'a spoonful of sugar helps the medicine go down', some adverse flavour may well help to remind the consumer of the presence of active compounds. Consumers may well expect taste penalties from the presence of functional ingredients and regard something indulgent as too good to be true.

A second question for good-tasting products is whether this will encourage over-consumption. This is an issue of particular importance for ingredients with a high degree of potency whose consumption should not be *ad libitum*. The question of product safety we will return to later. However, this can be illustrated with current sugar-free products which contain significant amounts of sugar alcohols. Such ingredients can cause colic, windiness and even osmotic diarrhoea. Even where there are warnings on labels, not all consumers heed these, with sometimes a predictably unfortunate outcome where large amounts of a product are eaten in a short time. It would appear, however, that consumers quickly learn to take such warnings seriously and to supervise children carefully in their use of such products.

There are also concerns about over-consumption in relation to fortified confectionery aimed at children. Multivitamin preparations in the form of candy may be highly attractive to children, and an attractive vehicle for administering such preparations when deemed necessary. There is the possibility of over-consumption where such fortified sweets are self-administered. Clearly such candy has to be treated like regular vitamin pills with the key being proper control by guardians. It is unlikely that children would buy these sweets for themselves, given the cost and the likely points of sale (that is, pharmacy and health counters rather than standard confectionery retailers).

There will also be various other technical considerations which will affect the choice of format, for example the nature of the functional ingredient, many of which have already been referred to. One aspect is the amount of functional ingredient that needs to be added. Where a large amount is necessary, a bar format may be the only option, particularly where a strict dosage is necessary. In this case, it may be preferable to choose a format where the dosage will be consumed in a single entity like a bar.

11.5.3 Marketing functional confectionery

The development of any new product entails a lot more than just getting the ingredient formula correct. The product has to get to the marketplace with a clear-cut proposition for consumers, and an obvious personality. Its benefits for consumers must be obvious. The target consumer must be identified, and where, when and in what circumstances it will be bought. The type of retail outlet must be identified, and how the product can be differentiated from competitors so as to attract the attention of consumers. Any new product will face fierce competition from existing products, even in respect of getting it onto shelves in the first place. It is not surprising therefore that the vast majority of new products have only a very short life.

A key issue facing new functional confectionery products is the question of branding. On the face of it, it would seem obvious that most functional confectionery will contain novel propositions, which will therefore require new brands to be created. However, the launch of new brands can be a very expensive and/or long-term process, as it can take costly advertising and promotion to sell the proposition to consumers (not to mention retailers who have to be persuaded to stock an untried product in the first place).

One way around this is to launch the product under the umbrella of an existing brand. This can be very successful if the manufacturer owns an appropriate brand. There are of course constraints with this approach, not least being the necessity for the functional product to fit in with the overall personality of the brand. Stretching a concept too far will lack credibility.

Another example of a successful launch of a functional confectionery under an existing brand is Mars' Milky Way Lite, in the USA. However, the success of Hershey's Sweet Escapes in that market demonstrates that it is possible to launch a new brand if the proposition is clear enough and understood by consumers. In this case, of course, the underlying health message has been abundantly publicised in the USA. Many functional concepts will be less well understood by the majority of consumers, and in these cases launching at a mass market will not be feasible.

11.5.4 Retail considerations

The manufacturer of a functional confectionery needs to target the type of retail outlet appropriate for the product. Many functional confectionery products will not gain access to the mass market confectionery counters such as those in supermarkets and convenience stores. The most likely contenders for these areas will be those functional products that are extensions of currently popular brands. Even so, retailers, especially supermarkets, will monitor performance to ensure that the product earns its place.

Products with a therapeutic purpose will often be targeted at pharmacies or pharmacy/health sections in supermarkets. Products with dietetic connotations, for example 'lite' products, may fit best with health and beauty counters.

Products whose concepts are only understood by innovators and early adopters may often be confined to specialist outlets like health food shops. Such products with limited outlets will imply low volumes, but success within this niche area may persuade larger retailers to stock such products. In this way, niche products can become mainstream. An example of this is Ricola's herb confectionery in Spain which extended to traditional outlets in 1996, having previously only sold through pharmacies, where it held a 64% share of the sector.[4]

An integral part of such retailing aspects is the question of price. This will have to be set at a level appropriate to the type of product and retail outlet. In most cases prices for functional confectionery will be higher than for standard confectionery. This reflects higher ingredient costs and the higher costs associated with specialist production, marketing and distribution. Consumers will usually be prepared to pay appropriately for a credible product that has desirable properties. However, products to be sold alongside conventional confectionery, for example sugar-free or 'lite' variants of existing brands, will generally have to be priced at around the same sort of level. The mass market will not usually accept higher prices even though the manufacturing costs for making a product with a positive benefit like reduced calories (compared to similar products) might be considerably higher, reducing profit margins below that of standard confectionery.

11.5.5 Product claims

A crucial part of a product identity is its 'proposition', that is, what it can do for the consumer. This needs to be clearly communicated. However, in many markets there are restrictions on claims. For example, in the EU, medicinal claims or even implied claims that a product can prevent, treat or cure a medical condition are prohibited unless the product holds a medical licence. This imposes strong restrictions on aspects of production and marketing. This will apply to many products in the cough sweet/throat soother categories. At the other end of the spectrum, claims about nutrient content are generally permitted, although rules about minimum content and other labelling aspects may apply. Thus it is relatively easy to fortify a product, to promote it, for example, 'with vitamin C'. It may be more difficult to make a nutrient function claim about the added vitamin and more difficult still to claim a nutrient–health relationship.

Such general health claims are difficult to make in many markets, for example being currently forbidden under EU legislation. It is increasingly being recognised that such restrictions are a bar to consumer understanding and also that they impede the development of functional products which may be of great benefit to consumers. The challenge that faces not only regulators but also manufacturers is how such claims should be made and regulated in the marketplace which, on the one hand, permit the development of products that enhance consumer health but at the same time protect the consumer against unwarranted or unsubstantiated claims. There are a number of initiatives under way around the world to address these issues. These regulatory aspects are crucial to the development of functional foods generally and are discussed in more detail elsewhere in this book.

At the present time, the effect of tight regulation is to impose restrictions on the type of products that can be launched to those with concepts already well understood by the consumer. Unless the consumer understands the proposition behind a product, then it will not be bought. For functional confectionery there will normally be insufficient resources available for the public education by advertisement or media material to explain new concepts. Even where the concept is understood, strict interpretation of current legislation will often not permit the use of explicit reference to the potential benefits of the product, so the manufacturer may have to resort to the use of implied benefits. In this case there is no differentiation from those products that are promoted on the basis of containing ingredients that are traditionally perceived as beneficial but for which hard scientific data in support are lacking.

11.5.6 Safety aspects of functional ingredients

A manufacturer who uses unusual ingredients with physiological activity needs to check safety data carefully, and, as with all ingredients, that its use is permitted by local regulation. Advice on this should be available from the supplier, but the manufacturer will need to double check. If the market becomes more receptive to unusual ingredients we are likely to see the use of an increasing variety of plant extracts. Not all of these will be innocuous at all doses or in all circumstances. Some may have unpleasant side-effects as well as beneficial ones. Assessing the strength of such ingredients may well be necessary as part of the review process. Furthermore, the manufacturer needs to keep aware of developments relating to the ingredient. An example of this is St John's Wort which has been an increasingly popular ingredient used for its effectiveness in treating depression. First, the strength of the preparations can vary enormously. This has implications for dosage. Second, there is evidence that St John's Wort may interact adversely when used in conjunction with medically prescribed anti-depressants,[16] raising the issue of the need for label warnings.

Where physiologically active ingredients are added to a product, some consideration needs to be given to the need for information on labels regarding overall consumption. For an ingredient well known to consumers, consumption may need to relate to existing products. For example, a product containing caffeine could relate the caffeine content to a cup of coffee.

In some cases, regulation may already exist. In the UK it is necessary to add labels to products that contain sugar alcohols, warning of the possibility of laxative effects in the event of over-consumption.

11.5.7 Legal aspects specific to confectionery

The developer of novel functional confectionery products may need to check regulations pertaining to this sector. Some regulations may hinder the development of new products. A specific instance of this relates to chocolate. Many countries have tight regulations covering what may or may not be termed chocolate. While this protection of the consumer has an admirable purpose, it can hold back development and marketing of low calorie, low fat or sugar-free chocolate. One product subject to this kind of legislation is the Cadbury Lite Bar, launched in Australia in 1992. In this product, sugar was replaced by isomalt and polydextrose and sweetened with aspartame. This could not be described as chocolate under Australian regulations.

11.6 Summary

Confectionery that could be described as functional has a history going back millennia into ancient Egyptian times. Such early functional confectionery had a therapeutic purpose, and this tradition is still apparent today with many confectionery-like products available to cure ailments such as coughs and sore throats. These products are available in most countries of the world. Compared to mainstream confectionery, the market for functional confectionery is small but growing as new types are brought onto the market.

Confectionery has traditionally contained the sugar, sucrose, as its characterising ingredient. This acts as a sweetener but it has many other technical virtues which make it a very versatile ingredient for this type of product. Other important ingredients of confectionery include other sugars and syrups, milk products, fats and oils, cocoa, cereal products, nuts, dried fruits as well as flavourings and a variety of gums, gelling agents and such-like. There are three main classes of confectionery: sugar confectionery (candy); bars (which may or may not contain chocolate); and chewing gum.

Confectionery can be made 'functional' either by addition of functional ingredients, or by substituting existing ingredients. Examples of both approaches can be found on the market today. The technical attributes of sucrose can sometimes be difficult to replace using alternative ingredients. Nevertheless, sugar-free confectioneries are increasingly being launched, usually as calorie-reduced or non-cariogenic products. Indeed, in Europe, the majority of chewing gum now sold does not contain sucrose, and many brands of sugar-free gum are promoted on dental health grounds. Reduction and replacement of fat in confectionery is more difficult to achieve. Functional ingredients can be incorporated into confectionery, but the format chosen will depend on a variety of technical and marketing factors.

The range of concepts found in functional confectionery products remains fairly limited at the present time. There are, however, many new concepts that could be developed and which are feasible from a technical standpoint. In general terms, however, the market in functional confectionery is very much in its infancy, with a wide variety of products being tried out in various countries, some with a degree of local success, but with no clear trends emerging. This can be partly ascribed to the very different local conditions and consumers' health preoccupations found around the world.

One brake on progress is that consumer understanding of the concepts behind functional products is often limited. In many cases the consumer will need to be educated about recent scientific findings. Advertisement about concepts may lack credibility in the eyes of consumers as being too commercially orientated. It may be important to disseminate concept ideas via more general media, particularly if this can be done by independent scientific experts. Claims in advertising and on product packaging are often prevented because food regulations are generally restrictive in the area of claims.

Another factor, which could hold back development of functional confectionery, is doubt as to the appropriateness of confectionery for this purpose. Although certain medicinal candies are well accepted by the consumer, in general there is only limited experience of consumer reaction to other types of functional confectionery. Confectionery is generally associated in the consumer's mind with pleasure and indulgence, and so many confectionery formats may be inappropriate for functional concepts.

It remains to be seen whether this is of importance as functional confectionery will usually be retailed away from mainstream confectionery. Many products will be niche products appealing to a minority of consumers, or to consumers in times of need (e.g. throat soothers). Furthermore, functional confectionery will be differentiated by higher price necessitated by high ingredient costs and low volumes of manufacture.

In spite of present uncertainties, it seems likely that the market for functional confectionery will continue to develop in the coming years into novel areas as consumers progressively understand the rationale behind functional products generally, and as regulatory requirements on health claims become more flexible.

11.7 References

1 LEES, R. *A History of Sweet and Chocolate Manufacture*, Surbiton, Specialised Publications Ltd, 1988.
2 MINTZ, S.W. *Sweetness and Power*, New York, Viking Penguin, 1985.
3 BIDLACK, W.R. *Phytochemicals: A New Paradigm*, Lancaster, Pennsylvania, Technomic Publishing, 1998.
4 PETTIT, B. *The International 'Healt hy' Confectionery Market*, 2nd edn, Leatherhead Food Research Association, 1999.
5 CAOBISCO, *International Statistical Review of the Biscuit, Chocolate and Sugar Confectionery Industries 1998*, Brussels, 1999.
6 HASLER, C. 'Functional foods: the Western perspective', *Nutrition Reviews*, 1996, **54**, S6–S10.

7 LONGMAN, B. *Strategies in Nutraceuticals: Functional Food and Drink, Reuters Business Insight*, London, Datamonitor plc, 1998.

8 JARDINE, N.J. 'Phytochemicals and Phenolics', in *Chocolate and Cocoa, Health and Nutrition*, I. Knight (ed.), Oxford, Blackwell Science, 1999.

9 Joint Health Claims Initiative, *Final Draft Code of Practice on Health Claims on Foods*, JHCI, 1998.

10 LEES, R. and JACKSON, E.B. *Sugar Confectionery and Chocolate Manufacture*, Glasgow, Leonard Hill, 1985.

11 BECKETT, S. *Industrial Chocolate Manufacture and Use*, Glasgow, Blackie A&P, 1994.

12 MINIFIE, B.W. *Chocolate, Cocoa and Confectionery: Science & Technology*, New York, AVI Publishing, 1982.

13 JACKSON, E.B. *Sugar Confectionery Manufacture*, Glasgow, Blackie A&P, 1990.

14 MANLEY, D. *Technology of Biscuits, Crackers and Cookies*, London, Ellis Horwood, 1991.

15 MALLENTIN, J. *The Newsletter for Functional Foods, Nutraceuticals and Healthy Living*, 21–4, December/January 1999.

16 Adwatch, *Food Labelling and Marketing Newsletter*, Sustain, October 1999.

12

Probiotic functional foods

T. Mattila-Sandholm and M. Saarela, VTT Biotechnology, Espoo

12.1 Introduction: the health benefits of probiotic foods

The area of food for health has been identified as a priority area for research in Europe. This is based on the recognition that there is enormous potential for improving health through food. Furthermore, diet is a major focus of public health strategy aimed at maintaining optimum health throughout life, preventing early onset of chronic diseases such as gastrointestinal disorders, cardiovascular disease, cancer and osteoporosis, as well as promoting healthier ageing. Although the highly complex relationship between food and health is still poorly understood, recent research advances in different disciplines provide promising new approaches to improve our understanding. The growing demand for 'healthy' foods is stimulating innovation and new product development in the food industry internationally. Indeed, the food industry has a central role in facilitating improved eating practices through the provision and promotion of healthy foods.

Probiotics are live microbial food supplements which benefit the health of consumers by maintaining or improving their intestinal microbial balance.[1] Due to their perceived health benefits probiotic bacteria have been increasingly included in yoghurts and fermented milks during the past two decades. Most commonly they have been lactobacilli such as *Lactobacillus acidophilus*, and bifidobacteria often referred to as 'bifidus' (see Table 12.1).[2] A major development in functional foods pertains to foods containing probiotics and prebiotics which enhance health-promoting microbial flora in the intestine. There is growing scientific evidence to support the concept that the maintenance of healthy gut microflora may provide protection against gastrointestinal disorders including gastrointestinal infections, inflammatory bowel diseases and

Table 12.1 Examples of fermented milk products containing probiotic bacteria available in food retail outlets in Europe. (Adapted from Daly and Davis, 1998.).[2]

Product	Brand name	Company (organism -10^7-10^8 viable LAB/ml)	Countries
Yoghurt	LC1	Nestlé (*Lb. johnsonii* LC-1)	France, Belgium, Spain, Switzerland, Portugal, Italy, Germany, UK
Yoghurt	Gefilus	Valio (*Lb. rhamnosus* GG)	Finland
Yoghurt	Vifit	Mona (*Lb. rhamnosus* GG)	Netherlands, Ireland
Yoghurt	Vifit	Sudmilch (*Lb. rhamnosus* GG)	Germany
Yoghurt drink	Yo-Plus	Waterford Foods (*Lb. acidophilus*)	Ireland
Yoghurt	Bio-Pot	Onken (Biogarde cultures)	Europe
Yoghurt	LA7	Bauer (*Lb. acidophilus*)	Germany
Fermented milk drink	Yakult	Yakult (*Lb. casei* Shirota strain)	Netherlands, UK, Germany
Cultures yoghurt-style product	Gaio	MD-Foods (*E. faecium*)	Denmark
Yoghurt	SNO	Dairygold (*Lb. acidophilus*)	Ireland
Yoghurt	Actimel Cholesterol Control	Danone (*Lb. acidophilus*)	Belgium
Fermented milk drink	Actimel	Danone (*Lb. casei*)	Europe
Yoghurt	Yoplait	Waterford-Foods (*Lb. acidophilus*)	Ireland
Fermented milk drink	Bra-Mjolk	Arla (*Bifidus, Lb. reuterii, Lb. acidophilus*)	Sweden
Fermented milk drink	Fyos	Nutricia (*Lb. casei*)	Netherlands
Yoghurt	Symbalance	Tonilait (*Lb. reuterii, Lb. casei, Lb. acidophilus*)	Switzerland
Yoghurt	Shape	St Ivel (*Lb. acidophilus*)	Ireland, UK

even cancer. The use of probiotic bacterial cultures stimulates the growth of preferred micro-organisms, crowds out potentially harmful bacteria and reinforces the body's natural defence mechanisms.

Before a probiotic can benefit human health it must fulfil several criteria: it must have good technological properties so that it can be manufactured and incorporated into food products without losing viability and functionality or creating unpleasant flavours or textures; it must survive passage through the upper gastrointestinal tract and arrive alive at its site of action; and it must be able to function in the gut environment. To study the probiotic strain in the gastrointestinal (GI) tract, molecular techniques must be established for distinguishing the ingested probiotic strain from the potentially thousands of other bacterial strains that make up the gastrointestinal ecosystem. Techniques are also required to establish the effect of the probiotic strain on other members of the intestinal microbiota and importantly on the host. This includes not only positive health benefits, but also demonstration that probiotic strains do not have any deleterious effects. Armed with this knowledge, the probiotics can then enter human clinical pilot studies that attempt to assess their clinical health benefits to consumers (Table 12.2).[3, 4]

12.1.1 Demonstration of Nutritional Functionality of Probiotic Foods (FAIR CT96-1028)

Europe has traditionally had a leading position on the probiotic market. Considerable confusion and scepticism, however, exists on the side of consumers, consumer organisations and certain quarters of the scientific community about the claims associated with probiotic products. This greatly hampers further exploitation of functional foods containing probiotic bacteria and weakens the market position of European producers in the face of competition. To eliminate these hurdles, to speed up adaptation of the probiotic food technology and to enhance the attractiveness of new probiotic foods, it is essential to demonstrate the up-to-date basis for marketable claims by presenting the health and nutritional benefits of probiotic bacteria and foods. Special emphasis should be put on intestinal integrity and immune modulation, exploitation of validated methods for the selection of novel probiotic bacteria and foods, and dissemination of the obtained knowledge to the extended audiences consisting of industries, authorities and consumers. The Probdemo project was initiated to demonstrate the value of probiotic products to European consumers. The project objectives were divided into four interactive tasks (Table 12.3):

1. To establish a scientifically based selection of probiotic bacterial strains currently available for functional foods. Six probiotic strains representing *Lactobacillus* and *Bifidobacterium* species were chosen for demonstration purposes.
2. To demonstrate the beneficial value of probiotic products in human pilot trials both in children and adults. Initial tests showed that probiotic strains did not have any deleterious effects in healthy children or adults. Furthermore, probiotic strains were shown to be effective in the treatment of infants with food allergy and small children with rotavirus diarrhoea. The effect of probiotics was also demonstrated in adults with inflammatory bowel disease (IBD).
3. To demonstrate and meet the functional and technological requirements essential for the industrial production of probiotics as functional foods. This has been established by studying probiotic strain properties *in vitro* and

Table 12.2   Clinical effects of some probiotic strains and yoghurt strains.

Strain	Clinical effects in humans	References
Lactobacillus rhamnosus GG	Adherence to human intestinal cells, lowering faecal enzyme activities, Prevention of antibiotic-associated diarrhoea, treatment and prevention of rotavirus diarrhoea, prevention of acute diarrhoea, immune response modulation	19, 43, 46, 57–69
Lactobacillus johnsonii (acidophilus) LJ-1 (LA-1)	Prevention of traveller's diarrhoea, modulation of intestinal flora, alleviation of lactose intolerance symptoms, improvement of constipation, immune enhancement, adjuvant in Helicobacter pylori treatment	70–74
Bifidobacterium lactis Bb-12	Prevention of traveller's diarrhoea, treatment of viral diarrhoea including rotavirus diarrhoea, modulation of intestinal flora, improvement of constipation, modulation of immune response	70, 71, 75–80
Lactobacillus reuteri ATCC55730	Colonisation of intestinal tract, shortening of rotavirus diarrhoea, treatment of acute diarrhoea, safe and well-tolerated in HIV-positive subjects	81–84
Lactobacillus casei Shirota	Modulation of intestinal flora, lowering faecal enzyme activities, positive effects on superficial bladder cancer	85–88
Lactobacillus plantarum DSM9843	Adherence to human intestinal cells, modulation of intestinal flora	29, 89
Saccharomyces boulardii	Prevention of antibiotic-associated diarrhoea, treatment of Clostridium difficile colitis, prevention of diarrhoea in critically ill tube-fed patients	90–92
Yoghurt strains (Streptococcus thermophilus & Lactobacillus bulgaricus)	No effect on rotavirus diarrhoea, no immune enhancing effect during rotavirus diarrhoea, no effect on faecal enzymes	58, 63

reflecting these results to the clinical situations. The main focus has been on demonstrating adhesion *in vitro* and *in vivo* using human biopsies, on demonstrating the technological criteria for probiotic products, and on pilot production of probiotic strains.

4.   To disseminate the knowledge and results to extended audiences consisting of industrial users, authorities and consumer organisations. This has been

Table 12.3 Tasks concerning the development and manufacturing of functional probiotic foods needed for demonstration. [5, 6]

NUTRITIONAL FUNCTIONALITY OF PROBIOTIC FOODS	
Task 1 *Selection and verification of probiotic strains*	

Task 2 *Clinical pilot testing on humans*	**Task 3** *Technological properties of probiotic foods*
Subtask 2.1 *Clinical pilot testing on children*	Subtask 3.1 *Probiotic properties*
Subtask 2.2 *Clinical pilot testing on adults and patients with GI-disorders*	Subtask 3.2 *Fermentative properties of probiotic foods*
Subtask 2.3 *Establishment of novel methodologies*	Subtask 3.3 *Large-scale production methods*

Task 4 *Dissemination of knowledge of probiotic products*

established by annual workshops (Workshop 1 was held on Safety of Probiotics in 1996, Workshop 2 on Probiotic Research Tools in 1997, Workshop 3 on Functional Food Research in 1998, Workshop 4 on Functional Foods in 2000).[5–8]

The project participants and institutes collectively have wide experience in this research area, building on the results of former EU programmes on lactic acid bacteria and probiotics. The industrial partners have long traditions in the markets of functional foods with special reference on probiotic products. VTT Biotechnology, Finland, has the role of coordination and dissemination of activities and demonstration tasks on probiotic strain properties, technological properties and clinical testing on adults. The University of Wageningen, Netherlands, has the key role of demonstrating the activity and viability of probiotic strains in human clinical trials by using molecular methods including PCR, *in situ* hybridisation and DGGE/TGGE. The Catholic University of Piacenza, Italy, has the role of showing the adhesive and aggregation properties of the strains to be demonstrated. The University of College Cork, Ireland, has profound expertise on human gastroenterology, clinical testing with adults and immune modulation activities of probiotics. University of Turku, Finland, has a long scientific tradition of clinical testing with children and the links between clinical pediatrics and functional foods. The industrial partners Valio Ltd. (Finland), Arla (Sweden), Nestlé (Switzerland) and Christian Hansen Laboratories (Denmark) have sound basis of industrial production of probiotic products and long experience on functional foods market as well as research in this area. This industrial role is of utmost importance in selecting the strains to be demonstrated, preparing the products to be developed and in verifying their beneficial effects.

12.2 Selecting probiotic strains

The theoretical basis for selection of probiotic micro-organisms illustrated in Table 12.4 and Fig. 12.1 includes:

* safety
* functional behaviour (survival, adherence, colonisation, anti-microbial production, immune stimulation, anti-genotoxic activity and prevention of pathogens such as *Helicobacter pylori, Salmonella, Listeria* and *Clostridium*)
* technological aspects (growth in milk, sensory properties, stability, phage resistance, viability in processes).

In general, strains for pilot testing should be selected based on established *in vitro* scientific data. Naturally, the safety of probiotic strains has been of prime importance and new guidelines have been developed.[9-13] Current safety criteria and functional properties for successful probiotics have been defined in recent reviews.[14-16] These include the following specifications:

* Strains for human use are preferably of human origin.
* They are isolated from healthy human GI tract.
* They have a history of being non-pathogenic even in immunocompromised hosts.
* They have no history of association with diseases such as infective endocarditis or GI disorders.

Table 12.4   Desirable properties of probiotic bacteria.[3]

Desirable properties	Desired effect
Human origin	Ability to maintain verified viability, species-specific effects on health
Acid and bile stability	Maintenance of viability in the intestine
Adherence to human intestinal cells	Maintenance of mild acidity in the intestine, antagonism against pathogens, competitive exclusion
Colonisation of the human gut	Maintenance of colonising properties, antagonism against pathogens, competitive exclusion
Production of anti-microbial substances	Antagonism against pathogens, competitive exclusion
Antagonism against pathogenic bacteria	Antagonism against pathogens, competitive exclusion (in intestinal tract and oral cavity)
Safety in human use	Tested safety in animal models and human use, accurate strain identification (genus, species)

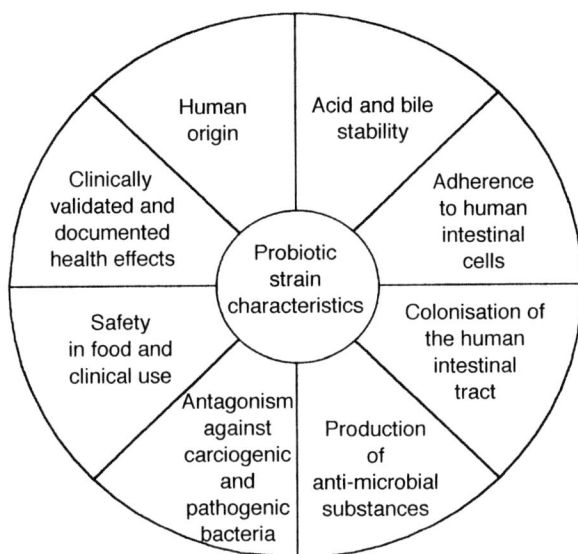

Fig. 12.1 The theoretical basis for selection of probiotic micro-organisms includes safety, functional (survival, adherence, colonisation, anti-microbial production, immune stimulation, anti-genotoxic activity and prevention of pathogens) and technological aspects (growth in milk, sensory properties, stability, phage resistance, viability in processes).

The significance of human origin has been debated recently, but most if not all current successful strains are indicated to be of human origin. Similarly, the importance of the ability to colonise the human gastrointestinal tract has been questioned. However, most current strains are reported to persist in humans at least temporarily as measured by faecal counts following ingestion. Acid and bile stability are self-evident properties for any strain expected to have effects in the intestinal tract. Ability to adhere and persist are also closely related to potential immune effects. It is likely that some mechanisms of adhering and/or binding to the intestinal cells are required. Thus controlled comparable studies on *in vitro* model systems, such as the Caco-2 cell line, are of importance.[17, 18] Adherent strains of probiotic bacteria are favoured since they are likely to persist longer in the intestinal tract and thus have better possibilities of showing metabolic effects than non-adhering strains. At least one of the commercial probiotic strains has been demonstrated to adhere to the colonic mucosae *in vivo*.[19]

To have an impact on colon flora it is important for probiotic strains to show antagonism against pathogenic bacteria via anti-microbial substance production or competitive exclusion. Enormous research efforts have focused on bacteriocin research. However, the mode of action and efficacy of bacteriocins in the gut is not known for probiotic bacteria. Although probiotic strains may produce bacteriocins *in vitro*, the role of bacteriocins in the pathogen inhibition *in vivo* can only be limited, since traditional bacteriocins have an inhibitory effect only against closely related species such as other *Lactobacillus* or on sporeformers such as *Bacillus* or *Clostridium*. However, low molecular weight metabolites (and secondary metabolites) may be more important since they show wide inhibitory spectrum against many harmful organisms like *Salmonella, Escherichia coli, Clostridium* and *Helicobacter*.[20–22]

12.2.1 Development of cultures aimed for functional probiotic foods

Probiotic dairy foods and cultures have a long history and large consumption in the Nordic diet. Industrial products, including cultured dairy products, and their probiotic properties have been studied for many decades. The objective of the Nordic programme (from 1994 to end of 1997) was to validate industrial probiotic strains with regard to *in vitro* functionality. Strains were provided by project participants Arla (Sweden), Christian Hansen (Denmark), Norwegian Dairies (Norway) and Valio Ltd (Finland). Strains studied included the following: *Lactobacillus paracasei* subsp. *paracasei* strains E-94506 and E-94510, *Lactobacillus rhamnosus* strains E-94509 and E-94522, *Lactobacillus acidophilus* E-94507, *Lactobacillus plantarum* E-79098, *Lactococcus lactis* subsp. *lactis* E-90414, *L. lactis* subsp. *cremoris* E-94523, *Bifidobacterium animalis (lactis)* E-94508 and *Bifidobacterium longum* E-94505. The studies included research on the *in vitro* cytokine release effects, adhesive properties, anti-mutagenicity and behaviour in the gastrointestinal tract models (TNO gastrointestinal tract model in the Netherlands, and the SHIME ecosystem at Ghent, Belgium). Also technological and production properties were assessed.

Assessment of adhesion properties
Adhesion of probiotic strains to human intestinal cells and the following colonisation of the human gastrointestinal tract has been suggested as an important prerequisite for probiotic action. Adhesion verifies the potential of the strain to inhabit the intestinal tract and to grow in intestinal conditions. Adhesion also provides an interaction with the mucosal surface facilitating contact with gut-associated lymphoid tissue mediating local and systemic immune effects. Thus, only adherent probiotics have been thought to induce immune effects and to stabilise intestinal mucosal barrier.[23] The Nordic programme project results of *in vitro* adhesion assays gave a clear indication of differences and variation between assays and different strains.[24, 25] It was evident that in addition to Caco-2 cell line experiments, other test systems were also needed to characterise the adhesion potential and different adhesion mechanisms. The adhesion system was also used to study the anti-invasion potential of probiotic stains. Different probiotic strains show relatively different behaviour in invasion inhibition and novel methodologies are needed to assess these properties in a way that relates them to clinical situations. Adhesion experiments indicate clear differences in the colonisation potential of different probiotic strains and, when later connected with clinical data, may provide a useful basis for selection and method

development for future probiotic strains.[17, 18] Lately adhesion assays have also been applicated to human ileostomy glycoproteins (modelling for small intestinal mucus), showing once again different characteristics of the probiotic features.[26]

In vivo *adhesion studies using colonic biopsies*

Faecal samples have been used in most colonisation studies on probiotic bacteria.[27, 28] These, however, reflect only the bacteriological situation in faecal material and do not give an accurate picture about the situation in different parts of the gastrointestinal tract or in the mucosal layer of the gut. There are advantages in taking biopsy material from colonoscopy patients: in this way tissue samples have been obtained, not only from the rectal-sigmoidal region, but also from other parts of large intestine (ascending, transverse and descending colon). As a result the preferential adhesion of a commercial probiotic strain (*Lactobacillus GG*) to the descending part of large colon was detected by using biopsy material. This probiotic strain was shown to survive in the gut epithelium for several days after consumption of the probiotic preparation was stopped and even after the strain could no longer be detected in faecal samples.[19] Johansson and co-workers have also demonstrated the adhesion of different *Lactobacillus* strains to rectal mucosal biopsy samples obtained from volunteers who had consumed fermented oatmeal soup.[29]

Immunological assessment

Gut-associated lymphoid tissue may have contact with adhesive probiotic preparations and therefore adhesion is one way of provoking immune effects. The Nordic network studied the interactions of probiotic strains and dairy cultures (*Lactobacillus bulgaricus, Streptococcus thermophilus*) with cytokine production (human TNF-α, interleukin-6, interleukin-10, interleukin-12, TGF-β, and interferon-α). Probiotic strains which had passed through the *in vitro* TNO gastrointestinal tract model were also assayed for their ability to induce cytokine production (TNF-α, interleukin-6).[30] The main goal was to investigate whether probiotic strains stimulate the immune system *in vitro* through cytokines. IL-6 production showed considerable variation between experiments performed with live bacteria. Test strains were not observed to induce IL-10.[31] Efforts were made to develop new methods to measure early cytokine responses by detection of mRNA by Northern hybridisation. This method proved more sensitive than the ELISA and has demonstrated that probiotic strains indeed produce IL-10 and IL-1b. Further investigations focused on analysis of the pathway of cytokine induction by probiotics, estimation of the effect of serum proteins, interaction between probiotics and human cell surface molecules.[32]

Gastrointestinal models

The Nordic network experiments with the TNO gastrointestinal tract model focused on survival studies after gastric and ileal delivery. The SHIME-reactor was chosen to illustrate the population dynamics in the small and large intestine.

Parameters such as pH, redox state, NH_4, SCFA, gas composition, enzyme activities and major bacterial groups were determined. As indicated already in the discussion of adhesion, changes occurred in samples taken from different parts of the TNO model system. Some of the non-viable bacteria recovered from the TNO model also showed some immunological activity. Probiotic treatment was shown to increase temporarily the numbers of lactic acid bacteria in different parts of the SHIME ecosystem. Enterobacteriaceae decreased markedly during treatment. The results indicated that further studies are necessary in order to evaluate the repeatability of the SHIME system in the assessment of fatty acid and enzymatic profile changes (Table 12.5).[33]

Anti-mutagenicity properties
Lactic acid bacteria or cultured dairy products have been reported to reduce the mutagenicity of known chemical mutagens in *in vitro* tests.[34] In *in vivo* trials probiotic strains have occasionally been associated with the reduction of faecal enzymatic activities involved in mutagen or carcinogen activation.[35] Results have been somewhat contradictory in trials studying the effects of orally ingested probiotic strains on actual faecal mutagenicity. Lidbeck and co-workers detected a decrease in faecal and urinary mutagenicity as a result of *Lactobacillus acidophilus* NCFB 1748 consumption.[36] No such effect was seen in similar tests with another probiotic.[37]

12.2.2 The Probdemo strains

One of the first tasks of the Probdemo project was to establish selection criteria for probiotic strains, and then apply these specific criteria for selecting the project strains. The preliminary selection criteria included stability in *in vitro* models simulating conditions in the upper gastrointestinal tract, where probiotic bacteria are first exposed to an acidic and protease-rich environment in the stomach before encountering bile acids in the small intestine. Other selection criteria employed included the ability to adhere to intestinal mucosae, the ability to inhibit intestinal pathogens and safety to the consumers.[5, 11, 12] Application of these selection criteria resulted in the selection of the following probiotic strains:

Table 12.5 Study themes for which an *in vitro* model can be used.[94]

- Survival and effect of exogenous bacteria on the microbial ecology (probiotics and genetically modified micro-organisms)
- Survival and colonisation resistance of potentially pathogenic bacteria
- Factors controlling the homeostatis in the intestinal microbial ecosystem
- Slow release of (pro)drugs and foods
- Deliberate transformation of (pro)drugs and food components by the micro-organisms
- Effect of (pro)drugs and drugs such as antibiotics on the microbial ecosystem
- Effect of food components (prebiotics) on microbial ecology
- Fermentation pattern of food components
- Effect of chemicals in the environment on the microbial ecology after ingestion

---

L. rhamnosus GG, *Lactobacillus johnsonii* LJ-1, *Lactobacillus salivarius* UCC 118, *Lactobacillus crispatus* M247, *L. paracasei* F19, and *B. lactis* Bb-12. *Bifidobacterium longum* UCC 35624 was later included in the study due to its promising positive influence on inflammatory bowel diseases.

Further characterisation of these strains, both at the phenotypic and genotypic level, continued throughout the project. This led to the discovery of new mechanisms for colonisation in the human intestinal tract such as expression of co-aggregation proteins.[38, 39] In safety studies it was demonstrated that the genes encoding vancomycin resistance in *L. rhamnosus* GG were distinct from the transferable genes in *Enterococcus*, indicating that they do not pose a safety concern in this strain.[40] The probiotic properties of the strains are now known to be chromosomally encoded rather than being coded on potentially unstable plasmids. Further research on the probiotic mechanisms of the project strains (including molecular studies to determine how and where they adhere to intestinal mucosae, inhibit pathogens and induce immunomodulation in the host) has been performed, yielding further insights into how probiotic bacteria can be selected and can benefit human health.

12.3 Pilot testing in clinical human trials

Probiotic strains should be safe and clinically tested prior to commercial human use. Although this is an important aspect, no firm guidelines exist for safety criteria. Examples of clinical and safety criteria for probiotic foods are listed in Tables 12.6 and 12.7.[16, 41]

Guidelines for probiotic clinical trials (Probdemo approach) stem from the trial design using volunteers (healthy or diseased in case of demonstration). In a trial design volunteers should be randomly selected from a panel of a specific population group targeted for the trial. A number of exclusion criteria were employed when choosing the original healthy volunteer panel. These exclusion criteria were the following:

- antibiotic treatment during the last month
- strong chronic intestinal disorders
- chronic inflammatory diseases
- chronic viral illness
- current drug therapy

Table 12.6 Requirements for good clinical studies for probiotic bacteria.[32]

◆ Defined and well-characterised strains of bacteria
◆ Well-defined strains, well-defined study preparations
◆ Double-blind, placebo controlled
◆ Randomised
◆ Results confirmed by different groups
◆ Publication in peer review journals

Table 12.7 Recommendations for safety of probiotic cultures and foods (Probdemo approach).[16]

1. The producer that markets the food has the ultimate responsibility for supplying a safe food. Probiotic foods should be as safe as other foods.

2. When the probiotic food turns out to be a novel food it hence will be subject to the appropriate legal approval (EU directive for novel foods).

3. When a strain has a long history of safe use, it will be safe as a probiotic strain and will not result in a novel food.

4. The best test for food safety is a well-documented history of safe human consumption. Thus when a strain belongs to a species for which no strains are known that are pathogenic and for which other strains have been described that have a long history of safe use, it is likely to be safe as a probiotic strain and will not result in a novel food.

5. When a strain belongs to a species for which no pathogenic strains are known but which do not have a history of safe use, it may be safe as a probiotic strain but will result in a novel food and hence should be treated as such.

6. When a new strain belongs to a species for which strains are known that are pathogenic, it will result in a novel food.

7. Proper state-of-the-art taxonomy is required to describe a probiotic strain. Today it includes DNA–DNA hybridisation and rRNA sequence determination. This reasoning specifically applies to mutants of a probiotic strain.

8. In line with recommendation 1, strains that carry transferable antibiotic resistance genes, i.e. genes encoding proteins that inactivate antibiotics, should not be marketed.

9. Strains that have not been properly taxonomically described using the approaches as indicated above under recommendation 7 should not be marketed. Strains should also be deposited in an internationally recognised culture collection.

- pregnancy
- particular nutritional regimen (i.e. vegetarian)
- diagnosis of GI cancer
- known allergies to dairy products
- participation in other current trials.

In addition, a premature study end was considered if the volunteer:

- proceeded to take antibiotics or laxatives
- consumed other fermented products during the study period (>3 times overall)
- was non-compliant with the intake of the study product (>3 days overall).

The clinical trials on probiotics should regularly run for at least several weeks in total (usually several months, Fig. 12.2). Throughout the study the volunteers are required to refrain from other fermented dairy products. The trial

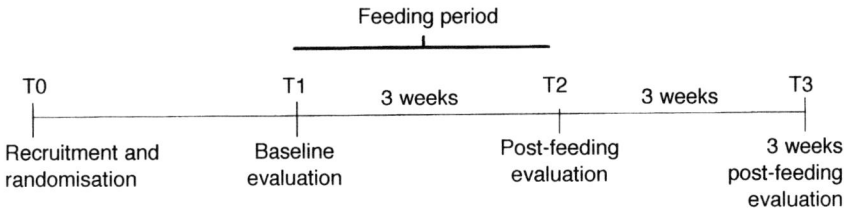

Fig. 12.2   Example of a feeding trial for a probiotic product.[3, 47]

Table 12.8   Parameters for probiotic feeding trial analysis[3, 47]

In faeces	1. Microbial numbers (i.e. probiotic strain, total lactobacilli, coliforms, *Bifidobacterium*, *Clostridium*, *Bacteroides*, *Enterococcus*). 2. Total and probiotic-specific secretory IgA.
In blood	1. General haematology, i.e. blood cell numbers, haemoglobin levels. 2. Phagocytic cell (granulocyte, monocyte) activity assessed by measuring FITC-labelled *E. coli* uptake by flow cytometry. 3. Total serum antibody levels (IgG, IgM, IgE). 4. Probiotic-specific antibodies (measured by agglutination, RIA, ELISA and flow cytometry). 5. Inflammatory markers, i.e. Erythrocyte Sedimentation Rate (ESR), C-active Protein (CRP). 6. Inflammatory cytokines, i.e. IFN-γ, TNF-α, IL-4, Sol. IL-2R, Sol. IL-6R.
In saliva	1. Total and probiotic-specific secretory IgA.

encompasses numerous important phases, the most important being a fixed time period during which predetermined test product is consumed daily by each volunteer (consisting of 10^8 to 10^{10} probiotic bacteria as a daily dosage), and dates when clinical samples (faecal, blood, saliva and urine) are taken from the volunteers for analysis (Table 12.8).

12.3.1 Clinical trials: Probdemo approach

Ultimately, the only way to demonstrate that a probiotic strain can influence human health positively is to conduct human clinical trials and measure an index of the health of the individuals during the trial. A number of pilot human trials were completed in the Probdemo project (Table 12.9). All of the trials were conducted using a randomised, double-blind, placebo-controlled design. An aim of each trial was to establish that the probiotic bacteria survive transit through the upper gastrointestinal tract and are viable and active in the colon. Strain-specific molecular probes and PCR-based molecular typing techniques developed within the project demonstrated that the project strains survive intestinal transit, and that viable probiotic bacteria can be identified in the faeces

Table 12.9 Clinical pilot testing carried out in the Probdemo project during the years 1996–2000.[5-8]

Clinical pilot testing	Strain
Healthy children	*Lactobacillus rhamnosus* (Valio)
	Bifidobacterium lactis (Chr. Hansen)
	Lactobacillus paracasei (Arla)
Children with atopic eczema	*Lactobacillus rhamnosus* (Valio)
	Bifidobacterium lactis (Chr. Hansen)
Children with rotavirus	*Bifidobacterium lactis* (Chr. Hansen)
Children with common cold	*Lactobacillus rhamnosus* (Valio)
Healthy adults	*Lactobacillus johnsonii* (Nestlé)
	Lactobacillus salivarius (UCC)
	Lactobacillus paracasei (Arla)
Adults with milk hypersensitivity, atopic dermatitis	*Lactobacillus paracasei* (Arla)
IBD (inflammatory bowel disease)	*Lactobacillus salivarius* (UCC)
	Bifidobacterium longum/infantis (UCC)
Elderly with *Helicobacter pylori*	*Lactobacillus paracasei* (Arla)

of volunteers consuming probiotic product.[42] Biopsy sampling showed that *L. rhamnosus* GG, *L. salivarius* UCC 118, *L. paracasei* F19 and *L. crispatus* M247 all adhere to and persist in the colonic mucosae.[6-8, 19, 43] Interestingly, *L. crispatus* MU5, an isogenic mutant of *L. crispatus* M247 lacking the co-aggregation protein, was unable to adhere to colonic mucosae in *in vitro* models to the same degree as the parent strain. The mutant strain also failed to colonise the colonic mucosae *in vivo*, demonstrating that the co-aggregation protein is important for this strain's ability to colonise the human GI tract.[39]

Molecular analysis (by temperature gradient gel electrophoresis (TGGE) technique) on the effect of probiotics on the population dynamics of the intestinal microbiota revealed that probiotic strains did not disturb the balance of the major bacterial population groups. TGGE technique was also used to show that the microbiota in infants was relatively undeveloped and in constant flux, but was complex and quite stable in healthy adults.[44]

There has long been speculation about stimulation of the immune system by consumption of probiotic bacteria. Human clinical trials in the Probdemo project have shown that probiotic bacteria can have positive effects on the immune system of their host. In two separate trials, both *L. johnsonii* LJ-1 and *L. salivarius* UCC 118 stimulated a mucosal IgA response and increased phagocytic activity. The immunomodulation mediated by these strains was not linked to an inflammatory response or general modification of immune responsiveness that could potentially have harmful effects, but was rather associated with transient alterations beneficial to the consumer.[7,45] Further evidence for immunomodulation by probiotic bacteria was provided by a trial involving children with severe atopic eczema resulting from food allergy. Children fed *L. rhamnosus* GG and *B. lactis* Bb-12 showed a significant improvement in clinical symptoms compared to the placebo group.[7,8] *B. lactis* Bb-12 was also tested for its ability to prevent diarrhoea in children attending day care centres in Denmark. The strain was fed in the form of freeze-dried powder in capsules, and although the probiotic did not reduce the incidence of diarrhoea in these children, it did reduce the duration of diarrhoea by, on average, one day.[8,46]

Inflammatory bowel disease (IBD) is a term used to cover a range of incurable diseases (including Crohn's disease, ulcerative colitis and pouchitis) with unknown aetiology that result in chronic relapsing inflammation of the gut. In addition to a genetic predisposition, the composition and activity of the intestinal microbiota have been proposed to play a role in these diseases.[47] Murine models for Crohn's disease and ulcerative colitis were used in the Probdemo project to investigate the effect of *L. salivarius* UCC 118 and *B. longum* UCC 35624 on these diseases. In both models, probiotic therapy significantly reduced disease severity compared to placebo control groups.[48] In preliminary human trials using biopsy sampling *L. salivarius* UCC 118 has been demonstrated to colonise both healthy and diseased intestinal tissue in patients with ulcerative colitis.[8]

The Probdemo project concluded in early 2000 and the final results were disseminated in the 4th Probdemo Workshop in Rovaniemi, Finland, February 2000.[8] This included the results of a number of clinical trials (Table 12.9). The effect of *L. rhamnosus* GG on diarrhoea and respiratory infections was examined in a trial involving 600 children in Finland. The preliminary results showed that the number of absences due to illness was lower in the *L. rhamnosus* GG milk group. The *L. rhamnosus* GG group also resisted the first respiratory infection longer than the control group.[49] *L. paracasei* F19 strain was fed to 63 small children for three weeks to study the faecal recovery of the strain and the possible side-effects caused by ingestion. Results of the trial showed that *L. paracasei* F19 product was readily ingested by infants and also well tolerated.[50] *L. paracasei* F19 was further trialled in elderly volunteers infected with the gastric pathogen *Helicobacter pylori* to study the effectiveness of the probiotic in improving these individuals' quality of life. The preliminary results indicate that fermented milk as such (with or without added probiotic) can have an impact on the *H. pylori* infection.[51] A trial examining the effect of *L. paracasei* F19 on milk hypersensitivity in young adults was also performed. The pilot study showed that milk products with *L. paracasei* F19 are safe and well tolerated in healthy and in milk-hypersensitive subjects.[52] Lastly, the previously mentioned human trials investigating the impact of *Lactobacillus salivarius* UCC 118 and *Bifidobacterium longum* UCC 35624 on controlling IBD and preventing relapse were completed in early 2000.[8]

12.4 Processing issues in developing probiotic foods

Functional foods with probiotics are now well established in the European market. Starting about 20 years ago, this product range has increased and is presently known to most consumers. This is a result of intensive research and development within the industry and the academic field. This process will go on and new probiotic strains representing mainly lactobacilli and bifidobacteria will be identified and introduced into new products together with strains already used today. To be successful the food industry has to satisfy the demands of the consumer. All foods should be safe and have excellent organoleptic properties. Probiotic foods should also retain specific probiotic strains at a suitable level during the storage time experienced by them. In examining existing products it has been suggested that this is not always the case.[53]

Before probiotic strains can be delivered to consumers, they must first be able to be manufactured under industrial conditions, and then survive and retain their functionality during storage as frozen or freeze-dried cultures, and also in the food products into which they are finally formulated. Additionally, they must be able to be incorporated into foods without producing off-flavours or textures. Tasks connected to safety and technological properties of probiotic foods formed an important part of the Probdemo project. Another part of technological studies was to produce and characterise products for testing in clinical trials. The industrial partners in the project collaborated to establish fermentation conditions for all project strains to obtain an acceptable cell yield and good performance and viability of the cultures. Strain-to-strain differences were observed in the storage stability of freeze-dried and frozen concentrates, but conditions enabling adequate survival of the bacteria during storage over a 12-month period could be established for most of the project strains. Additionally, project strains were used to produce highly acceptable and organoleptically good fermented dairy products containing probiotics in the order of 10^8 CFU/g even at the end of the shelf life of the products. It was demonstrated that during some conditions it was possible to use solely the probiotic strain as the acid-producing strain. However, usually the use of a supporter starter was a preferable way to produce high quality products. Some of the Probdemo strains are currently used in products on the market. It was shown that the technological properties of the commercial products could be further improved by industrial optimisation.[54] Today, research efforts are being made in incorporating probiotic encapsulation technology into foods to ensure the viability and stability of probiotic cultures.[55, 56]

The Probdemo project demonstrated that all the selected probiotic strains could be used to:[54]

- produce concentrated cultures of each specific strain in levels above 10^{10} CFU/g with good storage properties at low temperature
- produce probiotic foods with help of a supporter culture (yoghurt culture or a pure *Streptococcus* strain)
- ferment milk together with supporter cultures without inhibition of the growth of any of the added strains

- produce probiotic foods with levels of the specified probiotic strain within 10^6–10^8 CFU/g product
- produce probiotic foods with high and constant levels of the probiotic strain when stored at low temperature for three weeks
- produce probiotic foods with an acceptable taste and flavour during the storage time
- produce probiotic foods with acceptable stability and viscosity (in many cases even improved quality in comparison to using solely supporter cultures).

12.5 Future trends

Continuously increasing consumer health consciousness and exploding expenditure are socio-economic factors responsible for the expanding European and world-wide interest in functional foods. The success of functional foods will largely depend on convincing evidence for health claims, backed by solid basic science, as well as the efficient dissemination of accurate and comprehensible information to consumers. The present state-of-the-art issues can be concluded as follows:

- Functional probiotic/prebiotic foods have existed for a long time and, thanks to science, their objective benefits can today be proven and enhanced.
- Functional probiotic/prebiotic foods will meet increasing needs and demands from consumers including improvement of specific functions and general well-being, and help to prevent avoidable illnesses. However, indicators of functional benefits need to be validated.
- The food industry is capable of mass-producing a variety of functional foods that can benefit a large number of consumers. The consumers, however, need easy access to reliable, scientifically valid information in order to make the right choices.
- The European food industry already has certain advantages in the area of food and health, while the future EU research potential in the field of nutrition and food science will enable it to become significantly more competitive.

The recent EU projects have demonstrated that with a scientific approach to selecting and applying probiotics, functional food products can be developed with measurable health benefits for European consumers. Probiotic strains can be successfully manufactured and incorporated into highly acceptable food products where they can retain their viability and functionality. The Probdemo project has demonstrated that probiotic bacteria can survive passage through the upper gastrointestinal tract and can persist in the colon, including the mucosae. There are many strain-to-strain variations, not only in their technological properties, but also in their effects on human health. Some of the mechanisms that are involved in producing health benefits are slowly being elucidated, allowing better targeted screening regimes to select appropriate strains for probiotic use. The human trials finalised to date have demonstrated that probiotics can improve the intestinal microbiota and modulate consumers' immune systems with positive effects on health. The results of clinical trials will no doubt provide deeper insights into mechanisms of probiotic action and, it is to be hoped, further demonstrations of the health value of probiotic foods.

The probiotic/prebiotic concept is today widely spread in the scientific and industrial fields. However, further scientific input is required. The human intestine is highly involved in immune modulation and microflora are an important component in maintaining an immunological steady state in the gut. Important target research areas, including GI tract diagnostics and immunology, methodology, biomarkers and functionality, will lead to tools and scientifically sound methods for well-designed informative human studies. Clinical studies are essential for the socio-economic success of probiotic functional foods, and they should be tailored for specific population groups such as the elderly and babies. Future research on probiotic bacteria will centre on selecting new and more specific or disease-specific strains for the well-being of the host. It may well be that different regions of the gastrointestinal tract (e.g. colon, jejunum, duodenum, etc.) require different probiotic bacteria or mixtures of strains. This is particularly true with states such as colon cancer, prevention of colon cancer, rotavirus diarrhoea and gastritis caused by *Helicobacter pylori*. With carefully controlled studies on selected strains the future will provide targeted probiotic bacteria for different age groups and for prevention and treatment of specific diseases. Additionally, mixtures of different probiotics should be carefully studied in relation to colonic flora and also in terms of promoting and preserving the intestinal integrity and colonisation resistance.

The future scientific and technological research trends are as follows:[8]

- to inter-link the European expertise and scientific knowledge on food, GI tract functionality and human health
- to study the mechanisms of action of probiotics and prebiotics in the GI tract, and develop diagnostic tools and biomarkers for their assessment
- to evaluate the role of immunological biomarkers and probiotic applications thereof
- to examine the effects of probiotics on GI diseases, GI infections and allergies in different population groups
- to address the consumer aspects and trade-offs, and to ensure the stability and viability of probiotic product.

12.6 Sources of further information and advice

Partners in the Probdemo Demonstration Project (FAIR CT96-1028)

Partner 1   VTT Biotechnology
             PO Box 1500, FIN-02044 VTT, FINLAND
             Contact: Professor Tiina Mattila-Sandholm (probiotic technology, networks)
             tel: +358-50-5527243 fax:+358-9-4552028,tiina.mattila-sandholm@vtt.fi

Partner 2   Arla R & D
             Torsgatan 14, S-10456 Stockholm, SWEDEN
             Contact: Professor Rangne Fondén (probiotic starters, technology)
             tel:+46-8-6773237 fax:+46-8-203329,rangne.fonden@arla.se

Partner 3   Valio Ltd. Research and Development Centre
             PO Box 390, 00100 Helsinki, FINLAND
             Contact: Dr Maija Saxelin (probiotic starters, technology)
             tel:+358-103813111 fax:+358 103813019,maija.saxelin@valio.fi

Partner 4   University of Wageningen
             Department of Microbiology
             PO Box 8033,
             NL-6703 CT Wageningen, THE NETHERLANDS
             Contact: Professor Willem de Vos (molecular tools for probiotics)
             tel:+31-317-483100,fax:+31-317-483829,
             willem.devos@algemeen.micr.wau.nl

Partner 5   Instituto di Microbiologia
             Facoltá di Agraria U.C.S.C.
             Via Emilia Parmense 84, I-29100 Piacenza, ITALY
             Contact: Professor Lorenzo Morelli (strain properties, adhesion,
             aggregation) tel:+39-523599248, fax:+39 523 599246, morelli@pc.unicatt.it

Partner 6   University College Cork
             Department of Microbiology
             Western Road, Cork, IRELAND
             Contact: Professor Kevin Collins (clinical trials, immunology)
             tel:+353-21-902642,fax:+353-21-275934, dydm8006@ucc.ie

Partner 7   Nestlé Research Center – Nestec Ltd
             PO Box 44
             CH-100 Lausanne 26, SWITZERLAND
             Contact: Dr Stephanie Blum, Dr. Eduardo Schiffrin (immunology,
             adhesion), Dr Roberto Reniero (technology)
             tel:+41-21-7858208, fax:+41-21-7858925, roberto.reniero@chlsnr.nestrd.ch

Partner 8   Chr. Hansen A/S
             10–12 Bøge Allé, DK-Hørsholm, DENMARK
             Contact: Benedikte Grenov (probiotic starters, technology)
             tel:+45-45-747474, fax:+45-45-748994,beg.dk@chr-hansen.com

Partner 9   University of Turku
             Department of Biochemistry and Food Chemistry
             FIN-20014 Turku, FINLAND
             Contact: Professor Seppo Salminen, Dr Erika Isolauri (clinical trials,
             allergies, immunology) tel:+358-400-601394,
             fax:+358-2-3336860,sepsal@utu.fi

12.7 References

1 FULLER, R. 'Probiotics in man and animals', *J Appl Bacteriol*, 1989, **66**, 365–78.

2 DALY, C. and DAVIS, R. 'The biotechnology of lactic acid bacteria with emphasis on applications in food safety and human health', *Agricult Food Sci Finland*, 1998, **7** (2), 219–50.

3 MATTILA-SANDHOLM, T. and SALMINEN, S. 'Up-to-date on probiotics in Europe', *Gastroenterol Int*, 1998, **11** (1), 8–16.

4 MATTILA-SANDHOLM, T., MÄTTÖ, J. and SAARELA, M. 'Lactic acid bacteria with health claims: interference and interactions with gastrointestinal flora', *Int Dairy J*, 1999, **9**, 25–35.

5 ALANDER, M. and MATTILA-SANDHOLM, T. (eds) 'Selection and safety criteria of probiotics', *1st Workshop, FAIR CT96-1028, PROBDEMO*, Helsinki, Finland, VTT Symposium 167, 55 pp., 1996.

6 ALANDER, M., KAUPPILA, T. and MATTILA-SANDHOLM, T. (eds) 'Novel methods for probiotic research', *2nd Workshop, FAIR CT96-1028, PROBDEMO*, Cork, Ireland, VTT Symposium 173, 70 pp., 1997.

7 MATTILA-SANDHOLM, T. and KAUPPILA, T. (eds) 'Functional food research in Europe', *3rd Workshop, FAIR CT96-1028, PROBDEMO*, Haikko, Finland, VTT Symposium 187, 125 pp., 1998.

8 ALANDER, M. and MATTILA-SANDHOLM, T. (eds) 'Functional foods for EU-health in 2000', *4th Workshop, FAIR CT96-1028, PROBDEMO*, Rovaniemi, Finland, VTT Symposium 198, 107 pp., 2000.

9 AGUIRRE, M. and COLLINS, M.D. 'Lactic acid bacteria and human clinical infection', *J Appl Bacteriol*, 1993, **75**, 95–107.

10 DONOHUE, D.C. and SALMINEN, S.J. 'Safety of probiotic bacteria', *Asia Pacific J Clin Nutr*, 1996, **5**, 25–8.

11 SAXELIN, M., RAUTELIN, H., SALMINEN, S. and MÄKELÄ, H. 'The safety of commercial product with viable *Lactobacillus* strains', *Inf Dis Clin Practice*, 1996, **5**, 331–5.

12 ADAMS, M.R. and MARTEAU, P. 'On safety of lactic acid bacteria from food', *Int J Food Microbiol*, 1995, **27**, 263–4.

13 SALMINEN, S., OUWEHAND, A.C. and ISOLAURI, E. 'Clinical applications of probiotic bacteria', *Int Dairy J*, 1998, **8**, 563–72.

14 LEE, Y.-K. and SALMINEN, S. 'The coming of age of probiotics', *Trends Food Sci Technol*, 1995, **6**, 241–5.

15 SALMINEN, S., VON WRIGHT, A., LAINE, M., VUOPIO-VARKILA, J., KORHONEN, T. and MATTILA-SANDHOLM, T. 'Development of selection criteria for probiotic strains to assess their potential in functional foods: a Nordic and European approach', *Biosci Microbiol*, 1996, **15** (2), 61–7.

16 SALMINEN, S., VON WRIGHT, A., MORELLI, L., MARTEAU, P., BRASSART, D., DE VOS, W., FONDEN, R., SAXELIN, M., COLLINS, K., MOGENSEN, G., BIRKELAND, S.-E. and MATTILA-SANDHOLM, T. 'Demonstration of safety of probiotics: a review', *Int J Food Microbiol*, 1998, **44** (1–2), 93–106.

17 LEHTO, E.M. and SALMINEN, S. 'Adhesion of two *Lactobacillus* strains, one *Lactococcus* and one *Probionibacterium* strain to cultured intestinal Caco-2 cell line', *Biosci Microflora*, 1997, **16**, 13–17.

18 TUOMOLA, E.M. and SALMINEN, S.J. 'Adhesion of some probiotic and dairy *Lactobacillus* strains to Caco-2 cell cultures', *Int J Food Microbiol*, 1998, **41**, 45–51.

19 ALANDER, M., KORPELA, R., SAXELIN, M., VILPPONEN-SALMELA, T., MATTILA-SANDHOLM, T. and VON WRIGHT, A. 'Recovery of *Lactobacillus rhamnosus* GG from human colonic biopsies', *Lett Appl Microbiol*, 1997, **24**, 361–4.

20 SKYTTÄ, E., HAIKARA, A. and MATTILA-SANDHOLM, T. 'Production and characterization of antibacterial compounds produced by *Pediococcus damnosus* and *Pediococcus pentosaceus*', *J Appl Bacteriol*, 1992, **72**, 134–42.

21 HELANDER, I., VON WRIGHT, A. and MATTILA-SANDHOLM, T. 'Potential of lactic acid bacteria and novel antimicrobials against gram-negative bacteria', *Trends Food Sci Technol*, 1997, **8** (5), 146–50.

22 NIKU-PAAVOLA, M.-L., LATVA-KALA, K., LAITILA, A., MATTILA-SANDHOLM, T. and HAIKARA, A. 'New types of antimicrobial compounds produced by *Lactobacillus plantarum*', *J Appl Microbiol*, 1999, **86**, 29–35.

23 SALMINEN, S., ISOLAURI, E. and SALMINEN, E. 'Probiotics and stabilisation of the gut mucosal barrier', *Asia Pacific J Clin Nutr*, 1996, **5**, 53–6.

24 TOBA, T., VIRKOLA, R., WESTERLUND, B., BJÖRKMAN, Y., SILLANPÄÄ, J., VARTIO, T., KALKKINEN, N. and KORHONEN, T.K. 'A collagen binding S-layer protein in *Lactobacillus crispatus*', *Appl Environ Microbiol*, 1995, **61**, 2467–71.

25 WESTERLUND, B. and KORHONEN, T. 'Bacterial proteins binding to the ammmalian extracellular matrix', *Mol Microbiol*, 1993, **9**, 687–94.

26 TUOMOLA, E.M., OUWEHAND, A.C. and SALMINEN, S. 'Human ileostomy glycoproteins as a model for small intestinal mucus to investigate adhesion of probiotics', *Lett Appl Microbiol*, 1999, **28**, 159–63.

27 HOLZAPFEL, W.H., HABERER, P., SNEL, J., SCHILLINGER, U. and HUIS IN'T VELD, J. 'Overview of gut flora and probiotics', *Int J Food Microbiol*, 1998, **41**, 103–25.

28 MARTEAU, P., POCHART, P., BOUHNIK, Y. and RAMBAUD, J.C. 'Fate and effects of some transiting micro-organisms in the human gastrointestinal tract'. *World Rev Nutr Diet*, 1993, **74**, 1–21.

29 JOHANSSON, M-L., MOLIN, G., JEPPSON, B., NOBAEK, S., AHRNÉ, S. and BENGMARK, S. 'Administration of different *Lactobacillus* strains in fermented oatmeal soup. *In vivo* colonization of human intestinal mucosa and effect on the indigenous flora', *Appl Environ Microbiol*, 1993, **59**, 15–20.

30 MIETTINEN, M., ALANDER, M., VON WRIGHT, A., VUOPIO-VARKILA, J., MARTEAU, P., HUIS IN'T VELD, J. and MATTILA-SANDHOLM, T. 'The survival and immune responses of probiotic strains after passage through a gastrointestinal model', *Microb Ecol Health Dis*, 1998, **10**, 141–7.

31 MIETTINEN, M., VUOPIO-VARKILA, J. and VARKILA, K. 'Production of human tumornecrosis factor alpha, interleukin-6 and interleukin-10 is induced by lactic acid bacteria', *Infect Immun*, 1996, **64** (12), 5403–5.

32 SALMINEN, S. and MATTILA-SANDHOLM, T. 'Screening of effective probiotic strains', *Biosci Microflora,* 1996, **15**, 61–7.

33 ALANDER, M., DE SMET, I., NOLLET, L., VERSTRAETE, W., VON WRIGHT, A. and MATTILA-SANDHOLM, T. 'The effect of probiotic strains on the microbiota of the Simulator of the Human Intestinal Microbial Ecosystem (SHIME)', *Microb Ecol Health Dis,* 1999, **46**, 71–9.

34 HOSONO, A., KASHINA, T. and KADA, T. 'Antimutagenic properties of lactic acid cultured milk on chemical and fecal mutagens', *J Dairy Sci,* 1986, **69**, 2237–42.

35 OUWEHAND, A.C. and SALMINEN, S. 'The health effects of cultured milk products with viable and non-viable bacteria', *Int Dairy J,* 1998, **8**, 749–58.

36 LIDBECK, A., ÖVERVIK, E., RAFTER, J., NORD, C.E. and GUSTAFSSON, J.-Å. 'Effect of *Lactobacillus acidophilus* supplementation on mutagen excretion in faeces and in urine in humans', *Microb Ecol Health Dis,* 1992, **5**, 59–67.

37 VON WRIGHT, A., KORPELA, R., RÄTY, K. and MYKKÄNEN, H. 'High fibre diet, *Lactobacillus* GG supplementation and fecal/urinary mutagenicity', Lactic Acid Bacteria Conference, Cork, Ireland, p. A14, 1995.

38 MORELLI, L., CESENA, C., LUCCHINI, F., CALLEGARI, M.L., ALANDER, M., MATTILA-SANDHOLM, T., VON WRIGHT, A., SALMINEN, S., LEHTO, E. and VILPPONEN-SALMELA, T. 'Role of cell aggregation protein in adhesion *in vitro* and *in vivo*', *Novel Methods for Probiotic Research. 2nd Workshop, FAIR CT96-1028, PROBDEMO,* VTT Symposium 187 (Alander, M., Kauppila, T., Mattila-Sandholm, T., eds), Cork, Ireland, 1997.

39 CESENA, C., MORELLI, L., ALANDER, M., SILJANDER, T., SATOKARI, R., MATTILA-SANDHOLM, T., VILPPONEN-SALMELA, T. and VON WRIGHT, A. '*Lactobacillus crispatus* and its non-aggregating mutant in human colonization trials', *J Appl Environ Microbiol,* in press.

40 TYNKKYNEN, S., SINGH, K.V. and VARMANEN, P. 'Vancomycin resistance factor of *Lactobacillus rhamnosus* GG in relation to enterococcal vancomycin resistance (*van*) genes', *Int J Food Microbiol,* 1998, **41**, 195–204.

41 SALMINEN, S., DEIGHTON, M., BENNO, Y. and GORBACH, S.L. 'Lactic acid bacteria in health and disease'. In S. Salminen and A. von Wright (eds), pp. 211–54, *Lactic Acid Bacteria: Microbiology and Functional Aspects,* New York, Marcel Dekker, 1998.

42 LUCCHINI, F., KMET, V., CESENA, C., COPPI, L., BOTTAZZI, V. and MORELLI, L. 'Specific detection of a probiotic strain in faecal samples by using multiplex PCR', *FEMS Microbiol Lett,* 1998, **158**, 273–8.

43 ALANDER, M., SATOKARI, R., KORPELA, R., SAXELIN, M., VILPPONEN-SALMELA, T., MATTILA-SANDHOLM, T. and VON WRIGHT, A. 'Persistence of colonization of human colonic mucosa by a probiotic strain, *Lactobacillus rhamnosus* GG, after oral consumption', *Appl Environ Microbiol,* 1999, **65**, 351–4.

44 VAUGHAN, E., MOLLET, B. and DE VOS, W. 'Functionality of probiotics and intestinal lactobacilli: light in the intestinal tract tunnel', *Food Biotechnol,* 1999, **10** (5), 505–10.

45 SCHIFFRIN, E., BRASSART, D., SERVIN, A.I., ROCHAT and DONNET-HUGHES, A. 'Immune modulation of blood leukocytes in humans by lactic acid bacteria: criteria for strain selection', *Am J Clin Nutr*, 1997, **66**, 15S–20S.

46 ISOLAURI, E., SALMINEN, S. and MATTILA-SANDHOLM, T. 'New functional foods in the treatment of food allergy', *Ann Med*, 1999, **31** (4), 299–302.

47 MARTEAU, P. and CELLIER, C. 'Rationale for trials using probiotics in inflammatory bowel disease', *Functional Foods for EU Health in 2000, 4th Workshop, FAIR CT96-1028, PROBDEMO*, VTT Symposium 198 (Alander, M., Mattila-Sandholm, T., eds), Rovaniemi, Finland, pp. 35–42, 2000.

48 DUNNE, C., MURPHY, L., FLYNN, S., O'MAHONY, L., O'HALLORAN, S., FEENEY, M., MORRISEY, D., THORNTON, G., FITZGERALD, G., DALY, C., KIELY, B., QUIGLEY, E.M.M., O'SULLIVAN, G., SHANAHAN, F. and COLLINS, J.K. 'Probiotics; from myth to reality – demonstration of functionality in animal models of disease and in human clinical trials', *Antonie van Leeuwenhoek*, 1999, **76**, 279–92.

49 HATAKKA, K., SAVILAHTI, E., SAXELIN, M., PÖNKÄ, A., POUSSA, T., MEURMAN, J.H., NÄSE, L. and KORPELA, R. 'The effect of long-term consumption of a probiotic milk containing *Lactobacillus* GG on the infections of children attending a day care centre', *Functional Foods for EU Health in 2000, 4th Workshop, FAIR CT96-1028, PROBDEMO*, VTT Symposium 198 (Alander, M., Mattila-Sandholm, T., eds), Rovaniemi, Finland, p. 78, 2000.

50 BENNET, R., NORD, C.-E. and MÄTTÖ, J. 'Faecal recovery and absence of side effects in children given *Lactobacillus* F19 or placebo', *Functional Foods for EU Health in 2000, 4th Workshop, FAIR CT96-1028, PROBDEMO*, VTT Symposium 198 (Alander, M., Mattila-Sandholm, T., eds), Rovaniemi, Finland, p. 72, 2000.

51 VIITANEN, M., NORD, C.-E., HAMMARSTRÖM, L., OHLSON, K. and FONDEN, R. '*Lactobacillus* F19 and *Helicobacter pylori* in elderly persons', *Functional Foods for EU Health in 2000, 4th Workshop, FAIR CT96-1028, PROBDEMO*, VTT Symposium 198 (Alander, M., Mattila-Sandholm, T., eds), Rovaniemi, Finland, p. 74, 2000.

52 PELTO, L., LAGSTRÖM, H., KANKAANPÄÄ, P., ISOLAURI, E., FONDEN, R. and SALMINEN, S. 'Safety and tolerance of *Lactobacillus paracasei* F19 in milk-hypersensitive subjects: a pilot study', *Functional Foods for EU Health in 2000, 4th Workshop, FAIR CT96-1028, PROBDEMO*, VTT Symposium 198 (Alander, M., Mattila-Sandholm, T., eds), Rovaniemi, Finland, pp. 75–6, 2000.

53 HAMILTON-MILLER, J., SHAH, S. and WINKLER, J. 'Public health issues arising from microbiological and labelling quality of foods and supplements containing probiotic microrganisms', *Public Health Nutrition*, 1999, **2**, 223–9.

54 FONDEN, R., GRENOV, B., RENIERO, R., SAXELIN, M. and BIRKELAND, S.E. 'Technological aspects for probiotics, industrial panel statements', *Functional Foods for EU Health in 2000, 4th Workshop, FAIR CT96-1028, PROBDEMO*, VTT Symposium 198 (Alander, M., Mattila-Sandholm, T., eds), Rovaniemi, Finland, pp. 43–50, 2000.

55 MYLLÄRINEN, P., FORSSELL, P., VON WRIGHT, A., ALANDER, M. and MATTILA-SANDHOLM, T. 'The use of starch as a capsulation material for lactic acid bacteria', *Functional Food Research in Europe, 3rd workshop, FAIR CT96-1028, PROBDEMO,* VTT Symposium 187 (Mattila-Sandholm, T., Kauppila, T., eds), Haikko, Finland, p. 91, 1998.

56 MYLLÄRINEN, P., FORSSELL, P., WRIGHT, A., ALANDER, M., MATTILA-SAND-HOLM, T. and POUTANEN, K. 'The use of starch as a capsulation material for lactic acid bacteria', *International Meeting of Production and Uses of Starch,* Wellesbourne, Edinburgh, Warwick Association of Applied Biologists, 1998.

57 SIITONEN, S., VAPAATALO, H., SALMINEN, S., GORDIN, A. SAXELIN, M., WIKBERG, R. and KIRKKOLA, A.L. 'Effect of *Lactobacillus* GG yoghurt in prevention of antibiotic associated diarrhea', *Ann Med,* 1990, **22**, 57–9.

58 GOLDIN, B., GORBACH, S.L., SAXELIN, M., BARAKAT, S., GUALTIERI, L. and SALMINEN, S. 'Survival of *Lactobacillus* species (strain GG) in human gastrointestinal tract', *Dig Dis Sci,* 1992, **37**, 121–8.

59 KAILA, M., ISOLAURI, E., SOPPI, E., VIRTANEN, E., LAINE, S. and ARVILOMMI, H. 'Enhancement of the circulating antibody secreting cell response in human diarrhea by a human *Lactobacillus* strain', *Pediatr Res,* 1992, **32**, 141–4.

60 HOSODA, M., HE, F., HIRAMATU, M., HASHIMOTO, H. and BENNO, Y. 'Effects of *Lactobacillus* GG intake on fecal microflora and defecation in healthy volunteers', *Bifidus,* 1994, **8**, 21–8.

61 ISOLAURI, E., JUNTUNEN, M., RAUTANEN, T., SILLANAUKEE, P. and KOIVULA, T. 'A human *Lactobacillus* strain (*Lactobacillus casei* sp. strain GG) promotes recovery from acute diarrhoea in children', *Pediatrics,* 1991, **88**, 90–7.

62 ISOLAURI, E., KAILA, M., MYKKÄNEN, H., LING, W.H. and SALMINEN, S. 'Oral bacteriotherapy for viral gastroenteritis', *Dig Dis Sci,* 1994, **39**, 2595–600.

63 MAJAMAA, H., ISOLAURI, E., SAXELIN, M. and VESIKARI, T. 'Lactic acid bacteria in the treatment of acute rotavirus gastroenteritis', *J Pediatr Gastroenterol Nutr,* 1995, **20**, 333–8.

64 RAZA, S., GRAHAM, S.M., ALLEN, S.J., SULTANA, S., CUEVAS, L. and HART, C.A. '*Lactobacillus* GG promotes recovery from acute nonbloody diarrhea in Pakistan', *Pediatr Infect Dis J,* 1995, **14**, 107–11.

65 HILTON, E., KOLAKOWSKI, P., SINGER, C. and SMITH, M. 'Efficacy of *Lactobacillus* GG as a diarrhea preventative', *J Travel Med,* 1997, **4**, 41–3.

66 SHORNIKOVA, A.V., ISOLAURI, E., BURKANOVA, L., LUKOVNIKOVA, S. and VESIKARI, T. 'A trial in Karelian republic of oral rehydration and *Lactobacillus* GG for treatment of acute diarrhoea', *Acta Paediatr,* 1997, **86**, 460–5.

67 PELTO, L., ISOLAURI, E., LILIUS, E.M., NUUTILA, J. and SALMINEN, S. 'Probiotic bacteria down-regulate the milk-induced inflammatory response in milk-hypersensitive subjects but have an immunostimulatory effect in healthy subjects', *Clin Exp Allergy,* 1998, **28**, 1474–9.

68 RAUTANEN, T., ISOLAURI, E., SALO, E. and VESIKARI, T. 'Management of acute diarrhoea with low osmolarity oral rehydration solution and *Lactobacillus*

strain GG', *Arc Dis Child,* 1998, **79**, 157–60.

69 ARVOLA, T., LAIHO, K., TORKKELI, S., MYKKÄNEN, H., SALMINEN, S., MAUNULA, L. and ISOLAURI, E. 'Prophylactic *Lactobacillus* GG reduces antibiotic-associated diarrhea in children with respiratory infections: a randomized study', *Pediatrics,* 1999, **104**, e64.

70 LINK-AMSTER, H., ROCHAT, F., SAUDAN, K.Y., MIGNOT, O. and AESCHLIMAN, J.M. 'Modulation of a specific humoral immune response and changes in intestinal flora mediated through fermented milk intake', *FEMS Immunol Med Microbiol,* 1994, **10**, 55–63.

71 SCHIFFRIN, E.J., ROCHAT, F., LINK-ANGLER, H., AESCHLIMANN, J.M. and DONNET-HUGHES, A. 'Immuno-modulation of human blood cells following the ingestion of lactic acid bacteria', *J Dairy Sci,* 1995, **78**, 491–7.

72 MARTEAU, P., VAERMAN, J.P., DEHENNIN, J.P., BORD, S., BRASSART, D., POCHART, P., DESJEUX, J.F. and RAMBAUD, J.C. 'Effects of intrajejunal perfusion and chronic ingestion of *Lactobacillus johnsonii* strain La1 on serum concentrations and jejunal secretions of immunoglobulins and serum proteins in healthy humans', *Gastroentérologie Clinique et Biologique,* 1997, **21** 293–8.

73 MICHETTI, P., DORTA, G., WIESEL, P.H., BRASSART, D., VERDU, E., HERRANZ, M., FELLEY, C., PORTA, N., ROUVET, M., BLUM, A.L. and CORTHESY-THEULAZ, I. 'Effect of whey-based culture supernatant of *Lactobacillus acidophilus (johnsonii)* La1 on *Helicobacter pylori* infection in humans', *Digestion,* 1999, **60**, 203–9.

74 DONNET-HUGHES, A., ROCHAT, F., SERRANT, P., AESCHLIMANN, J.M. and SCHIFFRIN, J.E. 'Modulation of nonspecific mechanisms of defense by lactic acid bacteria: effective dose', *J Dairy Sci,* 1999, **82**, 863–9.

75 BLACK, F.T., ANDERSEN, P.L., ORSKOV, J., ORSKOV, F., GAARSLEV, K. and LAULUND, S. 'Prophylactic efficacy of lactobacilli on traveller's diarrhoea'. In *Travel Medicine,* 1st Conference on international travel medicine, April 1988, Zurich, Switzerland, Berlin, New York, Springer-Verlag Company, 1989, 333–5.

76 BLACK, F., EINARSSON, K., LIDBECK, A., ORRHAGE, K. and NORD, C.E. 'Effect of lactic acid producing bacteria on the human intestinal microflora during ampicillin treatment', *Scand J Infect Dis,* 1991, **23**, 247–54.

77 MARTEAU, P., POCHART, P., FLOURIE, B., PELLIER, P., SANTOS, L., DESJEUX, J.F. and RAMBAUD, J.C. 'Effect of chronic ingestion of a fermented dairy product containing *Lactobacillus acidophilus* and *Bifidobacterium bifidum* on metabolic activities of the colonic flora in humans', *Am J Clin Nutr,* 1990, **52**, 685–8.

78 ALM, L., RYD-KJELLEN, E., SETTERBERG, G. and BLOMQUIST, L. 'Effect of a new fermented milk product "Cultura" on constipation in geriatric patients', 1st Lactic Acid Bacteria Computer Conference, 1993.

79 SAAVEDRA, J.M., BAUMAN, N.A., OUNG, I., PERMAN, J.A. and YOLKEN, R.H. 'Feeding of *Bifidobacterium bifidum* and *Streptococcus thermophilus* to infants in hospital for prevention of diarrhea and shedding of rotavirus',

Lancet, 1994, **344**, 1046–9.

80 FUKUSHIMA, Y., KAWATA, Y., HARA, H., TERADA, A. and MITSUOKA, T. 'Effect of a probiotic formula on intestinal immunoglobulin A production in healthy children', *Int J Food Microbiol*, 1998, **42**, 39–44.

81 WOLF, B.W., GARLEB, D.G. and CASAS, I. 'Safety and tolerance of *Lactobacillus reuteri* in healthy adult male subjects', *Microb Ecol Health Dis*, 1995, **8**, 41–50.

82 SHORNIKOVA, A.V., CASAS, I.A., MYKKÄNEN, H. and VESIKARI, T. 'Bacteriotherapy with *Lactobacillus reuteri* in rotavirus gastroenteritis', *Pediatr Infect Dis*, 1997, **16**, 1103–7.

83 SHORNIKOVA, A.V., CASAS, I., ISOLAURI, E., MYKKÄNEN, H. and VESIKARI, T. '*Lactobacillus reuteri* as a therapeutic agent in acute diarrhea in young children', *J Ped Gastroenterol Nutr*, 1997, **24**, 399–404.

84 WOLF, B.W., WHEELER, K.B., ATAYA, D.G. and GARLEB, K.A. 'Safety and tolerance of *Lactobacillus reuteri* supplementation to a population infected with human immunodeficiency virus', *Food Chem Toxicol*, 1998, **36**, 1085–94.

85 ASO, Y. and AKAZAN, H. 'Prophylactic effect of a *Lactobacillus casei* preparation on the recurrence of superficial bladder cancer', *Urol Int*, 1992, **49**, 125–9.

86 TANAKA, R. and OHWAKI, M.A. 'Controlled study on the ingestion of *Lactobacillus casei* fermented milk on the intestinal microflora, its microbiology and immune system in healthy adults', *Proceedings of XII Riken Symposium on Intestinal Flora*, Tokyo, Japan. pp. 85–104, 1994.

87 ASO, Y., AKAZAN, H., KOTAKE, T., TSUKAMOTO, T., IMAI, K. and NAITO, S. 'Preventive effect of a *Lactobacillus casei* preparation on the recurrence of superficial bladder cancer in a double-blind trial', *Eur Urol*, 1995, **27**, 104–9.

88 SPANHAAK, S., HAVENAAR, R. and SCHAAFSMA, G. 'The effect of consumption of milk fermented by *Lactobacillus casei* strain Shirota on the intestinal microflora and immune parameters in humans', *Eur J Clin Nutr*, 1998, **52**, 899–907.

89 JOHANSSON, M.-L., NOBAEK, S., BERGGREN, A., NYMAN, M., BJÖRCK, I., AHRNE, S., JEPPSSON, B. and MOLIN, G. 'Survival of *Lactobacillus plantarum* DSM 9843 (299v), and effect on the short-chain fatty acid content of faeces after ingestion of a rose-hip drink with fermented oats', *Int J Food Microbiol*, 1998, **42**, 29–38.

90 SURAWICZ, C.M., ELMER, G.W., SPEELMAN, P., MCFARLAND, L., CHINN, J. and VAN BELLE, G. 'Prevention of antibiotic-associated diarrhea by *Saccharomyces boulardii*. A prospective study', *Gastroenterol*, 1989, **84**, 981–8.

91 MCFARLAND, L.V., SURAWICZ, C.M. and GREENBERG, R.N. 'A randomised placebo-controlled trial of *Saccharomyces boulardii* in combination with standard antibiotics for *Clostridium difficile* disease', *JAMA*, 1994, **271**, 1913–18.

92 BLEICHNER, G., BLEHAUT, H., MENTEC, H. and MOYSE, D. '*Saccharomyces boulardii* prevents diarrhea in critically ill tube-fed patients. A multicenter, randomized, double-blind placebo-controlled trial', *Intensive Care Med*, 1997, **23**, 517–23.

93 MOLLY, K. 'Development, validation and application of a simulation of the gastrointestinal microbial ecosystem', PhD thesis, University of Ghent. Appl. Biol. Sciences, Section Cell- and Genebiotechnology, 1995.

13

Dietary fibre functional products

F. Guillon (URPOI, Centre de Recherches INRA, Nantes),
M. Champ (UFDNH, Centre de Recherches INRA, Nantes),
J.-F. Thibault (URPOI, Centre de Recherches INRA, Nantes)

13.1 Introduction

The term 'dietary fibre' was first coined in 1953 by Hispley to describe plant cell wall components of foods, which he suggested to be protective against toxemia during pregnancy. However, the dietary fibre hypothesis really emerged in the 1970s from medical workers working on the relationships between diet and incidence of chronic disease, in particular the role of polysaccharides in the diet (Walker 1974, Burkitt 1983, Burkitt and Trowell 1975). For more than two decades, data regarding the beneficial effects of dietary fibre have been accumulating. These materials may participate in the regulation of the gastrointestinal motility, influence glucose and lipid metabolism, promote faecal ouput, stimulate bacterial metabolic activity, detoxify the colon luminal contents and contribute towards maintaining the equilibrium of the colon ecosystem and integrity of intestinal mucosa (FAO/WHO 1997, Cherbut *et al.* 1995, Guillon *et al.* 1998a, Kritchevesky and Bonfield 1995, Rémésy 1996, Schweizer and Edwards 1992, Southgate *et al.* 1991). In this respect, dietary fibre can fit the definition of functional food by the fact that it can affect one or more targeted functions in the body in a positive manner (Diplock *et al.* 1999).

However, despite the tremendous amount of work carried out all over the world, the mechanisms of actions on the functions of the body are not fully understood. A major finding is that it is not only the amount but also the type of dietary fibre that influences physiological response to intake, although emphasis remains on increased dietary fibre intake. The physicochemical properties of dietary fibre and their digestive fate have been shown to play a key role in gut function. These properties are related to the source, the processing history of fibre and the form by which it is ingested. Dietary fibre may be present in the diet as plant cell walls or as isolated molecules, endogenous or supplement constituents of food. The chemical structure of dietary constituents and the way the molecules assemble are important in determining their properties. During processing, major changes can occur in the architecture of plant cell walls and in structural features of individual molecules, which can markedly affect fibre properties, food properties and dietary response.

13.2 Defining dietary fibre

The definition of dietary fibre has been a matter of controversy and, today, it is still not fully agreed upon by experts in the field. Over the years, several definitions have been used based on different concepts (Tables 13.1 and 13.2). These definitions can be grouped into three main views. The first relies on a 'botanical' view; and regards dietary fibre as mainly plant cell walls constituents. The second group of definitions is based on a chemical view and

Table 13.1   Different definitions of dietary fibre (from Dysseler 1997)

Authors	Polymers included in the definition
Trowell 1972	Cellulose, lignin, hemicelluloses, pectins (skeletal remains of plant cells)
Trowell 1974	Cell wall polysaccharides + lignin + unavailable associated substances (cutin, suberin, phytic acids)
Trowell *et al.* 1976	Unavailable storage polysaccharides + cell-wall polysaccharides + lignin
Southgate *et al.* 1978	Unavailable polysaccharides + lignin
Southgate *et al.* 1981	Non-starch polysaccharides + lignin
Cummings and Englyst 1987	Non-starch polysaccharides

Table 13.2   Suggested definition by organisation or countries (from Dysseler 1997)

Organisation or countries	Definition and constituents of dietary fibre
COST (1994)	Lignin, inositolphosphate, resistant starch, oligosaccharides, plant cell-wall polysaccharides, inulin, polydextrose
CIAA (1992)	Organic constituents non-hydrolysed by human digestive enzymes
CEEREAL (1993)	Indigestible polysaccharides + lignin
Belgium (1993)	Indigestible oligo + indigestible polysaccharides + lignin
Croatia, Germany, Norway and Sweden (1993)	Indigestible polysaccharides + lignin
Scientific Committee for Foods (1994)	Oligosaccharides and polysaccharides and hydrophilic derivatives that are not digested and not absorbed in the upper gut of humans, including lignin

on related methods used for the measurement of dietary fibre in food. It includes mostly non-starch polysaccharides. The last is based on the physiological and nutritional consequences of eating dietary fibre; the definition includes all polysaccharide and lignin that resist digestion in the upper gastrointestinal tract. Recently, this definition has been expanded to include oligosaccharides not digested in the small intestine.

This last definition seems to be the most consensual, although it is difficult to formalise in a precise legalistic sense. It includes a wide array of compounds (Table 13.3) that vary in chemical structure, and properties: non-starch polysaccharides from plant cell walls, lignin but also gums, microbial polysaccharides, inulin, resistant starch and oligosaccharides.

Resistant starch (RS) is a particular case. The definition suggested by the group of experts relies on a physiological concept. RS is defined as the sum of starch and the products of starch degradation not absorbed in the small intestine of healthy individuals (Asp 1992, Asp et al. 1996). As a matter of fact there are many reasons why starch may be incompletely digested and absorbed during passage through the digestive tract. It can be divided into extrinsic or intrinsic factors. Extrinsic factors are related to the environment of starch in food, for example enclosure in intact cells. Intrinsic factors refer to the characteristics of the starch, resistant native starch granules, chemically modified starches, and retrograded starch occurring in processed foods. The predominant methods used for determination of total dietary fibre (TDF) (AOAC 1995) lead to an underestimation of resistant starch. Alternative analytical methods have been proposed to predict the ileal digestibility of starch in healthy subjects. They have been validated on the basis of in vivo data (Champ et al. 1999) or ileostomates (Asp et al. 1996). These methods are not exempt from criticism and none of them presently available has been shown to measure all RS.

Non-digestible oligosaccharides, also referred to as resistant oligosaccharides, are defined based on physiological (they resist hydrolysis by acid and enzymes in the upper gut due the nature of their glycosidic linkages) and chemical criteria (degree of polymerisation). The precise boundary between oligosaccharides and polysaccharides is arbitrary but generally oligosaccharides are defined as saccharides containing from 3 to 10 monosaccharides (< 10: FAO/WHO 1997; 10: Asp et al. 1992, Cho et al. 1999, Voragen 1998). This definition includes oligosaccharides with prebiotic properties with a degree of polymerisation in the range 3–10. Some of the most important oligosaccharides are fructoligosaccharides and alpha galactosides. The predominant methods used for the determination of total dietary fibre do not measure oligosaccharides because of their ethanol/water solubility. Specific enzymatic or HPLC methods have been employed to measure oligosaccharides directly in foods (Coussement 1999). Adaptations of the AOAC method have been applied with success to determine oligofructosaccharides in foods (Dysseler et al. 1999).

Table 13.3 Classification and chemical characteristics of the main dietary fibres. (Adapted from Lineback 1999, Dreher 1999.)

Class	Components	Structure (bonds backbone) in	Main sources
Polysaccharides of cell walls in higher plants	Cellulose	β-D- glucan (4-linked)	No fractionated plant material
	Hemicelluloses	Xyloglucans (4-linked D-glucans with attached side chains)	Dicotyledons
		Xylans (β-D-4 linked)	Dicotyledons
		Arabinoxylans-Glucuronoarabinoxylans	Monocotyledons
		Mixed linkage β-D-glucan (3- and 4-linked)	Monocotyledons, more abundant in barley, oat grains
	Pectic substances	Galacturonans and rhamnogalacturonans Arabinan(alpha-L-5 linked, with attached side chains) Arabinogalactan 1 (beta-D-4 linked galactan with attached side chains)	Dicotyledons
Other molecules	Lignin	Complex polyphenolic polymer	Mature plants
Hydrocolloids from seaweed extracts	Carageenans	Sulfated polymers composed of galactose and anhydrogalactose	Red seaweeds, mainly *Chondrus crispus*
	Alginates	Polymers of D-mannuronic and L guluronic acids, monomers occur in blocks	Brown seaweeds; mainly *Laminaria digitata, Stipes of Laminaria hyperborea, Ascophyllum nodosum Fucus serratus*
Microbial sources	Xanthan gum	Backbone identical to cellulose with trisaccharide side-chains composed of alpha D mannose, beta-D-glucuronic acid and a terminal beta-D mannose	*Xanthomonas campestris*

Category	Name	Structure	Origin
	Gellan gum	Linear backbone composed of 1,3-beta-D-glucose, 1,4-beta-D-glucuronic acid, 1,4 beta-D-glucose and 1,4-alpha D rhamnose	*Pseudomonas elodea*
Plant exudates	Gum arabic	Structure close to arabinogalactan of type II with more complex side chains	From different species of acacia
	Gum Karaya	Structure close to pectins; side chains containing glucuronic acid	*Sterculia*
	Gum tragacanth	Pectic and arabinogalactan II structures	*Astragalus gummifer*
Seeds extracts	Guar gum	Galactomannan, ratio D-galactose to D-mannose : 1 : 2	Endosperm of leguminosae seeds *Cyamopsis teragonolobus*
	Locust bean (carob) gum	Galactomannan, ratio D-galactose to D-mannose : 1 : 4	*Cerotona siliqua*
	Psyllium	Polysaccharide composed of arabinose, xylose and galacturonic acid	*Plantago ovata*
Roots extracts	Konjac	Acetylated glucomannan	*Amorphophallus konjac*
Modified cellulose and pectins	Modified cellulose	Carboxymethyl cellulose Methyl cellulose Hydroxypropylmethyl cellulose	
	Pectins	Low and high methyl esterified Amidated pectins	Apple pomace, citrus peel
Resistant starches	Physical trapped starches	Alpha1-4,1-6-linked glucose units	Whole grains, legume seeds and cereals

Table 13.3 Continued

Class	Components	Structure (bonds backbone) in	Main sources
	Resistant starch granules	Native starches having a B-type X ray diffraction pattern	Raw potato, green banana; high amylose starches
	Retrograded amylose		High amylose starch
Oligosaccharides	Fructo-oligosaccharides	Oligosaccharides mainly composed of fructose, (Glucosyl (fructosyl)$_n$ fructose)	Extracted from chicory roots (Raftilose®) or enzymatically synthesised from saccharose (Actilight®, Neosugar)
	α-galactosides (raffinose, stachyose, verbascose)	Saccharose (galactose)$_n$ = from 1 to 3	Pulse (beans, lentils, peas)

13.3 Sources of dietary fibre

Within food systems, dietary fibre is found in two main forms: as intrinsic constituents of various plant foods or as additions as a supplement. As supplements, they can be used as ingredients (> 5%) or additives (< 5%).

13.3.1 Endogeneous

Cereals and cereal products, roots, tubers, vegetables, nuts and fruits are all sources of dietary fibre. When considering dietary fibre in these foods, it is mainly the role of cell walls that is being considered. The cell wall is a dynamic complex structure surrounding the plant cells, exterior to the plasmalemma. The composition and the properties are constantly adapted to growth, differentiation and variations in the environment of the cell. Schematically, cell walls can be divided into two classes: primary cell walls are those deposited by growing plant cells; they are thin and hydrated. The primary cell wall of most flowering plants is a composite polymeric structure in which crystalline cellulose interlocked with xyloglucans is embedded in a matrix of pectic polysaccharides, with a small amount of the structural proteins intercalated in the matrix (Carpita and Gibeaut 1993, Cosgrove 1997, Selvendran and Robertson 1990).

The individual macromolecules are held together by covalent, ionic, hydrogen bonds and van der Waals forces. Physical enmeshment may also be involved. Cellulose plays a major role in determining the strength of the cell wall; xyloglucans may bind tightly to the surface of cellulose and act as a lubricating agent to prevent cellulose aggregation. Pectins are thought to determine the porosity of the cell walls and thus limit the diffusion of molecules through the walls; they may control the charge environment of microdomains in the cell walls; they may be involved in the defence response of the plant against invading organisms. Primary cell walls can vary in composition, thickness and morphology, depending on the source and physiological stage of the plant. This type of wall is found in parenchymatous tissue, which is the major tissue of the pulp of fruits and vegetables. In grasses, the branched arabinoxylans and mixed linked beta glucans are thought to play the role that xyloglucans play in dicotyledons (Carpita and Gibeaut 1993).

As primary cell walls cease growth, the walls become thicker by deposition of more layers of matrix polysaccharides and cellulose. They can be impregnated with lignin to form stiff and uncompressible walls. The cells with thickened walls have specialised functions, providing rigidity, transporting water and nutrients or protecting the plant from desiccation or predators. They are part of the epidermis, collenchyma, sclerenchyma and vascular conducting tissues. These tissues generally may contribute a small amount of the plant material ingested but may also play a major role in the physical effects of fibre.

Some substances such as cutin, suberin, complex internal ester of hydroxy aliphatic acids may be deposited at the epidermal or subepidermal surface of organs (stems, leaves or roots, tubers). They prevent water loss and impede microbial digestion of the external walls.

Physically inaccessible starch found in partly milled grains and seeds and starchy foods cooked and cooled can be regarded as a natural source of RS. Fructans such as inulin and fructoligosaccharides occur as photosynthetic products of storage in a number of plants such as Jerusalem artichokes, onions, asparagus, chicory, leek, garlic. In Jerusalem artichokes and onions, they may account for up to 60–70% of the dry matter.

Another example of naturally occurring oligosaccharides are the alpha galactosides (Voragen 1998). Alpha galactosides derived from sucrose (raffinose, stachyose, verbascose) are mainly in leguminous seeds. They account for 2–8% of the dry matter. Another group of alpha galactosides in legumes are glucose galactosides (melibiose and mannitriose) and inositol galactosides (galactinol, galactopinitol, ciceritol). Ciceritol has been reported as the major alpha galctosides in chickpeas (Quemener and Brillouet 1983, Bernabé et al. 1993). In seeds, the exact role(s) of alpha galactosides is not clearly established. It has been suggested that they may be storage molecules as they disappear at the onset of sprouting. They can also participate in the protection of seed against desiccation and freezing. There are some differences between flatulence-inducing potential alpha galactosides. Ciceritol may be less flatogenic than sucrose galactosides (Fleming 1981).

We consume different organs of the plant, and each contain a range of different tissues and cell types (Table 13.4). These different levels of organisation must be taken into account to further understand the behaviour of fibre under processing and their physiological implications.

13.3.2 Supplements

Concentrates

Fibre concentrates arise mainly from the processing of fruit, vegetable, legume or cereal sources (Guillon and Thibault 1996). Fibre concentrates are, by definition, fibre enriched. Concentrated sources of dietary fibre from fruits and vegetables can be obtained through dehydration processes. These concentrates potentially can be used as ingredients for high fibre products. The appearance of the ingredient and its functionality will depend on the fibre matrix and changes induced by the treatments. Heated force air dehydration can lead to some collapses of the cell walls while freeze-drying, or instant controlled depression can better preserve the walls and thus the appearance and texture of the product.

Concentrates can also be co-products of agricultural and food by-products. They result from mechanical treatment aiming at separating different tissues in plant material or from extraction processes for isolating particular components such as pectins, starch, proteins or juice.

Bran from cereals is the coarse outer layer of the kernel and is generally separated from cleaned and scoured grains during milling. In parboiled rice, the harvested rice is subjected to soaking and steaming before being dried and milled. Oat bran is probably the most popular bran product. It has been introduced, with success, into reduced-calorie breads, baked goods, beverages

Table 13.4 Structure of plant foods. (Adapted from Southgate 1995.)

Plant foods	Main tissues present
Cereal foods	
Flours, product derived from flours	Thin wall structures from the endosperm extensively broken
Whole grains	Grains almost intact; the cellular structure is retained
Brans	Thicker, more lignified walls (pericarp, seed coat, nucellar layer) with small amounts of endospermal walls (aleurone, layer, some amount of the starch endosperm)
Fruits	For the most part undifferentiated parenchymatous tissues with small amount of lignified vascular tissues. Outer skin cutinised
Leafy vegetables	Parenchymatous tissues and variable amounts of vascular and support tissues.
Leaves, petioles, stems and associated structures such as flowers	Outer tissues cutinised and may be suberinised
Seed legumes	Thick, not lignified seed coats which are cutinised
	The cotyledons (or endospermal tissues) with rather thick walls compared to those encountered in the cereal endosperm
Tubers	Suberinised skin; thin wall undifferentiated cells with storage polysaccharides. Vascular lignified tissues in small amount
Roots	Outer tissues often suberinised; most of the time undifferentiated tissues except in mature roots where vascular lignified tissues may be significantly developed

and meat substitutes. Rice bran may be as effective as oat bran in lowering blood cholesterol and this has stimulated interest for the product. It can be added to baked goods, breads, snacks and extruded foodstuffs. Seed legumes are also a source of fibre concentrate, obtained from milled or dehulled seeds fractionated to obtain starch and protein concentrates. Two types of fibre with distinct characteristics are generated: from the hulls and the residual cotyledons.

Sugar fibre can derive from sugar beet pulp, co-product from the sugar beet industry or directly produced from the beet root as starting material. In the first two cases, the roots are first washed to eliminate the bulk of sand and process to extract sucrose. In the latter case, the process is adapted to minimise or avoid colour and odour formation during processing. In the first case, the beet pulp is further treated to remove taste, colour and odour. Then the fibre is dried. Several processe have been patented and sugar beet fibre is now available on the market under various trade names.

The precursors of fruit fibre concentrates correspond mostly to the tissues produced upon expression of fruit juice. The pulp is generally extensively washed to remove residual sugars and then dried. Generally they exhibit unique flavour and taste.

The composition and properties of these fibres depend on the major constitutive tissues, and preservation of the cell integrity on the processing (Table 13.5) they are going through. Concentrates are generally incorporated into foods to increase the dietary fibre content of food. Fibre ingredients that exhibit high water retention capacity can be used as bulking agents or fat replacers (Table 13.6). Depending on their end use, many of the fibre ingredients are undergoing further processing to improve their functionality and, therefore, extend their use.

Isolates
Isolates are obtained either by extraction in liquid medium, purification and recovery of one type of polysaccharides (pectins, alginates, carrageenans, beta glucans inulin, alpha galactosides), by drying and grinding of native exsudates (arabic, ghatti gums) or by organic synthesis (polydextrose). The extraction conditions differ according to the polysaccharides extracted. Guar and carob gum flours are prepared from milled cotyledons. Beta glucan preparations (oat gum) can be obtained by wet milling of oat grain. Many of the isolated polysaccharides find industrial applications as techno-functional ingredients (thickening agents or emulsion stabilisers) (see Table 13.6). In this context, they are used at set concentrations (usually 0.5–2.0%). The incorporation in high amounts of polysaccharides with texturing properties, apart from necessitating adaptation of the formulation and technology, may have detrimental effects on the organoleptic properties of the end products.

The major products sold as cellulose fibre preparation are derived from woody plants through pulping and bleaching process. The bleached cellulose pulp is a white product, which may then be dried and mechanically sized (Ang and Miller 1991). The manufacturing processes likely differ between

Table 13.5 Chemical composition of some fibre concentrates

Fibre	TDF	Rha-Fuc	Ara	Xyl	Man	Gal	Glc*	Uronic acid	Lignin	Starch	Proteins	Ashes
Wheat bran[1]	50.4	nd	9.6	16.5	1.3	1.2	11.0 (98%)	6.6	2.6	18.6	15.8	4.0
Oat bran[2]	86.2	nd	4.1	26.3	0.1	1.2	45.2 (83%)	nd	14.9	nd	4.5	5.6
Maize bran[2]	71.9	nd	4.5	8.6	0.1	1.2	56.4 (94%)	nd	1.2	nd	8.8	2.1
Barley bran[2]	72.6	nd	6.3	21.7	0.1	0.7	33.5 (84%)	nd	10.4	nd	9.4	6.9
Apple fibre[3]	83.3	1.1	6.8	4.9	1.3	4.0	22.2	20.6	nd	7.0	6.2	1.2
Citrus fibre[3]	76.0	1.3	8.0	2.7	2.0	6.0	20.6	30.0	nd	traces	7.0	5.1
Soy fibre (cotyledon)[4]	79.8	3.6	12.9	4.7	1.2	27.0	12.4	15.8	nd	nd	nd	nd
Soy fibre (hull)[4]	75.6	1.3	5.7	9.4	5.4	2.8	39.9	10.2	nd	nd	nd	nd
Sugar beet[3]	76.8	1.0	19.5	1.4	1.4	4.1	18.0	19.0	1.8	traces	9.6	4.7
Pea fibre (hull)[5]	91.5	0.9	4.2	14.6	1.0	1.2	45.1	12.7	nd	0.0	3.8	1.7

Notes:
[1] Ralet et al. 1990;
[2] Schimberni et al. 1982;
[3] Cloutour, 1995;
[4] Lo, 1989;
[5] Ralet et al. 1993
* non-starch glucose. () percentage of cellulosic glucose, nd: not determined

Table 13.6 Some examples of fibre preparations used as ingredients

Fibres	Reference	Supplier	Characteristics	Physiological effects
Oat fibre	Oat fibre herbacel HF 01-HF 07	Herbafood Nahrungsmittell	88–98% total dietary fibre, mainly insoluble Colour: white Flavour: neutral Available in different particle size Water retention capacity: 7g H2O g/g dry matter Application: bakery goods, meat products With a combination of low viscosity pectins in beverages	
Wheat fibre	Vitacel wheat fibre	JRS	98% total dietary fibre Colour: white Flavour/taste: neutral Available in different particle size Water retention capacity: from 3.5 to 7.4g H2O g/g dry matter according to the particle size Applications: baked goods, processed meat, fish, pasta extruded product, sausage	
Orange fibre	Vitacel orange fibre	JRS	60% dietary fibre, about half as soluble Colour: bright yellow Flavour and taste: slightly bitter Available in different particle size Water retention capacity: about 8 g H2O g/g dry matter Applications: fruit preparations, snacks, dry baked goods, fruit and candy bars, muesli bars; fine particle size: beverages, sauces	
Soy fibre	Fibrarich	VaessenSchoemaker Chemische Industrie	50% dietary fibre Colour: light cream Aroma/flavour: bland	

Source	Product	Company	Properties	Effect
Carob fibre		Carob General Applications	High water retention capacity. Applications: structure improver in a wide range of cooked products. Insoluble fibre. Many applications	Hypocholesterolemic effect
Apple	Pomelite	Val de Vire	Soluble fibre. Colourless. Brings viscosity to the final products (less than commercial pectins at the same concentration). Stability maximal at pH 4 at low temperature. Applications: fruit beverages, dairy products, fresh dessert, apple sauce, compotes and fruit desserts	Regulation of carbohydrate assimilation
Pectins	HerbapektSF50	Herbafood Nahrungsmittell	Pectins with low viscosity. Up to 5–10%	
Acacia gum	Fibregum	CNI	Soluble fibre. Tasteless. Low viscosity. Resistance to hot temperature, acidic medium	
Acacia gum	Valfibre	Valmar	80% of dietary fibre. Soluble. Odourless. Tasteless. Low viscosity	Non-cariogenic. Low-calorie ingredients
Inulin	Frutafit	Sensus	Soluble fibre	
Fructologosaccharides	Raftilose	Orafti Active Food Ingredients	Soluble fibre. Application: biscuits, dairy products, ice cream	

manufacturers resulting in final product with distinct chemical or physical properties. Variations of the final product also may be ascribed to differences in the starting material. Powdered cellulose can be promoted for reducing calories in foods, while maintaining the texture, structure and mouth feel of the product. Cellulose can be chemically modified to produce water-soluble cellulose gums. The chemically modified celluloses include carboxymethyl cellulose, methyl cellulose and hydroxypropylmethyl cellulose. They are generally used as additives and can improve stability in baked goods and sauces. Because of filming properties, some cellulose derivatives are used as binders in food matrices and may serve as oil barrier for fried products.

Several patents have been filed over the last few years for the production of RS (Würsch 1999). Generally, starch is heated in water more than 100°C to hydrate and gelatinise and then cooled for a sufficient time to retrograde and form RS. The yield of RS mainly depends on the amylose content, and amylose-rich starches (amylomaize, high amylose pea or barley starches) are generally preferred as starting materials. The yield of RS can be increased by playing on various processing steps (debranching of the gelatinised starch and fractionation, extrusion cooking after high temperature gelatinisation) and conditions (concentration, temperature, storage time). Yield can be finally improved by subsequent hydrolysis of the unretrograded starch with enzymes. The final product is a bland white powder with no flavour or taste. RS can be incorporated into foods as bulking agent, dietary fibre or fat mimetic.

Polydextrose is prepared by vacuum thermal polymerisation of glucose using sorbitol as a plasticiser and citric acid as catalyst (Craig *et al.* 1999). The average degree of polymerisation is about 12. It can be used in foods as functional ingredients (sugar and partial fat replacer, humectant, cryoprotectant, freezing point depression) or as dietary fibre.

Fructo-oligosaccharides are prepared enzymatically from inulin (enzymatic hydrolysis) or sucrose (transglycosylation) (De Leenheer 1996, Coussement 1999). They are mainly used as dietary fibres (prebiotic effects). As a technological agent, they can help to reduce sucrose and fat content while maintaining texture and mouth feel of the product (dairy products, ice cream, sorbet). Enzymatic hydrolysis processes can also be applied to produce oligosaccharides from plant cell wall polysaccharides (Voragen 1998).

13.3.3 Amounts of dietary fibre in some foods

The main difficulty with determining the amount of fibre in food is to reconcile various chemical groups with a division of carbohydrates that reflects physiology (Asp *et al.* 1992). Until recently, mainly two types of methods have been used for the measurement of dietary fibre in foods, namely enzymatic gravimetric methods whereby the fibre is isolated and weighed (AOAC methods) and component analysis methods in which individual dietary fibre saccharides are determined more or less specifically (Englyst *et al.* 1994). Moreover, the methods rely on different definitions of dietary fibre. In the

Table 13.7   Dietary fibre content of some foods (g/100 g edible portion) (FAO/WHO 1997)

Food	Moisture	Dietary fibre content	
		Non-starch polysaccharides[1]	Total fibre[2]
Banana	75.1	1.1	1.6
French beans	13.3	4.7	nd
Beans, green	11.3	17.0	40.0
Lentils, green	10.8	8.9	nd
Potatoes	79.0	1.3	1.8
Wheat	14.0	9.0	12.6
Maize	12.0	nd	11.0
Rice	11.8	2.0	3.5
Oat	8.9	6.8	10.3

Notes:
[1] NST = Non-starch polysaccharides (Englyst *et al.* 1994);
[2] TDF = total dietary fibre (AOAC 1995)

Englyst methods, lignin and RS are excluded. With the AOAC method, lignin (+ cutins, tannins, Maillard products) and part of the RS are included (Table 13.7). Oligosaccharides are not recovered.

Table 13.8 presents some values of dietary fibre amount in foods. These foods are natural sources of dietary fibre as there are no available data for industrial foods where fibre preparations are added for their functional properties. The analytical values were obtained by the AOAC method (1995).

Table 13.8 shows that foods generally regarded as good sources of fibre, fresh vegetables and fruits, are in fact low fibre foods. These foods contain large amounts of water and even if rich on a dry weight basis, their contribution to fibre intake is relatively low. Expressed on a dry weight basis the most fibre-concentrated foods are brans (mainly breakfast cereals), vegetables, fresh and dried fruits, legume seeds, muesli and wholemeal breads.

13.4 Processing dietary fibre ingredients

Many fibre supplements are age-old familiar and have been modified in some way to improve their functionality (all the parameters that make food acceptable for processing and to the consumer) while still providing an enhanced level of dietary fibre. For example, gums, algal polysaccharides and pectins have been used for years to thicken – to impart viscosity to aqueous phase in food systems. They provide texture and mouth feel. They can stabilise suspensions, emulsions, foams, impart freeze/thaw stability and control syneresis. Because of their impact on the texture and sensory property of the end products, they are generally used in low amounts. Insoluble fibre or composite (mixture of soluble and insoluble) preparations are mainly used as texturing and/or bulking agents.

Table 13.8   Dietary fibre content of some foods (g/100 g edible portion*) (Dreher 1999)

| | Moisture | Dietary fibre content | | |
		Tot.	Insol.	Sol.
French bread	29.2	2.7	1.9	0.8
White sourdough bread	37.1	1.9	1.3	0.6
Wholewheat sourdough bread	39.7	8.1	7.0	1.1
Cookies: brownies	12.8	2.5	1.7	0.8
Cookies: butter	4.7	2.4	1.6	0.8
Croissants	20.4	2.3	1.4	0.9
Cornflakes: plain	2.8	2.0	1.7	0.3
Puffed rice	6.5	1.4	1.0	0.4
Muesli	5.0	12.0		
Wheat bran (breakfast cereals)	2.9	35.3	32.8	2.5
Wheat flakes	2.4	11.4	9.6	1.8
Barley bran	3.5	70	67.0	3.0
Parboiled rice: cooked	77	0.5		
Rice: cooked	77.5	0.7	0.7	0
Brown rice: cooked	73.1	1.7		
Pasta: macaroni	69.6	2.0	1.7	0.3
Boiled potatoes	79.5	1.3	1.0	0.3
French fried potatoes	48.6	3.0	1.5	1.5
Peas, green, canned	80.7	4.5	3.6	0.9
Peas, green, boiled	76.9	6.7	5.0	1.7
Peas frozen, boiled	81.6	4.4	3.2	1.2
Beans, green, canned		2.1	1.4	0.7
Beans, green, boiled		2.5	1.5	1.0
Carrots, raw	88.5	2.4	1.1	1.3
Carrots, cooked	90.5	2.7	1.2	1.5
Lettuce	96.0	0.7	0.5	0.2
Tomatoes, raw	94.5	1.2	0.8	0.4
Apple	84.6	1.5	1.3	0.2
Bananas	75.7	1.7	1.2	0.5
Kiwi	83.0	3.4		
Prunes, dried	26.2	7.3	31	4.2

Note:
* Mainly analysed by the AOAC (1995)

The physicochemical properties of fibre preparation play a key role in their functionality: fibre dimensions, hydration-rheological properties and fat binding/retention properties. The colour and flavour are also of importance.

A second generation of fibres with optimised properties for targeted applications has been emerging. Our purpose here is to examine the impact of some processes on the properties of some fibre preparations.

13.4.1 Grinding

Most of the fibre concentrates are available at different particle sizes. Partitioning may be done and fractions with different chemical compositions obtained, depending on the origin and history of the cell wall material (Auffret *et al.* 1994). Brans, which contain different tissues, are particularly affected (Heller *et al.* 1977). For example, glucan-enriched fraction from oat can be easily obtained by mechanical separation because the beta glucans are concentrated in the outermost endosperm layer (the subaleurone). This is not the case with barley as the beta glucans are more or less evenly distributed throughout the whole kernel.

Grinding can also affect the physical characteristics of fibre. The milling process used can be of importance (Sidiras *et al.* 1990). Ball milling not only reduces particle size but can also severely disrupt the crystalline order of cellulose. The effect is proportional to the time of ball milling. Hammer mill has no effect on cellulose crystallinity.

Grinding may affect hydration characteristics of the fibres as well as texture (Table 13.9). However, the most marked changes concern the kinetics of water uptake; the ground fibre is instantaneously hydrated compared to the raw fibre (Auffret *et al.* 1994). However, extensive milling can lead to a decrease in the specific surface area. Atmospheric humidity can provoke agglomeration of particles and collapse of some cellular structures, thus decreasing porosity (Fan *et al.* 1980, Gharpuray *et al.* 1983).

Grinding can also affect the binding properties of the fibre (Ryden and Robertson 1995). These effects are mainly related to changes in the physical structure of the fibre and in particular to increased specific surface area.

13.4.2 Heat treatments

As previously mentioned, fibre concentrates are generally supplied in a dry form. It improves the fibre shelf life without the addition of chemicals and reduces package size. Different drying methods are used in the food industry: convection, under vacuum, freeze drying, etc. The characteristics of the fibre products must be taken into account to design the procedure that minimises adverse effects. For example, agglomeration, deformation or darkening of the products must be avoided or at least minimised. It is also important to maintain or improve hydration properties of the fibre if they are to be used as texturing and bulking agents. Drying, most of the time depresses swelling and water retention capacities of the sample (Table 13.10) (Larrauri 1999, Femenia *et al.* 1999). Moreover, a partial modification of some dietary fibre components may also occur. This can be observed with a sample exposed to variable periods of temperature treatments while at a relatively high moisture. Femenia *et al.* (1999) found no changes in solubility of non-starch polysaccharides for fresh, freeze-dried and 40°C dried fibre from cauliflower but a decrease in sample dried at 75°C. The lowest swelling and water retention capacities were also obtained with samples dried at 75°C. Close association between polysaccharides within the cell walls in dehydrated samples could reduce pore volume and restrict the extent of rehydration (Table 13.11). Similar results have been observed with sugar beet and submitted to pectin extraction prior to drying (Table 13.11). Freeze-drying led to a maintenance or increase of swelling and water retention

Table 13.9   Hydration characteristics of some fibre concentrates

Source of fibre	Particle size (µm)	Swelling (ml g^{-1})	Water retention (g water g^{-1} dry pellet)	Water absorption (ml water g^{-1} dry fibre)	Reference
Sugar beet fibre	500–200 µm	11.5	26.5		1
		19.3	32.9		2
	390	14.7	19.7		3
	385	21.4	22.6	8.8	4
	205	15.9	19.2	7.3	4
	540	11.0	26.6		5
	660	13.5	7.2		6
Citrus fibre		15.7	11,2	5.2	7
	540	15.7	10.4	7.0	4
	235	13.3	8.6	7.0	4
	420	14.7	10.4		6
	139	10.4	10.7	4.6	8
Apple fibre	540	9.6	6.9	3.8	6
	250	8.6	5.5	4.6	6
	133	7.4	5.4		8
Pea hull	500	6.0	7.1	2.4	9
	80	5.6	7.1	2.7	9
	950	9.9	4.3	1.9	4
	300	7.8	6.2	2.8	4
	560	6.2	4.2	2.7	6
	100	6.5	3.9	3.3	6
	67	6.6	3.8	3.7	8
Wheat bran	500–250		6.4	2.7	10
	900	11.9	6.8	1.0	4
	320	5.9	3.0	0.9	4
	1000–500	7.0	7.0		5
	Coarse	7.4	5.6		11
	Ground	6.4	6.6		11
Maize bran		5.7	2.4		12
Oat bran		5.53	3.5		12
Resistant starch	40	5.6	3.5	3.0	8
	84	7.4	3.1	3.9	

Sources:
1. Bertin *et al.* 1988; 2. Ralet *et al.* 1991; 3. Auffret *et al.* 1993; 4. Auffret *et al.* 1994; 5. Renard *et al.* 1994; 6. Cloutour 1995; 7. Thibault *et al.* 1988; 8. Robertson *et al.* in press; 9. Ralet *et al.* 1993; 10. Ralet *et al.* 1990; 11. Ponne *et al.* 1997; 12. Ponne *et al.* 1998.

capacity while drastic drying at high temperature resulted in a decrease of these properties (Guillon *et al.* 1998b, Cloutour 1995).

The wall is a strong mechanical component of living cells. It allows high turgor pressure and gives the cell its shape. However, when stress overpasses mechanical resistance of the wall, an irreversible deformation of the cell is obtained. This type of deformation occurs in most drying processes, except in the case of freeze-drying. Blanching prior to drying contributes towards increasing the permeability of the cell walls and induces an increase of the

Table 13.10 Effect of processing on the hydration properties of some dietary fibres

Dietary fibre	Treatment	Swelling (ml g^{-1})	Water retention capacity (g water g^{-1})	Reference
Sugar beet fibre	Native	10.8	6.1	1
	Depectinated – soft drying	27.6	14.0	1
	Depectinated – drastic drying	7.2	4.1	1
	Native	19.3	32.9	2
	Extruded	14.4	28.2	2
Cauliflower-based fibre supplements	Native (fresh)	22.9	19.9	3
	Freeze-dried	19.4	18.7	3
	Boiled	27.4	24.6	3
	Dried 40°C	16.9	12.8	3
	Dried 75°C	4.2	5.7	3
Apple fibre	Dried 50°C	32.0	13.9	4
	Dried under vacuum (80°C, 13 mbar)	54.4	22.2	4
	Freeze-dried	50.6	20.5	4
	High rate freezing + dried under vacuum	56.7	17.9	4
	CID + dried under vacuum	46.8	18.6	4
Pea hull	Native	6.2	4.2	5
	Mercerised + freeze-drying	8.6	6.0	5
	Depectinated + freeze-drying	11.7	7.2	5
	Depectinated + mercerised + freeze-drying	9.7	6.8	5
	Native	6.0	7.1	2
	Extruded	5.2	4.3	2
Wheat bran	Native	7.0	7	6
	Delignified	11.0	10.4	6
	Native	nd	6.4	7
	Extruded	nd	6.0	7

Sources:
1. Guillon et al. 1998b; 2. Thibault et al. 1988; 3. Femenia et al. 1999; 4. Guillon, personal communication; 5. Cloutour 1995; 6. Renard et al. 1994; 7. Ralet et al. 1990

Table 13.11 Porosity of sugar beet fibre and pea hulls; effect of processing

Dietary fibre	Particle size (μm)	Chemical treatment	Drying	Pore volume (ml g⁻¹)			
				Total	$>1\,\mu m^3$	$<5\,nm^4$	$5\,nm{-}1\,\mu m^5$
Sugar beet[1]	480			14.9	10.4	2.9	1.6
	100			13.8	8.8	2.9	2.1
	190	Partially depectinated	Solvent exchange + oven drying 40°C	18.3	14.1	3.3	0.9
	90	Depectinated	Pilot air-drying 100°C	6.1	3.6	2.2	0.3
Pea hull[2]	1500			6.7	3.5	ND	ND
	560			5.4	1.9	1.56	1.94
	100			5.2	2.8	ND	ND
	520	Mercerisation		8.6	3.2	1.6	3.8
	450	Mercerisation	Solvent exchange + oven drying	6.8	1.7	1.3	3.8

Notes:

ND: not determined

[1] Guillon *et al.* 1998b; [2] Cloutour 1995; [3] Volume accessible to bacteria estimated from microporosity measurement; [4] Volume inaccessible to enzyme estimated from macroporosity measurement; [5] Volume accessible to enzyme but not to bacteria.

Sugar beet fibre: When pectin extraction followed mild drying, the total pore volume and volume accessible to bacteria increased. The removal of pectins possibly increased pores between adjacent cells. In contrast, harsh drying induced a noticeable decrease in the total pore volume and especially in pore volume accessible to bacteria. This change was ascribed to distortion and shrinking of cells during drying.

Pea hull: Treatment of mercerisation increased the macroporosity but poorly affected the microporosity of pea hull. Removal of xylans and small amounts of pectins probably caused this increase but because much pectin remained, the treatment was not efficient in changing the cellulose crystallinity profile and thus, the microporosity.

deformation. The drying conditions have a strong impact on shrinking. Products rapidly dried generally contain more void volumes and show a lower density than products slowly dried.

Drying can also affect certain bioactive compounds in fruit and vegetable products (Larrauri 1999). A decrease of polyphenol contents of red grape pomace peels was observed on drying at a temperature above 100°. Carotenoids seem sensitive to high temperature and losses occur during dehydration of carrots at 60°C.

13.4.3 Thermo-mechanical treatment
Fibre-rich preparation may be extrusion cooked to modify its functionality. The results on different fibres show that extrusion cooking has a moderate effect on the hydration properties of pea hull brans, sugar beet or lemon fibre (Table 13.10). In contrast, extrusion cooking can influence solubility of the fibres. Wheat bran and other cereals need a high amount of energy, and about 15% of soluble material is obtained (Ralet *et al.* 1990). Less energy is required for the hulls and a similar amount of material is solubilised (Ralet *et al.* 1993). Feroylated heteroxylans and glucans are solubilised from wheat bran, and arabinans, heteroxylans and pectins from pea hull. The main effect of extrusion cooking of sugar beet pulp, lemon and apple fibre is to increase by up to 40% the water solubility of pectins in cold water (Thibault *et al.* 1995). The soluble pectins can have high molecular weight and high degree of methylation. They can form gel as other high methoxy (HM) pectins (Ralet *et al.* 1994).

A new process has been developed to fit the industrial demand for products with preserved nutritional quality and improved functionality. This process is named 'instant controlled depression' and associates texturation and drying processes (Louka and Allaf 1998). It consists of submitting the material to thermal processing at high pressure for a short time and then flash expansion. The operation interpolated after the pre-drying stage permits expansion of the dried products, by self-vaporisation of the residual water. As a result, the product recovers its original shape. Its organoleptic properties are close to those of freeze-dried products. The colour is preserved and its ability to rehydrate safeguarded. The quality of the end product depends on the operating conditions and on the characteristics of the raw material. The energy cost compared to freeze-drying is low. This process has been applied with success to small cubes of fruits and vegetables.

13.4.4 Chemical treatments
Hydration properties of fibre can be altered substantially by treating them with solvents, oxidants, acid or alkaline. The action of these chemicals is mainly to extract more or less selectively compounds such as pectins, hemicelluloses and lignins. The extent of extraction depends on the concentration of the chemical and on the temperature conditions.

At the laboratory scale, it has been demonstrated that substantial removal of pectins by relatively mild chemical treatment leads to an increase of the pore volume of sugar beet fibre, and thus of the water hydration properties (Table 13.10) (Auffret *et al.* 1993, Guillon *et al.* 1998b). Similar results have been obtained with pea hull (Weightman *et al.* 1994). However, if the chemical treated fibre undergoes harsh drying, its hydration properties become limited, probably because of structural collapse of the fibre matrix (Table 13.10) (Auffret *et al.* 1993, Guillon *et al.* 1998b).

Removal of compounds is not necessarily a prerequesite to increase the hydration properties. The swelling action of water on cellulosic material is enhanced by the breakdown of intra- and interchain bonds by alkaline agent or phosphoric acid (Sinitsyn *et al.* 1991).

Bleaching can be used to lighten fibre material. For this purpose, hydroxide peroxide treatment has been applied (Gould *et al.* 1989). Phenolic compounds and other phytochemicals may be lost. Peroxide can induce the release of carbohydrates bound to phenolic compounds. This treatment can increase the fibre ability to absorb water, soften and swell when hydrated. For example, treated wheat straw can be used as high substitute for a portion of flour in cakes without introducing undesirable sensory characteristics or causing deterioration of the baking performance (Jasberg *et al.* 1989).

13.4.5 Enzymatic treatment

Endogenous phytase activity in wheat grain can be used to reduce phytate levels but exogenous enzyme can also make a significant contribution (Jayarajah *et al.* 1997). The endogenous phytase activity results in destruction of phytate without accumulation of inositol phosphate intermediates, and at low moisture levels, without modification of the fibre components through polysaccharidase activities which may be present in bran.

Enzymatic treatments can be applied to improve the functionality of fibre preparations. The properties mainly concerned are the hydration properties and solution viscosity. Oat beta glucans and guar gum may be hydrolysed to provide grades developing different viscosity in solution. The treatment results in a decrease of molecular weight and yield products with generally improved resistance to thermal, pH, and shear degradation when compared to the high molecular weight parents.

Treatment of pea hull and apple fibres with pectinolytic and cellulolytic enzymes has been found to increase the proportion of water-soluble fibre and confer the matrix with a softer texture, making easier its incorporation into foods (Caprez *et al.* 1987).

Xylanase preparations find widespread use in the baking industry to improve handling characteristics of the dough, loaf volume and crumb structure of the bread, especially bread containing high amount of dietary fibre (Poutanen 1997). The enzymes degrade *in situ* the water-insoluble arabinoxylans present in discrete endosperm cell wall particles, thus causing a substantial enrichment in the water-soluble arabinoxylans with corresponding increase in viscosity of the aqueous phase (Poutanen *et al.* 1998). The improving action of pentosanases on the volume of bread may be compared to those reported when high molecular weight soluble pentosans or guar gum are added to flour ingredients. Of course when added in excess, enzymes induce an extensive depolymerisation of the water-soluble arabinoxylans, thus causing a decrease in viscosity and a deterioration of the dough quality.

13.5 Processing foods containing dietary fibre

Most foods are processed for consumer convenience in the food industry or at home. Industrial processing is applied to prolong shelf life of the products or to produce foods ready to eat or easy to prepare while preserving their quality, i.e. texture, colour, flavour, palatability and nutritional quality. Industrial processing mainly includes heat treatments, thermo-mechanical and non-thermal treatments.

13.5.1 Heat treatment

Wet heat treatment mainly includes blanching, boiling, canning, steaming and microwaving. The major consequences of processing are release of cell contents and the solubilisation of labile dietary fibre components, i.e. pectins, beta glucans, arabinoxylans, oligosaccharides. The extent of solubilisation of the cell wall polysaccharides depends on the chemical nature of the polysaccharide and its association with other macromolecules within cell walls, and on the processing parameters (temperature, duration, etc). During cooking and processing, there can be extensive breakdown of pectic polysaccharides through a beta-eliminative degradation. This results in significant reduction of the molecular weight and thus increases solubilisation (Anderson and Clydesdale 1980, Varo *et al.* 1984, Stolle-Smits *et al.* 1995, Svanberg *et al.* 1997). The viscosity of the water-soluble dietary fibre decreases following intense heat treatment, in accordance with a shift towards a lower molecular weight (Svanberg 1997). As a result of partial solubilisation of cell wall components, the insoluble fibre matrix can exhibit higher swelling because of a looser and more porous network. Depending on the pore size distribution, the water retention capacity may be increased or decreased. For leafy vegetables, the tissues become softer. In seed legumes, pectins cementing the cells are solubilised, leading to separation of cotyledon cells. Blanching applied to inactive enzymes, although it can also cause some solubilisation. For example, blanching carrots leads to a deesterification of pectic polysaccharides (Plat *et al.* 1991), and the change has been mainly ascribed to enzyme activity rather than beta elimination. Pectin methyl esterase is known to remain active at increased temperatures (Lopez *et al.* 1997), and activity can be affected by intracellular cations release during cell metabolism or disruption (Alonso *et al.* 1997). It can influence the texture or tissue firmness in vegetables (Wu and Chang 1990). Microwave cooking is generally considered as a mild form of heat treatment. Applied to green beans, microwaving slightly affected the total dietary fibre content but a shift toward lower molecular weight of the water-soluble fibre was observed (Svanberg 1997). Only severe microwaving (repeated treatment) decreased the total fibre content (Svanberg 1997). The polysaccharides in cereal fibres are not susceptible to beta elimination during cooking or processing. Moreover, the presence of phenolic compounds may limit the extractability of arabinoxylans.

Dry heat treatment such as baking or roasting, does not significantly alter the dietary fibre composition. In extreme conditions, a significant increase in the lignin content and a decrease in water hydration properties can be observed (Camire 1999). This could be ascribed to the formation of Maillard products. Maillard products arise from the reaction of sugars and proteins, often leading to browning and development of flavour. They are not digested by endogenous enzymes in the small intestine and therefore can contribute towards increased amount of total dietary fibre.

Heat treatment followed by a cooling period can induce the formation of RS in starchy foods. The amount will depend on the botanical source, the ratio of amylose to amylopectin, processing parameters (temperature, amount of water, cooling) and storage conditions. The RS content of common food cereals food like breads, breakfast cereals, pasta and rice is generally below 3%, potato 4–5%, potato flakes 3% (Asp et al. 1996). In the case of cooked cereal products (rice, pasta, bread), RS does not seem to increase during storage or freezing (Würsch 1999). In contrast, deep-fat frying or storing cooked potato in the cold increases by up to about 12% the starch into RS. Repeated heating and cooling can lead to an accumulation of RS but the increase in absolute is relatively small compared to amount generated on the first heating/cooling cycle. Starch lipid and starch protein complexes can also be formed during cooking and these are more resistant to alpha amylase (Holm et al. 1983).

13.5.2 Thermo-mechanical treatment

Extrusion cooking is nowadays currently used by the food industry for various types of snacks, ready-to-eat cereal products, etc. In a typical twin extruder, the product is fed in and transported by rotation of the screws. Here, the product is submitted to heat and shear. At the end of extruder, the product is forced to pass through a die, and then water can be vaporised leading to an expanding product.

Extrusion of wheat or rye flour under normal conditions does not induce the formation of high amount of RS (Bjorck et al. 1984, Lue et al. 1990). No changes in these conditions are observed in the total amount of dietary fibre and a slight increase in the amount of soluble fibre at the expense of the insoluble fraction is reported (Varo et al. 1983, Bjorck et al. 1984). While under drastic conditions, an increase in the amount of total fibre and a significant conversion of insoluble to soluble fractions has been found (Bjorck *et al.* 1984). This increase in total dietary fibre is not ascribed to an increase of RS.

Popping and flaking only slightly change the composition of cereals. Soluble carbohydrates fractions are generally only a little enhanced by the treatments. The treatments bring disorganisation of the endosperm of grains, but the outer layers (aleuron and adjacent layer) are generally preserved. Popping of maize grains causes heterogeneous reactions within the grain (Farber and Gallant 1976). In the unpopped peripheral zones, starch granules are partly swollen while the inner part of the endosperm shows an alveolar structure where starch is completely gelatinised and pushed against the remnant cell walls. Steam flaking, especially with maize, generally produces a disorganisation of the cell structure: the cell walls are broken, and content of the cell more or less dispersed. Starch granules appear slightly deformed, partly gelatinised and fissured. Intensive mechanical/thermal treatments generally increase the accessibility and digestibility of starch. In the case of legumes, flaking compared to cooking results in a lower amount of resistant starch. In the case of beans, 9–11% of total starch was resistant in flake beans (Schweizer *et al.* 1990) against 16.5% in cooked beans (Noah *et al.* 1998).

13.5.3 Freezing

Enzyme activities and, in particular, pectinolytic activities are only slowed at freezer temperature. This means that in long storage periods, pectin solubilisation and degradation may occur. Starch can retrograde in frozen foods, leading to the formation of RS. Freezing can be accompanied by ice crystal formation, which can lead to disruption of the cell walls. This phenomenon can increase the release of cell content and the solubilisation of cell wall polysaccharides on cooking (Rahman *et al.* 1971). The formation and size of ice crystals depends on the temperature and rate of freezing. Preservation of the quality of products requires rapid freezing.

13.5.4 Fermentation

Fermented legumes are an integral and significant part of the diet in developing countries. It has been suggested as an economical method of processing and preserving foods. Fermentation has been shown to enhance the nutritive value of legumes, reduces some anti-nutritional endogenous compounds and improves consumer acceptability. It increases vitamins, removes some anti-nutritional factors such as trypsin inhibitors and eliminates alpha galactosides, compounds related to flatus production.

13.5.5 Germination

Malting is a well-established process used to produce cereal substrates for fermented beverages. Malted cereals may be used to formulate nutritious products, including infant and weaning foods. Grain germination is associated with water uptake. Subsequently, an activation process signalled by hormones arising from the embryonic axis results in synthesis and secretion of hydrolytic and other enzymes. These enzymes depolymerise cell polysaccharides, and the protein and starch reserves of the endosperm. Thus, germination induces chemical and biochemical changes in the seed. It can decrease the amount of alpha galactosides, lectins, trypsin inhibitors and phytate. Substantial solubilisation and degradation of some cell wall polysaccharides by endogenous enzymes may occur. For example, during malting endogenous beta glucanase is synthesised, which results in the depolymerisation of beta barley glucans, thus decreasing their capacity to increase viscosity of aqueous solution (Fincher and Stone 1986). Extensive degradation of cell arabinoxylans, the other major components of cereal endosperm cell walls, also occurs in germinating wheat grain (Fincher and Stone 1986).

Thus, although the amount of dietary fibre may be quantitatively equivalent in cooked/processed to that in raw material, their properties may be altered.

13.6 The physiological effects of dietary fibre

While the amount and source of fibre may be important for dietary responses, it is equally important to describe properties of fibre used if mechanisms responsible for fibre activity(s) are to be understood. Physical and chemical properties will determine local responses (direct effects as the result of the presence of dietary fibre in the digestive tract) and associated systemic responses which may be expected with ingestion of a particular fibre (Fig. 13.1). These properties include viscosity for soluble fibre, water retention, binding/adsorption properties, particle size. The fermentation of dietary fibre through the products

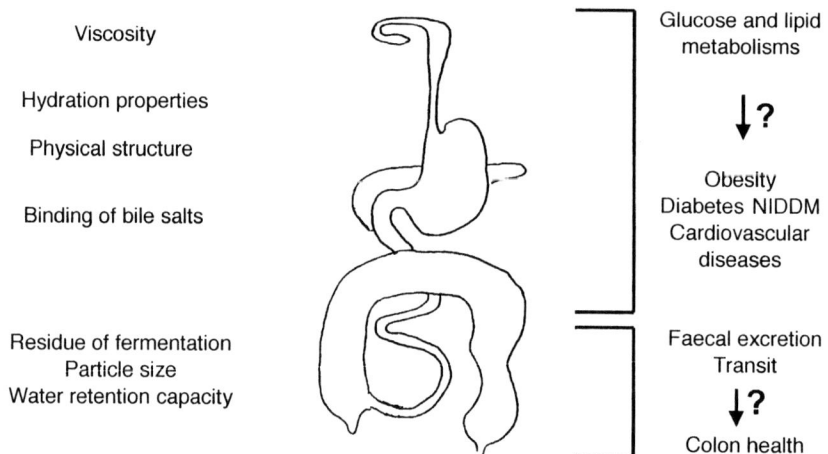

Viscosity

Hydration properties

Physical structure

Binding of bile salts

Residue of fermentation
Particle size
Water retention capacity

Glucose and lipid metabolisms

↓?

Obesity
Diabetes NIDDM
Cardiovascular diseases

Faecal excretion
Transit

↓?

Colon health

Fig. 13.1   Dietary fibre and its effect on the gastrointestinal tract.

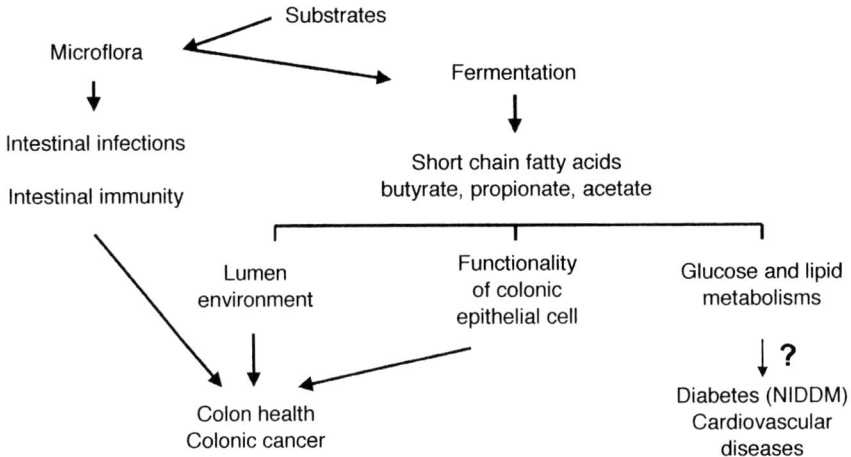

Fig. 13.2   Fermentation and its effects on colonic physiology.

and residues of fermentation and impact on the microflora also play a key role in the effects ascribed to dietary fibre (Fig. 13.2).

13.6.1 Physicochemical properties involved in the physiological effects of dietary fibre

Water-soluble polysaccharides and viscosity

Some water-soluble polysaccharides such as pectins and gums may form viscous solutions. Inclusion of these polysaccharides in a meal can increase the volume and viscosity of digesta in the upper gut. They can delay gastric emptying in the stomach, which can promote satiety. This can also reduce emulsification of dietary lipids in the acid medium of the stomach and subsequently lower the extent of lipid assimilation. In the lumen of the small intestine, viscosity can resist the effects of gastrointestinal motility. It can impede the diffusion of digestive enzymes towards their substrates, which slows down digestion. It can also slow down the release and transit of the products of hydrolysis towards the absorptive surface of the mucosa. The direct systemic response is a steady rate of nutrient delivery in the circulation resulting in lower post-prandial level.

Viscosity is imparted by the chemical structure of the polysaccharides (amount of space occupied by the macromolecules generally characterised by intrinsic viscosity) and also by the cross-linkages between the macromolecules (Morris 1990). Concentration temperature, ionic concentration, pH, association with proteins, and shear forces are all involved (Fig. 13.3).

Treatments that induce hydrolysis of pectins, beta glucans or various gums into lower molecular weight molecules will contribute towards reduced capacity of these molecules to increase the viscosity of digesta. In contrast, some treatments such as extrusion cooking can increase the amount of water-soluble

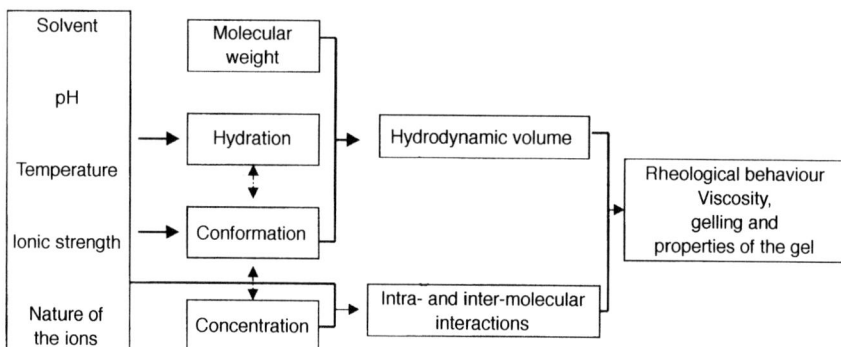

Fig. 13.3   Factors that determine the rheological properties in macromolecules (adapted from Blond and Le Meste 1988).

molecules without extensively splitting them. Thus, it is important to consider the property of fibre in food as it is eaten.

Moreover, although not digested by endogenous enzymes in the upper gut, macromolecules can undergo significant degradation. For example, pectins can be solubilised through disruption of calcium bridges under acidic conditions (in the stomach) or through beta elimination at a near neutral pH (e.g. in the small intestine). The extent and location of this degradation could have a nutritional impact. Changes in ionic environment and pH throughout the gastrointestinal tract can also influence the solubility and viscosity of polysaccharides. This is generally observed with polyelectrolytes (pectins, alginates). For example, at a high concentration alginate can form a gel in the stomach and may be soluble in the small intestine. The concentration in the lumen may be different from that in ingested food. In particular, the total volume of digesta may adapt in response to ingestion of viscous solution, partly offsetting the difference in initial viscosity.

As a consequence, the viscosity of fluid digesta may vary within the gut. This means that the measured viscosity of a fibre source may bear little relationship to the viscosity in the digestive segments of interest. At least the concentration, structure and molecular weight of the polymer (degree of space occupancy by the polymer) must be documented in the segment of the digestive tract under consideration for interpreting the data. Because most of the polysaccharides exhibit shear thinning, only one value at a single shear rate has no meaning. Morris (1990, 1992) recommends measuring the viscosity at a few shear rates and then derive the maximum viscosity (ho) at low shear rates and the shear rate ($g_{1/2}$).

Adsorption/binding ions and bile acids
The ability of certain fibre to adsorb or entrap bile acids and phospholipids has been suggested as a potential mechanism by which dietary fibre, containing uronic acids or phenolic acids, may increase faecal excretion of bile acids. An increased bile acid excretion results in higher cholestrol turnover from the body.

The exact mechanisms by which fibre sequesters bile acids are unclear; hydrophobic (fibre-containing phenolics) and ionic interactions (fibre-containing uronic acids) have been suggested (Thibault *et al.* 1992). *In vivo*, some fibre preparations (Wolever 1995) increase ileal and faecal excretions of sterols and lipids, but which help adsorption or increase of the fluid digesta viscosity account for this effect is still questionable.

Fibre consisting of lignified or coarse tissues such as rice straw are identified as neutraceuticals with binding properties (Robertson 1998).

Milling, relieving the constraint on accessibility to the binding surface and allowing a greater partitioning of compounds to fibre, can increase the affinity for some toxic heterocyclic amines in foods (Robertson 1998).

Adsorption has often been measured by methods similar to those used for water retention capacity, and both absorption and entrapment in the cell wall matrix can account for the retention. The prevailing chemical environment and characteristics of the fibre fractions in the small intestine must be taken into account for physiogically reliable measurements of the binding capacity .

Water absorption/retention properties

Insoluble fibre can absorb, swell and entrap water within its porous matrix. Water retention properties contribute towards the bulking effect of fibre in the colon. They can take part in the dilution of cytotoxic substances in the large intestine, thus reducing potency.

The hydration properties depend on the chemistry of the individual components of fibres, the way they are assembled in the cell walls, the anatomy and the particle size of the fibres (Fig. 13.4). Fibre mainly composed of primary cell walls exhibits general higher values than fibre with secondary cell walls (Table 13.9) (Thibault *et al.* 1992, Thibault *et al.* 1994).

Hydration properties depend on:

- Chemical structure
  - Polymers/hydrophilic/hydrophobic regions
  - Charged polymers
  - Polymers/amorphous/crystalline regions

- Physical structure
  - Porosity
  - Particle size

- Physico-chemical environment
  - pH, temperature, ions, other molecules

- History of the product
  - Processing
  - Drying

Fig. 13.4 Factors that determine the hydration properties of dietary fibre.

Environmental conditions such as pH, ionic strength and nature of the ions can influence the hydration values of fibres containing polyelectrolytes (charged groups such as carboxyl in fibre rich in pectins, carboxyl and sulfate groups in fibres from algae) (Thibault *et al.* 1992, Thibault *et al.* 1994).

Processes, such as grinding, drying, heating or extrusion cooking for example, provided that they modify the composition and the physical properties of the fibre matrix, will strongly affect the hydration properties (Thibault *et al.* 1992). Fibres with high values for hydration properties are generally well fermented, probably because bacteria and their secreted enzymes can rapidly diffuse and reach their substrates (Auffret *et al.* 1993, Cloutour 1995, Guillon *et al.* 1998b). In the colon, the most effective stool bulkers are low fermented fibres, because they retain a proportion of their matrix and thus are still able to bind water. Wheat bran and ispaghula are the reference fibres for this effect.

Different aspects of fibre hydration can be distinguished and a need was identified for a clear definition. In particular there should be a distinction between absorption, uptake, holding and binding. The definition of hydration properties arising from the European PROFIBRE project (Robertson 1998) are:

- *Swelling*: 'the volume occupied by a known weight of fibre under the condition used'
- *Water retention capacity*: 'the amount of water retained by a known weight of fibre under the condition used' – it is preferred to either water-holding capacity or water-binding capacity
- *Water absorption*: 'the kinetics of water movement under defined conditions'.

Swelling and water retention capacity provide a general view of fibre hydration and can provide information useful for fibre-supplemented foods. Water absorption can provide more information on the fibre, in particular its substrate pore volume. It will help our understanding of the behaviour of fibre in foods or during gut transit.

For each parameter, several methods have been proposed for their measurement but not always with a clear picture of what is being measured. Generally, swelling is measured as settled bed volume and water retention capacity as the amount of water retained after centrifugation by the insoluble substrate (pellet). Water absorption is measured using a Baumann apparatus or using osmotic pressure/dialysis techniques. Within PROFIBRE, protocols for each method were standardised and were evaluated for their levels, experimental variation or statistical tolerance (Robertson *et al.* in press).

When assessing the behaviour of fibre in food and in the digestive tract from the hydration properties, the physical fibre matrix properties as well as the physicochemical conditions prevailing in their environment in food or gut lumen should be taken into account. Hydration properties of the fibre matrix before ingestion may bear little relationship to the fibre in the colon as the result of fibre fermentation.

Disruptibiliy of the cell walls

In food with intact cells, the release of nutrients can be related to resistance of cell walls to disruption. Nutrients entrapped within the cellular structure cannot be digested until the cell walls have been damaged. In the case of starchy foods, the amount of starch escaping digestion and reaching the large intestine is increased in foods with intact cell walls.

Factors that influence cell wall disruptibility are structure, lignification and mechanical and thermomechanical treatments. Secondary cell walls are generally more resistant to mechanical stress. This means, for example, that the outer layer of cereal kernel or legume seeds will be more preserved than cell walls of the starchy endosperms. The physical structure of food can also be significantly disrupted in the mouth, due to chewing. The extent of disruption, depends on the food rheological properties. The physical degradation of food results in an increase of the available surface to enzymes. Thus, it can significantly affect the overall process of digestion and postprandial blood response.

Light microscopy can be used to examine the physical structure of food. Again, the main difficulty is to evaluate damages occurring within the digestive tract. In this respect, more *in vivo* data are required.

Particle size

Particle size can play a role in controlling a number of events occurring in the digestive tract (e.g. transit time, fermentation and faecal excretion). The rate of fermentation is proportional to the external surface area in contact with the bacteria for fibres with a low porosity such hulls and brans. Coarse wheat bran is more effective in regulating transit time than fine bran. Particles can induce an increased excitation of colonic mechanoreceptors, stimulating contractile activity in favour of a higher propulsion of digesta (Cherbut 1995, Edwards 1995). The decrease of intestinal transit time associated with these fibres protects the colon from prolonged exposure to cytotoxic substances which may also be carcinogenic.

Particle size is related to the processing history of the fibre product. Mechanical treatment such as grinding but also chewing decreases the particle size. Wet heat treatments that release a large amount of pectins through weakening the middle lamella can induce a concomitant loss of intercellular adhesion. Degradation of the fibre matrix by colonic bacteria can lead to an almost complete disintegration of the particles.

Particle size distribution can be measured by different methods, like sieving, or methods based on the change in resistivity of a conducting medium, or optical methods (laser diffraction, microscopy and image analysis computer) (Allen 1988). All of these methods are based on different principles. They will give different values for the same material but classification for a range of materials will be preserved. All have some drawbacks and limitations. The form of the fibre, wet or dry, is of importance as some fibres may swell in solution and as a consequence, their particle size increases. The measurement of particle size in a wet form of residue of fermentation may be more relevant when assessing the bulking effects of fibre in the large intestine. In any case, when giving particle size values, the methods used and the form of the fibre must be clear.

13.6.2 Fermentation patterns

Dietary fibre makes a substantial contribution as a substrate for fermentation. It has been found in the ileostomy model that the mean excretion of dry weight and energy were 50g/d and 800kJ/d, respectively on a low fibre diet, and 88g/d and 1700kJ/d on a high fibre diet (Langkilde and Andersson 1998). Effects of dietary fibre on bowel function like faecal mass, stool frequency, regulation of colonic pH and salvage of energy from non-digestible foods are directly related to their fermentation pattern (Cherbut 1995, Edwards 1995). Poorly fermented fibres contribute towards increased bulk in the large intestine, thereby reducing the risk for constipation and possibly also colonic cancer. Highly fermentable fibres, through the products of metabolism, are involved in physiological effects on the colon mucosa (Bingham 1990, Cummings 1995, Higginson 1995, McIntyre *et al*. 1993, Sakata 1995) and colon function (Edwards 1995) as well as post-absorptive actions on the liver and other tissues (Wolever 1993, Darcy-Vrillon and Duée 1995, Demigné *et al*. 1995, Topping and Pant 1995). They contribute towards maintaining the ecosystem equilibrium (Salminen *et al*. 1998). In addition, some fibre sources such as fructoligosaccharides can selectively stimulate the growth of health-promoting bacteria, including bifidobacteria and lactobacilli (Salminen *et al*. 1998, Van Loo *et al*. 1999). They may be the main genera responsible for the protective barrier function and for stimulating healthy immune response in adults.

All dietary fibres are not fermented to the same extent or at the same rate (Table 13.12). Factors controlling fermentation are related to the substrates available for fermentation, the microflora and its activity, and the host (Fig. 13.5).

Microbial degradation requires the contribution of a different group of bacteria linked in a trophic chain. Polysaccharide-degrading bacteria hydrolyse polymers into smaller fragments that can be used by saccharolytic species. The rate and extent of fermentation depends on the physical structure of the fibre matrix (access of bacteria to their substrates) and on the chemical structure of the individual polysaccharides (Fig. 13.6) (Guillon *et al*. 1996). Fibre products rich in secondary tissues (bran, hull) are poorly fermented compared to fibre mainly composed of parenchyma tissue (fruits, vegetables). Soluble poly-saccharides are fermented at a higher rate than equivalent polysaccharides within cell walls. Highly and randomly branched polysaccharides are generally fermented at a lower extent than blocked branched polysaccharides. Some polysaccharides such as carrageenans and ulvan are not degraded by colonic bacteria while their constitutive monomers or dimers are (Bobin-Dubigeon *et al*. 1997, Mathers *et al*. 1998). It has been suggested that bacteria do not possess the enzymatic equipment necessary for their breakdown. Polysaccharidase synthesis

Table 13.12 Factors affecting the fermentation pattern of dietary fibre. Percentage of sugar disappearance after *in vitro* batch incubation

Sources	Treatment	Particle size μm	WRC g H_2O/ g dry pellet	Apparent sugar disappearance 4 h*–6 h**	Apparent sugar disappearance 24 h	Reference
Beet fibre	Commercial fibre	660	7.2	14 ± 0**	70 ± 1	1
Citrus fibre	Commercial fibre	420	10.4	44 ± 2**	81 ± 1	1
Pea fibre (hull)	Commercial fibre	1950	4.8	6 ± 1**	22 ± 7	1
Pea fibre	Grinded	560	4.2	3 ± 1**	22 ± 2.0	1
Pea fibre	Grinded	115	3.3	10 ± 1**	41 ± 2	1
	Treated with pectinolytic enzymes + cellulase	30	nd	1 ± 3**	10 ± 3	1
	Mercerised	520	6.0	5 ± 0**	10 ± 2	1
	Partial removal of pectins	950	7.2	17 ± 2**	26 ± 0	1
	Extensive removal of pectins	650	6.8	29 ± 1**	29 ± 2	1
Apple fibre	Commercial fibre	540	6.9	13 ± 2**	51 ± 4	1
	Grinded	250	5.5	31 ± 4**	67 ± 2	1
	Partial removal of pectins	264	8.5	40 ± 1**	73 ± 2	1
Carrageenans				6 ± 6**	29 ± 4	2
Alginates				31 ± 1**	83 ± 1	2
Acacia gum					49 ± 12	3
Actilight					74 ± 11	3
Novelose (RS : 61.4, type B)	Removal of digestible starch			5*	87	4
Hylon®7 (RS : 27.4, type B)	Removal of digestible starch			8*	57	4

Sources:
1. Cloutour 1995; 2. Bobin-Dubigeon 1996; 3. Michel *et al.* 1998; 4. Martin *et al.* 1998.

Substrate

Chemical nature
Chemical structure
Physico-chemical properties

Fermentation

Micro-organisms
Enzyme activities

Colonic bacteria

Mucus
Transit time
...

Digestive environment

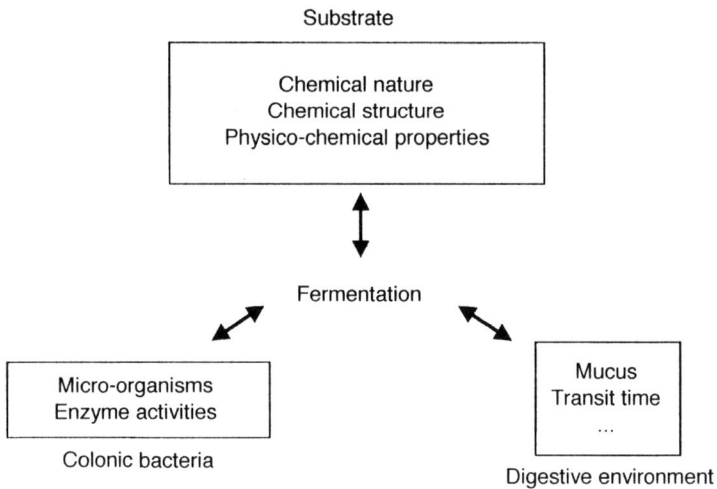

Fig. 13.5   Control process in fermentation in the large intestine.

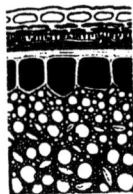

Accessibility
Range of tissues, range of composition
Surfaces cutinised or suberinised
Lignified tissues
Pore volume accessible to bacteria
Particle size

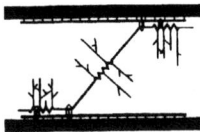

Accessibility
Range of macromolecules, range of composition
Soluble/insoluble polysaccharides
Lignification
Crystallinity of cellulose
Pore volume accessible to enzymes

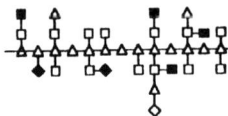

Specificity of enzymatic hydrolysis
Range of monomers,
Linear/branched molecules
Substituents
Degree of polymerisation

Δ

Metabolisation by bacteria
Nature of the monomers

Fig. 13.6   Factors related to fibre, which control its rate and extent of fermentation.

is generally induced by exposure to the substrates and repressed by the products of reaction (Macfarlane and Degnan 1996). In addition, the course of fermentation depends on the microflora composition, which varies from one individual to another, and intra-individually in the cell population densities of the principal taxonomic groups (Macfarlane and Macfarlane 1993). The main bacteria reported to be able to hydrolyse polysaccharides are *Bacteroides, Bifidobacterium, Ruminococcus* and some species of *Eubacterium* and *Clostridium. Bacteroides* is the bacterial genus presenting the highest degree of metabolic versality and is predominant in the microflora.

Some substrates (e.g. fructoligosaccharides, inulin), known as prebiotics, can promote selectively the growth and/or the activity of one or a limited number of bacteria in the colon.

End products of fermentation include short chain fatty acids (SCFA), mainly acetate, propionate and butyrate and gases (H_2, CO_2 and in some cases CH_4). The amount and molar ratios of the three main SCFAs vary substantially, depending on the substrate type (Table 13.13). The nature of the monomers seems not to play a major role in the determination of SCFA profiles. Acetic acid is the major SCFA produced, whatever the substrate. The highest proportion is seen with pectin-type material. Starch is generally associated with a large proportion of butyrate while the highest proportion of propionic acid is observed with arabinogalactan, guar gum and galacto-oligosaccharides. Botham *et al.* (1998) showed that different glucans yielded different SCFA profiles; fermentation of cellulose produced mainly acetate while pea starch generated less acetate (47%) but more butyrate (36%) and more propionate (15%).

Table 13.13   Short chain fatty acid profile of some dietary fibres

Substrates rich in	Example	Short fatty acid profiles
Cellulose		High amount of acetate
Mixed β-glucans	Oat bran	High amount of butyrate and relatively low amount of acetate*
Resistant starch	Retrograded or native Eurylon®, Hylon®, Crystalean®	High amount of butyrate and relatively low amount of acetate
Wheat bran		High amount of butyrate
Fructoligosaccharides	Actilight	High amount of lactate and relatively high amount of acetate
Inulin		High amount of propionate and acetate*
Pectins		High amount of acetate
Galactomannans		High amount of propionate

Source:
* excerpted from Botham *et al.* 1998

SCFAs are mainly absorbed and stimulate salt and water absorption. They are metabolised by the colon epithelium, liver and muscle. Among them, butyrate is the preferred substrate for colon cells and may be involved in the protective effects of fibre against colon cancer. Acetic acid is the only SCFA that can be detected in peripheral blood. Propionic acid is mainly metabolised in the liver and is mainly discussed in relation to effects on carbohydrate and cholesterol metabolisms.

The mechanism by which butyrate may exert a protective role against colonic cancer is not fully understood. It has been suggested that butyrogenic fibres may interfere with immunoprophylaxis of bowel cancer since butyrate enhances the immunogenicity of the colonocyte (Pierre *et al.* 1997; Perrin *et al.* in press). Such an effect may be sufficient to generate rejection of early aberration of the colonic mucosa. In the case of more advanced lesions (Min mice model) a significant additional thrust on the local immunity via the flora may be necessary. In this respect, butyrogenic and prebiotic materials, would be very promising. RS, because of its butyrogenic character, also stimulates a great deal of research. RS encompasses substances with different characteristics and which differ in the rate and extent of fermentation. There is a major impetus in developing RS that will ferment in the distal part of the large bowel. More information on the fermentation profile of resistant starch *in vivo* is required to progress the field.

While the amount of fibre may be important for dietary response it is equally important to describe its source and properties if mechanisms responsible for fibre activity(s) are to be understood. Numerous mechanisms of action have been identified which are related to physicochemical properties and fermentation patterns in the large intestine. The fact that fibre sources differ in their susceptibility to undergo modification during cooking and processing must be considered. The physicochemical environment prevailing in different areas of the digestive tract as the changes occurring within the fibre matrix during passage must also be taken into account. More *in vivo* data are still required. Moreover, methods for measurement of the physicochemical properties that are relevant from a physiological point of view are still needed.

The relationships between target function of the body and improved state of health and/or reduced risk of disease remain to establish. Moreover, most of our knowledge is derived from studies where model fibres were used at doses that were not always realistic. More data are needed with food as eaten, and as part of a complex diet to confirm attributes of fibres.

13.7 Recommended intakes of dietary fibre

The document entitled 'Dietary fibre intakes in Europe' and published in 1993 by the European Community within the framework of COST 92 provides a record of fibre intake in the different member states of the European Union. The range value is from 21 to 25.3g/day. It is obvious that the data are obtained by different methods of intake calculation but also of food analysis, which makes comparison difficult. The contribution of food containing added fibre for technological or functional purposes is not taken into account. Cereals, followed by vegetables, including pulses and potato, are the main food group contributors to dietary fibre intake. Of course, there are variations between countries. For example, consumption of cereals is highest in North Europe and lowest in South Europe (Table 13.14).

Nutritional recommendations about fibre intake in the different countries relies on the same analytical basis (Table 13.15). In agreement with a proposal from Organisation Mondiale de la Santé (World Health Organization), Dupin (1992) suggests in France a daily intake of 30–40 g dietary fibre. Several other countries, such as Denmark and Sweden, suggest a lower intake, namely 25–30 g dietary fibre/day. The Netherlands and USA express their recommendation as g fibre/MJ or 2000 Kcal.

Recommendations are based on what hitherto has been known about fibre. Most of the time, the guidelines are qualitative. They emphasise the need to eat more fruit and vegetables, and to avoid fat. Dietary diversity is encouraged more than precise nutritional guidelines.

13.8 Conclusions and future trends

Dietary fibre has been accepted in the prevention and management of disease in Western society. Dietary fibre exerts its direct physiological effect throughout the gastrointestinal tract in addition to metabolic activities.

The food industry has the opportunity to improve the health of customers and/or to reduce their risk of disease through foods with added activities. One difficulty for food companies when dealing with dietary fibre is to meet both nutritional and technological requirements; and most often, a compromise must be found (Fig. 13.7). In the last few years, ingredient suppliers have been engaged in research aimed at further improving the quality of fibre, which in part determines how much fibre can be added to foods and contribute towards their quality and nutritional attributes. It is important to further understand the effects of cooking and processing on fibre functionality and to take major notice of them. Novel generations of fibre (modified or mixtures of fibres with complementary properties) with optimised properties for specific application of final products have been developed. However, food companies still need to establish and develop innovative ways to bring dietary fibre into more products. Fibre supplementation of foods remains a largely empirical process. Predictive models for the mechanisms involved in successful incorporation of fibre in foods must be developed.

Well-validated relevant biomarkers to physiological functions and health end points are crucial to demonstrate accurately that food is truly effective. If appealing and believable, fibre-rich products will contribute significantly to dietary guidelines.

Table 13.14 Dietary intake in some countries

Country	Surveys	Analytical methods	Intake (g/j)	Reference
France	Household food survey	Unavailable carbohydrates	15.9 (year 1989)	Baghéri & Debry (1990)[1]
	Surveys of individuals	Unavailable carbohydrates	17.9–26.4	Le Quintrec & Gendre (1986)[2]
	Surveys of individuals	Unavailable carbohydrates	18.2 (13.6–22.8)	Several references[1]
	Household surveys	NSP, Unavailable carbohydrates	15.9–17.5	Several references[1]
	Food balance sheet	Unavailable carbohydrates	25.3	Bright-See, MacKeown-Eyssen (1984)[1]
Belgium	Surveys of individuals	TDF	21.0 (H), 19 (F)	Joossens et al. (1989)[1]
UK	Food frequency questionnaire	NST	15.5–16.4 (M, 40–69 years old)	Emmett et al. (1993)[2]
			14.3–15.1 (F, 25–69 years old)	
		Unavailable carbohydrates	23.2–25.3 (M, 40–69 years old)	
			21.6–23.3 (F, 25–69 years old)	
	Dairy record/7d	Unavailable carbohydrates	19 ± 7 (1980–83)	O'Neill and Fehili (1999)[2]
			21 ± 9 (1990)	
Germany	Dairy record/3 months	Unavailable carbohydrates	24 ± 8.4 (students)	Kasper et al. (1980)[2]
			22.0 ± 5.5 (manual labour)	
			21.7 ± 5.5 (teachers)	
			17.6 ± 4.6 (office workers)	
Italy	Food frequency questionnaire	Unavailable carbohydrates TDF	32.4	Turrini et al. (1995)
USA	USDA – survey 89–91 Children – adolescent	TDF	15.6 (20 years old)	Mueller et al. (1997)
Japan	Nutrition survey Aomori	Unavailable carbohydrates TDF	23.7 ± 8.4	Nakaji et al. (1993)
			22.2 ± 8.5	

Sources:
[1] Cummings and Frølich (1993); [2] mentioned by Cho et al. (1999a)

Notes:
NSP: non-starch polysaccharides; TDF: total dietary fibre. AOAC method: Unavailable carbohydrates: Southgate method; M. F: male. female.

Table 13.15 Dietary fibre daily intake recommendation. (Adapted from Cho et al. 1999.)

Country	Recommended intake	Basis	Source of recommendation
World-wide	27–40 g	TDF	World Health Organization
	16–24 g	NSP	
France	25–30 g	DF	French gastroenterologist – unpublished
Belgium	26–38 g (male)	DF	National Council for Nutrition (unofficial)
	19–28 g (female)		
UK	18 g	NSP	Department of Health Committee on Aspect of Food Policy, Department of Health Dietary Reference Values, report
Germany	30 g	DF	German Society of Nutrition
Italy	19 g	TDF	National Nutrition Institute
USA	25 g/2,000 kcal (adult)	DF	American Health Foundation
	3–20 years of age		
	0.5 g/BDW up to 25 g/day (adolescent)	DF	American Academy of Pediatrics
Japan	20–25 g	TDF	Ministry of Health and Welfare

Notes:
* DF: dietary fibre (method not indicated); TDF: total dietary fibre (AOAC, 1995); NSP: non-starch polysaccharides (Englyst et al. 1982)

- Positive image in the eyes of the consumer with regard to source, wholesomeness, etc.
- Be concentrated so that minimum amount can have a maximum physiological effect
- Bland in taste, colour, texture and odour
- Compatible with processing
- Good shelf life that does not adversely affect that of food to be added
- Have the expected physiological effects
- Be reasonable in price.

Fig. 13.7   A model for dietary fibre (from Larrauri 1999).

The success of foods for cholesterol reduction and for well-balanced intestinal flora are examples of possible success with this approach (Table 13.16). Modern research on dietary fibre has been ongoing for almost 30 years. There is no doubt that further development regarding effects of dietary fibre and associated substances will be important for the development of nutritious foods and for improved public health.

Table 13.16   Claims and dietary fibre

Dietary fibre content	Recommended intake	Source of recommendation
Source	3 g/100 g or 1.5 g/100 kcal	Codex Alimentarius
High	6 g/100 g or 3 g/100 kcal	Codex Alimentarius
Functional	Fructoligosaccharides induce an increase in the number and/or activity of bifidobacteria and lactic acid bacteria in the human intestine	CNHPF
Health		
Psyllium	Decrease the risk of cardiovascular disease	CNHPF
Sources of soluble beta glucans (barley bran, barley flour)	Reduction of blood cholesterol	FDA
Diet rich in cereal products (wholemeal), fruits and vegetables	Low fat and high fibre diet food containing cereals, fruits and vegetables may reduce the risk of some types of cancer, a multi-factor disease	FDA

Note:
Adapted from Cho *et al.* (1999a)

13.9 Bibliography

ALLEN, T. 'Granulométrie', *Technique de l'Ingénieur*, 1988, 1040–66.

ALONSO, J., HOWELL, N. and CANET, W. 'Purification and characterisation of two pectinmethylesterase from persimmon (*Diospyros kaki*)', *J Sci Food Agric*, 1997, **75**, 352–8.

ANDERSON, N.E. and CLYDESDALE, F.M. 'Effects of processing on the dietary fibre content of wheat bran, pureed green beans, and carrots', *J Sci*, 1980, **45**, 1533–7.

ANG, J.F. and MILLER, W.B. 'Multiple functions of powdered cellulose as a food ingredient', *Amer Assoc Cereal Chem*, 1991, **36** (7), 558–64.

Anonymous, 'Ingrédients "santé": une forme pétillante', *RIA, Spécial FIE 99*, HS Juillet–août: 97–108, 1999.

AOAC INTERNATIONAL, 'Total, soluble and insoluble dietary fiber in foods. AOAC official method 991.43', 1995, *Official Methods of Analysis*, 16th edn.

ASP, N.G. 'Resistant starch. Proceedings from the second plenary meeting of EURESTA: European FLAIR Concerted Action No. 11 on physiological implications of the consumption of resistant starch in man', *Eur J Clin Nutr*, 1992, **46** Supp. (2), S1.

ASP, N.G., VAN AMELSVOORT, J.M.M. and HAUTVAST, J.G.A.J. 'Nutritional implication of resistant starch', *Nutr Res Rev*, 1996, **9**, 1–31

ASP, N.G., SCHWEIZER, T.F., SOUTHGATE, D.A.T. and THEANDER, O. Dietary fibre analysis'. In: T.F. Schweizer and C.A. Edwards (eds), pp. 57–101, *Dietary Fibre: A Component of Food*, ILSI Human Nutrition Reviews, London, Springer-Verlag, 1992.

AUFFRET, A., BARRY, J.-L. and THIBAULT, J.-F. 'Effect of chemical treatments of sugar beet fibre on their physico-chemical properties and on their *in vitro* fermentation', *J Sci Food Agric*, 1993, **61**, 195–203.

AUFFRET, A., RALET, M.-C., GUILLON, F., BARRY, J.-L. and THIBAULT, J.-F. 'Effect of grinding and experimental conditions on the measurement of hydration properties of dietary fibres', *Lebensm Wiss U Technol*, 1994, **27**, 166–72.

BERNABÉ, M., FENWICK, R., FRIAS, J., JIMÉNEZ-BARBERO, J., PRICE, K., VALVERDE, S. and VIDAL-VALVERDE, C. 'Determination by NMR spectroscopy of the structure of cicerotol, a pseudotrisaccharide isolated from lentils', *J Agri Food Chem*, 1993, **41**, 870–2.

BERTIN, C., ROUAU, X. and THIBAULT, J.-F. 'Structure and properties of sugar beet fibres', *J Sci Food Agric*, 1988, **44**, 15–29.

BINGHAM, S.A. 'Mechanisms and experimental and epidemiological evidence relating dietary fibre (non-starch polysaccharides) and starch to protection against large bowel cancer', *Proc Nutr Soc*, 1990, **49**, 153–71.

BJORCK, I., NYLAN, M. and ASP, N.G. 'Extrusion cooking and dietary fiber: effects on dietary fiber content and on degradation in the rat intestinal tract', *Cereal Chem*, 1984, **61**, 174–9.

BLOND, G. and LE MESTE, M. 'Propriétés d'hydration des macromolécules, relation avec leurs propriétés fonctionnelles' In D. Lorient, B. Colas, and M.

Lemeste (eds), pp. 11–31, *Propriétés Fonctionnelles des Macromolécules Alimentaires. Les Cahiers de L'ENS.BANA*, Paris, Tec Lavoisier, 1988.

BOBIN-DUBIGEON, C. 'Caractérisation chimique, physico-chimique et fermentaire de produits alimentaires à base d'algues', thèse de doctorat, Université de Nantes, 1996, 194.

BOBIN-DUBIGEON, C., LAHAYE, M., GUILLON, F., BARRY, J.-L. and GALLANT, D.J. 'Factors limiting the biodegradation of *Ulva* sp cell wall polysaccharides', *J Sci Food Agric*, 1997, **75**, 341–51.

BOTHAM, R.L., RYDEN, P., ROBERTSON, J.A. and RING, S.G. 'Structural features of polysaccharides and their influence on fermentation behaviour', In F. Guillon, R. Amadó, M.T. Amara-Collaço, H. Andersson, N.G. Asp, K.E. Bach Knudsen, M. Champ, J. Mathers, J.A. Robertson, I. Rowland and J. Van Loo (eds), pp. 46–51, *Functional Properties of Non-digestible Carbohydrates*, Nantes, INRA, 1998.

BURKITT, D.O. 'The development of the fibre hypothesis', In G.G. Birch and K.J. Parker (eds), pp. 21–7, *Dietary Fibre*, London, Applied Science Publishers, 1983.

BURKITT, D.O. and TROWELL, H.C. *Refined Carbohydrates Foods and Disease: Implication of Dietary Fiber*, London, Academic Press, 1975.

CAMIRE, M.E. 'Chemical and physical modification of dietary fibre'. In S.S. Cho, L. Prosky and M. Dreher (eds), pp. 373–84, *Complex Carbohydrates in Foods*, New York, Marcel Dekker, 1999.

CAPREZ, A., ARRIGONI, E., NEUKOM, H. and AMADÒ, R. 'Improvement of the sensory properties of two different dietary fibre sources through enzymatic modification', *Lebens Wiss Technol*, 1987, **20**, 245–50.

CARPITA, N.C. and GIBEAUT, D.M. 'Structural models of the primary walls of flowering plant', *Plant J*, 1993, **3**, 1–30

CHAMP, M., MARTIN, L., NOAH, L. and GRATAS, M. 'Analytical methods for resistant starch'. In S.S. Cho, L. Prosky and M. Dreher (eds), pp. 169–87, *Complex Carbohydrates in Foods*, New York, Marcel Dekker, 1999.

CHERBUT, C. 'Fermentation et fonction digestive colique', *Cah Nutr Dièt*, 1995, **30**, 143–7.

CHERBUT, C., BARRY, J.-L., LAIRON, D. and DURAND, M. *Dietary Fibre: Mechanisms of Action in Human Physiology and Metabolism*, Paris, John Libbey Eurotex, 1995.

CHO, S.S. and PROSKY, L. 'Application of complex carbohydrates to food product fat mimetics'. In S.S. Cho, L. Prosky and M. Dreher (eds), pp. 71–111, *Complex Carbohydrates in Foods*, New York, Marcel Dekker, 1999.

CHO, S.S., O'SULLIVAN, K. and RICKARD, S. 'Worldwide dietary fiber intake: recommendations and actual consumption patterns'. In S.S. Cho, L. Prosky and M. Dreher (eds), pp. 411–29, *Complex Carbohydrates in Foods*, New York, Marcel Dekker, 1999.

CHO, S.S., PROSKY, L. and DREHER, M. *Complex Carbohydrates in Foods*, New York, Marcel Dekker, 1999.

CLOUTOUR, F. 'Caractéristiques des fibres alimentaires: influence sur leur fermentation *in vitro* par la flore digestive de l'homme', thèse de doctorat, Université de Nantes, 1995, 130.

COSGROVE, D.J. 'Assembly and enlargement of the primary cell wall in plants', *Annu Rev Cell Dev Biol*, 1997, **13**, 171–201.

COUSSEMENT, P. 'Inulin and oligofructose as dietary fiber: analytical, nutritional and legal aspects'. In S.S. Cho, L. Prosky and M. Dreher (eds), pp. 203–11, *Complex Carbohydrates in Foods*, New York, Marcel Dekker, 1999.

CRAIG, S.A.S., HOLDEN, J.F., TROUP, J.P., AUERBACH, M.H. and FRIER, H. 'Polydextrose as soluble fiber and complex carbohydrate'. In S.S. Cho, L. Prosky and M. Dreher (eds), pp. 229–48, *Complex Carbohydrates in Foods*, New York, Marcel Dekker, 1999.

CUMMINGS, J.H. 'Short chain fatty acids'. In G.R. Gibson and G.T. Macfarlane (eds), pp. 101–130, *Human Colonic Bacteria: Role in Nutrition, Physiology and Pathology*, Boca Raton, FL, CRC Press, 1995.

CUMMINGS, J.H. and FRØLICH, W. *Fibre Intakes in Europe. 1993. A Survey Conducted by Members of the Management Committee of COST 92. Metabolic and Physiological Aspects of Dietary Fibre in Food*, Luxembourg, Commission of the European Communities, 1993.

DARCY-VRILLON, B. and DUÉE, P.H. 'Fibre effect on nutrient metabolism in splanchnic and peripheral tissues'. In C. Cherbut, J.-L. Barry, D. Lairon and M. Durand (eds), pp. 83–94, *Dietary Fibre: Mechanisms of Action in Human Physiology and Metabolism*, Paris, John Libbey Eurotex, 1995.

DE LEENHEER, L. 'Production and use of inulin: industrial reality with a promising future'. In: H. van Bekkum, H. Röper and F. Voragen (eds), *Carbohydrates as Organic Raw Materials III*, NL-2509JC The Hague, CRF Cabohydrate Research Foundation, pp. 67–92, 1996.

DEMIGNÉ, C., MORAND, C., LEVRAT, A.-M., BESSON, C., MOUNDRAS, C. and RÉMÉSY, C. 'Effect of propionate on fatty acid and cholesterol synthesis and on acetate metabolism in isolated rat hepatocytes', *Br J Nutr*, 1995, **74**, 209–19.

DIPLOCK, A.T., AGGET, P.J., ASHWELL, M., BORNET, F., FERN, E.B. and ROBERFROID, R. 'Functional food science in Europe', Foreword, *Br J Nutr*, 1999, **81**, S1–S27.

DREHER, M. 'Food sources and uses of dietary fiber'. In S.S. Cho, L. Prosky and M. Dreher (eds) *Complex Carbohydrates in Foods*, New York, Marcel Dekker, pp. 327–71, 1999.

DUPIN, H., ABRAHAM, J. and GIACHETTI, I. *Apports nutritionnels conseillès pour la population française*, Paris, Editions Lavoisier Technique et Documentation, 1982.

DYSSELER, P. 'Fibres alimentaires: définition et sources de fibres alimentaires'. Conference: Propriétés et utilisation: intérêts fonctionnels et nutritionnels', Fibres Alimentaires, Ingrédients Fonctionnels et Nutritionnels. Résultats de trois programmes européens, Rennes, 14 March 1997.

DYSSELER, P., HOFFEM, D., FOCKEDEY, J., QUEMENER, B., THIBAULT, J.-F. and COUSSEMENT, P. 'Determination of inulin and oligofructose in food products (modified AOAC dietary fibre method)'. In S.S. Cho, L. Prosky and M. Dreher (eds), *Complex Carbohydrates in Foods*, New York, Marcel Dekker, pp. 213–27, 1999.

EDWARDS, C. 'Dietary fibre, fermentation and the colon'. In C. Cherbut, J.-L. Barry, D. Lairon and M. Durand (eds), *Dietary Fibre: Mechanisms of Action in Human Physiology and Metabolism*, Paris, John Libbey Eurotex, pp. 51–60, 1995.

ENGLYST, H., WIGGINS, H.S. and CUMMINGS, J.R. 'Determination of the non-starch polysaccharides in plant foods by gas liquid chromatography of constituent sugars as alditol acetate', *Analyst*, 1982, **107**, 307–18.

ENGLYST, H.N., KINGMAN, S.M. and CUMMINGS, J.H. 'Classification and measurement of nutritionally important starch fractions', *Eur J Clin Nutr*, 1992, **46** Supp. 2, S33–S50.

ENGLYST, H., QUIGLEY, M.E. and HUDSON, G.J. 'Determination of dietary fibre as non-starch polysaccharides with gas-liquid chromatographic, high-performance liquid chromatographic measurement of constituent sugars', *Analyst*, 1994, **119**, 1497–509.

FAN, L.T., LEE, Y.H. and BEARDMORE, D.H. 'Mechanism of enzymatic hydrolysis of cellulose: effects of major structural features of cellulose on enzymatic hydrolysis', *Biotechnol Bioeng*, 1980, **22**, 177–9.

FAO/WHO, 'Carbohydrates in human nutrition', FAO Food and Nutrition Paper 66. Report of a Joint FAO/WHO Expert Consultation, Rome, April 1997.

FARBER, B. and GALLANT, D.J. 'Evaluation de divers traitements technologiques des céréales', *Ann Zootech*, 1976, **25**, 13–30

FAVIER, J.C., IRELAND-RIPERT, J., TOQUE, C. and FEINBERG, M. *Répertoire général des aliments*, Paris, Technique et Documentation, INRA, Ciqual-Regal, 1995.

FEMENIA, A., SELVENDRAN, R.,R., RING, S.G. and ROBERTSON, J.A. 'Effect of heat treatment and dehydration on properties of cauliflower fiber', *J Agric Food Chem*, 1999, **47**, 728–32.

FINCHER, G.B. and STONE, B.A. 'Cell walls and their components in cereal grain technology'. In *Advances in Cereal Science and Technology*, vol. VIII, St Paul, MN, American Association of Cereal Chemists, pp. 207–95, 1986.

FLEMING, S.E. 'A study of relationships between flatus potential and carbohydrate distribution in legume seeds', *J Food Sci*, 1981, **46**, 794–803.

GHARPURAY, M.M., LEE, Y.-H. and FAN, L.T. 'Structural modification of lignocellulosics by pretreatments to enhance enzymatic hydrolysis', *Biotechnol Bioeng*, 1983, **25**, 157–72.

GOULD, J.M., JASBERG, B.K. and COTE, G.C. 'Structure–function relationship of alkaline peroxide treated lignocellulose', *Cereal Chem*, 1989, **66**, 213–17.

GUILLON, F., AMADÓ, R., AMARA-COLLAÇO, M.T., ANDERSSON, H., ASP, N.G., BACH KNUDSEN, K.E., CHAMP, M., MATHERS, J., ROBERTSON, J.A., ROWLAND, I. and VAN LOO, J. *Functional Properties of Non-digestible Carbohydrates*, Nantes, INRA, 1998.

GUILLON, F., AUFFRET, A., ROBERTSON, J.A., THIBAULT, J.-F. and BARRY, J.L. 'Relationships between physical characteristics of sugar-beet fibre and its fermentability by human faecal flora', *Carbohydrate Polymers*, 1998b, **37**, 185–97.

GUILLON, F., CLOUTOUR, F. and BARRY, J.-L. 'Dietary fibre: relationships between intrinsic characteristics and fermentation pattern'. In Y. Mälki and J.H. Cummings (eds) *Proceedings of COST Action 92, Espoo, Finland, Dietary Fibre and Fermentation in the Colon*, Brussels, European Commission, pp. 117–29, 1996.

GUILLON, F. and THIBAULT, J.-F. 'Les fibres alimentaires, additifs ou ingrédients alimentaires?' *Actualités en diététique*, 1996, **22**, 897–903.

HELLER, S.N., RIVERS, J.M. and HACKLER, L.R. 'Dietary fibre: the effect of particle size and pH on its measurement', *J Food Sci*, 1977, **42**, 436–9.

HIGGINSON, J.M.D. 'Fiber and cancer: historical perspectives'. In D. Kritchevsky and C. Bonfield (eds) *Dietary Fiber in Health and Disease*, St Paul MN, Eagan Press, pp. 174–90, 1995.

HISPLEY, E.H. 'Dietary fibre and pregnancy toxaemia', *Brit Med J*, 1953, **2**, 420–2.

HOLM, J., BJORCK, I., OSTROUSKA, S., ELIASSON, A.-C., ASP, N.-G., LARSSON, L. and LINDQUIST, I. 'Digestibility of amylose-lipid complexes *in vitro* and *in vivo*', *Starch*, 1983, **35**, 294–8.

JASBERG, B.K., GOULD, J.M. and WARNER, K. 'High fiber, noncaloric flour subtitute for baked foods: alkaline peroxide-treated lignocellulose in chocolate cake', *Cereal Chem*, 1989, **66**, 209–13.

JAYARAJAH, C.N., TRANG, H.-R., ROBERTSON, J.A. and SELVENDRAN, R.R. 'Dephytinisation of wheat bran and the consequences for fibre matrix non-starch polysaccharides', *Food Chem*, 1997, **58**, 5–12.

JOOSENS, J.V., GEBOERS, J. and KESTEOOT, H. 'Nutrition and cardiovascular mortality in Belgium', *Acta Cardiologica*, 1989, **XLIV**, 157–82.

KASPER, H., RABAST, U. and EHL, M. 'Studies on the extent of dietary fiber intake in West Germany', *Nutr Métabo*, 1980, **24**, 102–9.

KLEESSEN, B., STOOF, G., PROLL, J., SCHMIEDL, D., NOACK, J. and BLAUT, M. 'Feeding resistant starch affects fecal and cecal microflora and short-chain fatty acids in rats', *J Anim Sci*, 1997, **75**, 2453–62.

KRITCHEVSKY, D. and BONFIELD, C. *Dietary Fiber in Health and Disease*, St Paul MN, Eagan Press, 1995.

LAIRON, D. and BARRY, J.L. France. In J.H. Cummings and W. Frölich (eds), *Fibre Intakes in Europe. 1993. A Survey Conducted by Members of the Management Committee of COST 92. Metabolic and Physiological Aspects of Dietary Fibre in Food*, Luxembourg, Commission of the European Communities, pp. 49–52, 1993.

LANGKILDE, A.M. and ANDERSSON, H. 'Amount and composition of substrate entering the colon'. In F. Guillon, R. Amadó, M.T. Amara-Collaço, H. Andersson, N.G. Asp, K.E. Bach Knudsen, M. Champ, J. Mathers, J.A. Robertson, I. Rowland and J. Van Loo (eds), *Functional Properties of Non-digestible Carbohydrates*, Nantes, INRA, pp. 140–2, 1998.

LARRAURI, J.A. 'New approaches in the preparation of high dietary fibre powders from fruit by-products', *Trends in Food Sci and Technol*, 1999, **10**, 3–8.

LE QUINTREC, Y. and GENDRE, J.P. 'Consumption of dietary fiber in France'. In G.A. Spiller (ed.) *CRC Handbook of Dietary Fiber in Human Nutrition*, Boca

Raton, FL, CRC Press, pp. 425–32, 1986.

LINEBACK, D. 'The chemistry of complex carbohydrates'. In S.S. Cho, L. Prosky and M. Dreher (eds) *Complex Carbohydrates in Foods*, New York, Marcel Dekker, pp. 115–29, 1999.

LO, G.S. 'Nutritional and physical properties of dietary fiber from soybeans', *Cereal Foods World*, 1989, **34**, 530–4.

LOPEZ, P., SANCHEZ, A.C., VERCET, A. and BURGOS, J. 'Thermal resistance of tomato polygalacturonase and pectinmethyl esterase at physiological pH', *Food Res Technol*, 1997, **204**, 146–50.

LOUKA, N. and ALLAF, K. 'Improvement of the quality of dried vegetable product by controlled instantaneous decompression'. In F. Guillon, R. Amadó, M.T. Amara-Collaço, H. Andersson, N.G. Asp, K.E. Bach Knudsen, M. Champ, J. Mathers, J.A. Robertson, I. Rowland and J. Van Loo (eds) *Functional Properties of Non-digestible Carbohydrates*, Nantes, INRA, pp. 81–2, 1998.

LUE, S., HSIEH, F., PENG, I.C. and HUFF, H.E. 'Expansion of corn extrudates containing dietary fiber: a microstructure study', *Lebensm Wiss u Technol*, 1990, **23**, 165–73.

MACFARLANE, G.T. and DEGNAN, B.A. 'Catabolite regulatory mechanisms in relation to polysaccharide breakdown and carbohydrate utilization'. In Y. Mälki and J.H. Cummings (eds) *Proceedings of COST Action 92, Dietary Fibre and Fermentation in the Colon*, Brussels, European Commission, pp. 117–29, 1996.

MACFARLANE, G.T. and MACFARLANE, S. 'Factors affecting fermentation reactions in the large bowel', *Nutr Soc Proc*, 1993, **52**, 367–73.

MCINTYRE, A., GIBSON, P.R. and YOUNG, G.P. 'Butyrate production from dietary fibre and protection against large bowel cancer in a rat model', *Gut*, 1993, **34**, 386–91.

MARTIN, L.J.M., DUMON, H.J.W. and CHAMP, M.M.J. 'Production of short chain fatty acids from resistant starch in a pig model', *J Sci Food Agric*, 1998, **77**, 71–80.

MATHERS, J.C., ROPER, C.S., CHERBUT, C., HOEBLER, C., DARCY-VRILLON, B. and VAUDELADE, P. 'Physiological responses to polysaccharides: are rats and pigs good models for humans?'. In F. Guillon, R. Amadó, M.T. Amara-Collaço, H. Andersson, N.G. Asp, K.E. Bach Knudsen, M. Champ, J. Mathers, J.A. Robertson, I. Rowland and J. Van Loo (eds) *Functional Properties of Non-digestible Carbohydrates*, Nantes, INRA, pp. 110–12, 1998.

MICHEL, C., KRAVTCHENKO, T.P., DAVID, A., GUENEAU, S., KOZLOWSKI, F. and CHERBUT, C. '*In vitro* prebiotic effects of Acacia gums onto the human intestinal microbiota depends on the botanical origin and environment pH', *Anaerobe*, 1998, **4**, 257–66.

MORRIS, E.R. 'Shear thinning of random coil polysaccharides: characterisation by two parameters from a simple linear plot', *Carbohydr Polym*, 1990, **13**, 85–96.

MORRIS, E.R. 'Physico-chemical properties of food polysaccharides'. In T.F. Schweizer and C. Edwards (eds) *Dietary Fibre, A Component of Food: Nutritional Function in Health and Disease*, ILSI Europe, Berlin, Springer-Verlag, pp. 41–56, 1992.

NOAH, L., GUILLON, F., BOUCHET, B. BULÉON, A., MOLIS, C., GRATAS, M. and CHAMP, M. 'Digestion of carbohydrate from white beans (*Phaseolus vulgaris L.*) in healthy humans', *J Nutr*, 1998, **128**, 977–85.

PERRIN, P., PIERRE, F., PATRY, Y., CHAMP, M., BERREUR, M., PRADAL, G., BORNET, F. MÉFLAH, K. and MÉNANTEAU, J. 'Only fibers promoting a stable butyrate-producing colonic ecosystem decrease the rate of aberrant crypt foci in rats', *Gut*, in press.

PIERRE, F., PERRIN, P., CHAMP, M., BORNET, F., MEFLAH, K. and MÉNANTEAU, J. 'Short-chain fructo-oligosaccharides reduce the occurrence of colon tumors and develop gut-associated lymphoid tissue in Min mice', *Cancer Research*, 1997, **57**, 225–8.

PLAT, D., BEN-HALOM, N., LEVI, A., REID, D. and GOLDSCHMIDT, E. 'Changes in pectic susbtances in carrots during hydration with and without blanching', *Food Chem*, 1991, **39**, 1–12.

PONNE, C.T., ARMSTRONG, D.R. and LUYTEN, H. 'Food fibres as technological agents in foods'. In F. Guillon, G. Abraham , R. Amadò, H. Andersson, N.G. Asp, K.E. Bach Knudsen, M. Champ and J.A. Robertson (eds) *Plant Polysaccharides in Human Nutrition: Structure, Function, Digestive Fate and Metabolic Effects*, Nantes, INRA, pp. 6–12, 1997.

PONNE, C.T., ARMSTRONG, D.R. and LUYTEN, H. 'Influence of dietary fibres on textural properties of food'. In F. Guillon, R. Amadó, M.T. Amara-Collaço, H. Andersson, N.G. Asp, K.E. Bach Knudsen, M. Champ, J. Mathers, J.A. Robertson, I. Rowland and J. Van Loo (eds), *Functional Properties of Non-digestible Carbohydrates*, Nantes, INRA, pp. 61–5, 1998.

POUTANEN, K. 'Enzymes, an important tool in the improvement of the quality of cereal foods', *Trends Food Sci Techn*, 1997, **8**, 300–6.

POUTANEN, K., SUIRTTI, T., AURA, A-M, LUIKKONEN, K. and AUTIO, K. 'Influence of processing on the ceral dietary fibre complex: what do we know?' In F. Guillon, R. Amadó, M.T. Amara-Collaço, H. Andersson, N.G. Asp, K.E. Bach Knudsen, M. Champ, J. Mathers, J.A. Robertson, I. Rowland and J. Van Loo (eds), *Functional Properties of Non-digestible Carbohydrates*, Nantes, INRA, pp. 66–70, 1998.

QUEMENER, B. and BRILLOUET, J.-M. 'Ciceritol, a pinitol digalactoside from seeds of chickpea lentil and white lupin', *Phytochem*, 1983, **22**, 1745–51.

RAHMAN, A.R., HENNING, W.L. and WESTCOOT, D.E. 'Histological and physical changes in carrots as affected by blanching, cooking, freezing, freeze-drying and compression', *J Food Sci*, 1971, **36**, 500–2.

RALET, M.-C., AXELOS, M. and THIBAULT, J.-F. 'Gelation properties of extruded lemon cell walls and their water soluble pectins', *Carbohydr Res*, 1994, **260**, 271–82.

RALET, M.-C., DELLA VALLE, G. and THIBAULT, J.-F. 'Raw and extruded fibre from pea hulls. Part I: composition and physico-chemical properties', 17–23, 'Part II: structural study of the water-soluble polysaccharides', 25–34, *Carbohydrate Polymers*, 1993, **20**, 17–34.

RALET, M.-C., THIBAULT, J.-F. and DELLA VALLE, G. 'Influence of extrusion cooking on the physico-chemical properties of wheat bran', *J Cereal Science*, 1990, **11**, 249–59.

RÉMÉSY, C. 'Intérêt nutritionnel des fibres et des micronutriments apportés par les fruits et légumes', *Actualités en diététique*, 1996, **22**, 883–95.

RENARD, C.M.G.C., CRÉPEAU, M.-J. and THIBAULT, J.-F. 'Influence of ionic strength, pH and dielectric constant on hydration properties of native and modified fibres from sugar-beet and wheat bran', *Indus Crops Prod*, 1994, **3**, 75–84.

ROBERTSON, J.A. 'Application of plant-based byproducts as fiber supplements in processed foods', *Recent Res Devel in Agric Food Chem*, 1998, **2**, 705–17.

ROBERTSON, J.A., DE MONREDON, J.-F., DYSSELER, P., GUILLON, F., AMADÓ, R. and THIBAULT, J.-F. 'Hydration properties of dietary fibre and resistant starch: a European collaborative study', *Lebensm Wiss u Technologie*, in press.

RYDEN, P. and ROBERTSON, J.A. 'The effect of fibre source and fermentation on the apparent hydrophobic binding properties of wheat bran in preparations for the mutagen 2-amino-3, 8-dimethylimidazol 4, 5-F quinoxaline (MEIQX)', *Carcinogenesis*, 1995, **16**, 209–16.

SAKATA, T. 'Effects of short chain fatty acids on gastrointestinal epithelial cells'. In C. Cherbut, J.-L. Barry, D. Lairon and M. Durand (eds) *Dietary Fibre: Mechanisms of Action in Human Physiology and Metabolism*, Paris, John Libbey Eurotex, pp. 61–8, 1995.

SALMINEN, S., BOULEY, C., BOUTRON-RUAULT, M.-C., CUMMINGS, J.H., FRANCK, A., GIBSON, G.R., ISOLAURI, E., MOREAU, M.-C., ROBERFROID, M. and ROWLAND, I. 'Functional food science and gastrointestinal physiology and function', *British J Nutr*, 1998, **80** (Supp. 1), S147–S171.

SCHIMBERNI, M., CARDINALI, F., SODINI, G. and CANELA, M. 'Chemical and functional characteristics of corn bran, oat hull and barley hull flour', *Lebensm Wiss u Technol*, 1982, **15**, 337–9.

SCHWEIZER, T.F., ANDERSSON, H., LANGKILDE, A.M., REIMANN, S. and TORSDOTTIR, I. 'Nutrients excreted in ileostomy effluents after consumption of mixed diets with beans and potatoes. II. Starch, dietary fibre and sugars', *Eur J Cli Nutr*, 1990, **44**, 567–75.

SCHWEIZER, T.F. and EDWARDS, C.A. *Dietary Fiber: A Component of Food*, London, Springer-Verlag, pp. 41–5, 1992.

SELVENDRAN, R.R. and ROBERTSON, J.A. 'The chemistry of dietary fibre: an holistic view of the cell wall matrix'. In D.A.T. Southgate, K. Waldron, I.T. Johnson and G.R. Fenwick (eds) *Dietary Fibre: Chemical and Biological Aspects*, Royal Society of Chemistry Special Publication No. 83, Royal Society of Chemistry, pp. 27–43, 1990.

SIDIRAS, D.K., KOULAS, D.P., VGENPOULOS, A.G. and KOUKIOS, E.G. 'Cellulose crystallinity as affected by various technical processes', *Cellulose Chem Technol*, 1990, **24**, 309–17.

SINITSYN, A.P., GUSAKOV, A.V. and VLASENKO, A.E.Y. 'Effect of structural and physicochemical features of cellulosic substrates on the efficiency of enzymatic hydrolysis', *Appl Biochem Biotechnol*, 1991, **30**, 43–59.

SOUTHGATE, D.A.T. 'The structure of dietary fiber'. In D. Kritchevsky and C.

Bonfield (eds) *Dietary Fiber in Health and Disease*, St Paul MN, Eagan Press, pp. 26–36, 1995.

SOUTHGATE, D.A.T., WALDRON, K., JOHNSON, I.T. and FENWICK, G.R. 'Dietary fibre: chemical and biological aspects', Royal Society of Chemistry Special Publication No. 83, Cambridge, Royal Society of Chemistry, 1991.

STARK, A. and MADAR, Z. 'Dietary fiber'. In I. Goldberg (ed.) *Functional Foods, Designer Foods, Pharmafoods, Nutraceuticals*, New York, Chapman & Hall, pp. 183–201, 1994.

STOLLE-SMITS, T., BEEKHUIZEN, J.G., VAN DIJK, C., VORAGEN, A.G.J. and RECOURT, K. 'Cell wall dissolution during industrial processing of green beans (*Phaseolus vulgaris* L.)', *J Agri Food Chem*, 1995, **43**, 2480–6.

SVANBERG, M. 'Effects of processing on dietary fibre in vegetables', thesis, Department of Applied Nutrition and Food Chemistry, Lund Institute of Technology, Lund University, Lund, Sweden, 1997, p. 138.

SVANBERG, M., SUORTTI, T. and NYMAN, M. 'Effects of processing on physicochemical properties of dietary fibre in carrots'. In F. Guillon, G. Abraham, R. Amadò, H. Andersson, N.G. Asp, K.E. Bach Knudsen, M. Champ and J.A. Robertson (eds) *Plant Polysaccharides in Human Nutrition: Structure, Function, Digestive Fate and Metabolic Effects*, Nantes, INRA, pp. 13–19, 1997.

THIBAULT, J.-F., DELLA VALLE, G. and RALET, M.-C. 'Produits riches en parois végétales à fraction hydrosoluble accrue, leur obtention, leur utilisation et compositions les contenant', *Brevet français no 88–11601* 5 September 1988.

THIBAULT, J.-F., LAHAYE, M. and GUILLON, F. 'Physicochemical properties of food plant cell walls'. In T.F. Schweizer and C. Edwards (eds) *Dietary Fibre, A Component of Food. Nutritional Function in Health and Disease*, ILSI Europe, Berlin, Springer-Verlag, pp. 21–39, 1992.

THIBAULT, J.-F., RALET, M.-C., AXELOS, M.A.V. and DELLA VALLE, G. 'Effects of extrusion-cooking of pectin rich materials', *Pectins and Pectinases*, Wageningen (Pays-Bas), 3–7 December 1995.

THIBAULT, J.-F., RENARD, M.G.C. and GUILLON, F. 'Physical and chemical analysis of dietary fibres in sugar-beet and vegetable'. In J.F. Jackson and H.F. Linskens (eds) *Modern Methods of Plant Analysis*, vol. 16 *Vegetable and Vegetable Products*, Heidelberg, Springer-Verlag, pp. 23–55, 1994.

TOPPING, D.L. and PANT, I. 'Short-chain fatty acids and hepatic lipid metabolism: experimental studies'. In J.H. Cummings, J.C. Rombeau and T. Sakata (eds) *Physiological and Clinical Aspects of Short-chain Fatty Acids*, Cambridge, Cambridge University Press, pp. 495–508, 1995.

TROWELL, H. 'Dietary fibre and coronary heart disease', *Revue Européenne d'Etudes Cliniques et Biologiques*, 1972, **17**(4), 345–9.

VAN LOO, J., CUMMINGS, J.H., DELZENNE, N., ENGLYST, H., FRANK, A., HOPKINS, M., KOK, N. MACFARLANE, G., NEWTON, D., QUIGLEY, M., ROBERFROID, M., VAN VLIET, T. and VAN DEN HEUVEL, E. 'Functional food properties of non digestible oligosaccharides: a consensus report from the ENDO project' (DG XII AIRII-CT94-1095), *Br J Nutr*, 1999, **81**, 121–32.

VARO, P., LAINE, R. and KOIVISTOINEN, P. 'Effect of heat treatment on dietary fiber: interlaboratory study', *J Assoc Off Anal Chem*, 1983, **66**, 933–8.

VARO, P., VEIJALAINEN, K. and KOIVISTOINEN, P. 'Effect of heat treatment on the dietary fibre contents of potato and tomato', *J Food Technol*, 1984, **19**, 485–92.

VORAGEN, A.G.J. 'Technological aspects of functional food-related carbohydrates', *Trends in Foods Science and Technology*, 1998, **9**, 328–35.

WALKER, A.R.P. 'Dietary fibre and the pattern disease', *Ann Intern Med*, 1974, **80**, 663–4.

WEIGHTMAN, R.M., RENARD, M.G.C., GALLANT, D.J. and THIBAULT, J.-F. 'Structure and properties of the polysaccharides from pea hulls. Part II: Modification of the composition and physico-chemical properties of commercial pea hulls by chemical extraction of the constituent polysaccharides', *Cabohyd Polym*, 1994, **24**, 139–48.

WOLEVER, T.M.S. 'Short chain fatty acids and carbohydrate metabolism'. In H.J. Binder, J.H. Cummings and K.H. Soergel (eds) *Short Chain Fatty Acids, Falk Symposium 73*, Dordrecht, Kluwer Academic, 8–10 September, pp. 251–9, 1995.

WU, A. and CHANG, W.H. 'Influence of precooking on the firmness and pectic substances of three stem vegetables', *Int J Food Sci Technol*, 1990, **25**, 558–63.

WÜRSCH, P. 'Production of resistant starch'. In S.S. Cho, L. Prosky and M. Dreher (eds) *Complex Carbohydrates in Foods*, New York, Marcel Dekker, pp. 71–111, 1999.

Index